Normal Midwifery Practice

Sam Chenery-Morris
and Moira McLean

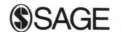

Los Angeles | London | New Delhi
Singapore | Washington DC

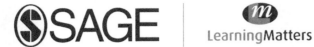

SAGE Publications Ltd
1 Oliver's Yard
55 City Road
London EC1Y 1SP

SAGE Publications Inc.
2455 Teller Road
Thousand Oaks, California 91320

SAGE Publications India Pvt Ltd
B 1/I 1, Mohan Cooperative Industrial Area
Mathura Road
New Delhi 110 044

SAGE Publications Asia-Pacific Pte Ltd
3 Church Street
#10-04 Samsung Hub
Singapore 049483

Editor: Becky Taylor
Development editor: Richenda Milton-Daws
Copy-editor: Amanda Crook
Production controller: Chris Marke
Project management: Diana Chambers
Marketing manager: Tamara Navaratnam
Cover design: Wendy Scott
Illustrations: David Woodroffe
Typeset by: Kelly Winter
Printed by: MPG Books Group, Bodmin, Cornwall

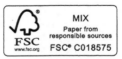

Library of Congress Control Number: 2012941847

British Library Cataloguing in Publication data

A catalogue record for this book is available from the British Library

ISBN 978 0 85725 757 4 (pbk)
ISBN 978 0 85725 862 5

Contents

Foreword

Welcome to this series on the practice of Midwifery. As a student midwife, you have commenced a journey that will equip you with knowledge and understanding of the breadth of information that you will require to facilitate normal birth as the lead professional, yet able to manage your role when interprofessional care is required, recognising women with complex health needs or the occurrence of adverse events in childbearing. At all times you will be working in partnership with the women and their families you have the privilege and honour to care for.

You may find this journey very demanding as attitudes and values are challenged, requiring you to draw on and develop your personal and professional strengths. However, this will be balanced with the exhilaration of supporting women and their families antenatally, during labour and as they welcome their new baby at birth, and also during the early postnatal period. For you, the outcome of this educational journey will mean you have demonstrated that you are 'Fit for practice', 'Fit for award' and 'Fit for purpose', and you can register as a midwife on Part 2 of the NMC Professional Register.

This series will address the requirements for midwifery education set out in the NMC Standards for Pre-registration Midwifery Education that include the Essential Skills Clusters (ESCs) and grading of practice (NMC, 2009). These Standards outline the baseline requirements of knowledge for safe and effective midwifery practice. They are designed to prepare you for contemporary midwifery practice in the UK, where midwifery care occurs in the context of a social model of care for normal childbirth. This is provided against a backdrop of government strategy and guidance (DH, 2004, 2007a, 2010; Marmot, 2010; CMACE, 2011), statutory midwifery regulation and adherence to professional standards of practice as a midwife (NMC, 2004) and the NMC *Code* (NMC, 2008a).

The current text will focus on the boundaries of normal midwifery practice throughout the childbirth continuum. It is essential that you fully understand the principles of care when the woman and her baby are fit and well. This will enable you to recognise when there is a deviation from the normal pattern of health in pregnancy and your role as a midwife when this occurs. You will therefore need to revisit the contents of this book as you develop your knowledge of complex care requirements, which will be found in other books in this series.

The interactive nature of this series will help develop your ability to reflect on and question your knowledge and practice. This will ensure that you progress professionally as a lifelong learner fully able to meet the demands of a midwifery career.

Judith Nabb
Series Editor

Acknowledgements

The authors and publisher are grateful to the following organisations:

Antenatal Screening Wales for permission to reproduce the table showing antenatal screening choices as Table 3.1 in this book. The original can be found at www.wales.nhs.uk

The National Institute for Health and Clinical Excellence for permission to adapt information from 'CG 37 Postnatal care: routine postnatal care of women and their babies', London: NICE, 2006, in Table 6.1. The original can be found at www.nice.org.uk

Every effort has been made to trace all copyright holders within the book, but if any have been inadvertently overlooked, the publisher will be pleased to make the necessary arrangements at the first opportunity.

About the authors

Sam Chenery-Morris is a senior midwifery lecturer at University Campus Suffolk (UCS), Ipswich. Initially Sam trained as a Registered Sick Children's Nurse and Registered General Nurse in Liverpool at the end of the 1980s. She undertook a diploma in midwifery in Norwich from 1994 to 1995 and worked as a midwife in all areas of practice. During this time she undertook a post-registration programme of study to achieve a BSc Midwifery Practice in 2000 and started the next phase of her midwifery career as a teacher in 2006. Since working in Ipswich she has gained an MA in Interprofessional Healthcare Education and has had several articles published on her research interest of student midwife assessments. She is currently studying for a PhD at the University of East Anglia (UEA). She enjoys teaching all aspects of midwifery and dedicates this book to her partner, children, and all the women and students who have inspired her.

Moira McLean is a senior lecturer in midwifery at De Montfort University in Leicester and Supervisor of Midwives. She is currently programme leader for BSc (Hons) Midwifery. Following initial nursing and midwifery training in Scotland, Moira has worked as a midwife and a lecturer in both Cambridge and Leicester. She has until recently had a small caseload of women, but she now continues to maintain her updating through working as a bank midwife in Cambridge and through her supervision activities. She continues to enjoy all aspects of teaching and has a particular interest in intrapartum care, bereavement and professional issues. Moira dedicates this book to her daughter Lorna and grandson Ewan, and all her students past, present and future who allow her to share her passion for midwifery.

Introduction

This new book for student midwives is the core book for a series aimed at equipping today's students with the ability to provide the best possible care for mothers and babies. For most women, pregnancy and birth are normal physiological events happening to a well population. However, these events also have huge emotional significance for the women and their partners. Giving birth is a rite of passage, and this special nature of the event must be recognised by all involved with women during pregnancy, labour and the postnatal period.

Book structure

Each chapter contains a summary of the key knowledge and ideas presented, and can be used as a quick reference guide or for revision. Chapter 1 sets the scene with an introduction to normal midwifery practice, thus providing a context for the rest of the book. Chapter 2 focuses on the importance of providing woman-centred care and explores the communication and inter-personal skills you will need to achieve this.

Chapters 3 and 4 look at antenatal care. Chapter 3 focuses on antenatal care in early pregnancy, and the antenatal booking interview, in particular, while Chapter 4 gives information about antenatal care in the second and third trimesters, and considers issues around antenatal education and planning for the birth. Chapter 5 focuses on the labour and birth itself, and includes a consideration of the place of birth as well as what to expect during each of the three stages of labour.

Chapter 6 is concerned with postnatal care, and Chapter 7 looks at care of the newborn and includes an important section on the establishment of breastfeeding. The book ends with a chapter looking at the midwife's role in medicines management.

Requirements for the NMC Standards for Pre-registration Midwifery Education and the Essential Skills Clusters

The Nursing and Midwifery Council (NMC) has established standards of competence to be met by all midwifery students in order to gain entry to the register, and these are the standards it considers necessary for safe and effective practice. In addition to the competencies, the NMC has set out specific skills that midwifery students must be able to perform at various points of an education programme. These are known as Essential Skills Clusters (ESCs). This book is structured so that it will help you to understand and meet the required competencies and ESCs.

The relevant competencies and ESCs are presented at the start of each chapter so that you can clearly see which ones the chapter addresses. The boxes refer to the latest Standards for Pre-Registration Midwifery Education published in 2009 (NMC, 2009).

Learning features

Case studies and scenarios

Examples from a range of midwifery contexts, including perspectives from women and their families, have been included to help you link theory to actual practice. Some include questions to help you to think critically about how you might react in a certain situation, and to improve your decision-making skills.

Activities

There are a wide range of activities in the text to help you to make sense of, and learn about, the material being presented by the authors. Some activities ask you to *reflect* on aspects of practice, or your experience of it, or the people or situations you encounter. Other activities help you develop key graduate skills such as your ability to *think critically* about a topic in order to challenge received wisdom; your ability to *research a topic and find appropriate information and evidence*; and your ability to *make decisions* using that evidence in situations that are often difficult and time-pressured. Communication and working as part of a team are core to all midwifery practice, and some activities ask you to carry out *group work activities* or think about your *communication skills* to help develop these.

All the activities require you to take a break from reading the text, think through the issues presented and carry out some independent study. Where appropriate, there are sample answers presented at the end of each chapter. Remember that academic study will always require independent work; attending lectures will never be enough to be successful on your programme, and these activities will help to deepen your knowledge and understanding of the issues under scrutiny and give you practice at working on your own.

You might want to think about including these activities as part of your personal development plan (PDP) or portfolio. When you have completed an activity, write it up in your PDP or portfolio in a section devoted to that particular skill, then look back over time to see how far you are developing. You can also do more of the activities for a key skill that you have identified as a weakness, which will help to build your skill and confidence in that area.

Research, theory and concept summaries

Summaries of key research, theories and concepts appear throughout the book to help you to get to grips with the evidence base in an easy-to-understand way.

Further reading and useful website suggestions

This book is intended as an introduction to normal midwifery and aims to provide you with a good framework from which to explore and learn further. You will be expected to read more widely, and the further reading and useful website suggestions at the end of each chapter should give you a useful starting point for further study.

Glossary

There is a glossary at the end of the book that explains specialist language in plain English. Words in the glossary appear in bold on the first instance that they appear in the text.

Chapter 1
Normal midwifery practice

Sam Chenery-Morris

NMC Standards for Pre-registration Midwifery Education

This chapter will address the following competencies:

Domain: Developing the individual midwife and others

Review, develop and enhance the midwife's own knowledge, skills and fitness to practise. This will include:

- making effective use of the framework for statutory supervision of midwives;
- meeting the NMC's continuing professional development and practice standards;
- reflecting on the midwife's own practice.

Domain: Achieving quality care through evaluation and research

Apply relevant knowledge to the midwife's own practice in structured ways which are capable of evaluation. This will include:

- critical appraisal of the midwife's own practice;
- gaining feedback from women and their families and appropriately applying this to practice.

NMC Essential Skills Clusters

This chapter will address the following ESCs:

Cluster: Communication

Women can trust/expect a newly qualified midwife to:

1. be attentive and share information that is clear, accurate and meaningful at a level which women and their partners and family can understand;
5. treat women with dignity and respect them as individuals;
8. be confident in their own role within a multi-disciplinary/multi-agency team.

Introduction

The origin of the word *midwife* can be traced back to the 1300s and translated as *with woman*. Although the dictionary offers definitions of *midwife* as a verb as well as a noun (**www.merriam-webster.com/dictionary/midwife**), it is most often used as a noun, to describe the person. This chapter sets the foundations of the book, and the translation *with woman* is the underlying philosophy for this series of books. *With woman* can be seen as an antidote to the medicalisation of birth – it respects each pregnancy and birth as individual and unique. It encourages interaction between women, their partners and families and midwives, putting the woman at the centre of her care and the decision-making processes related to her care.

In the UK, 700,000 women will give birth each year, and the majority of these women will see a midwife for some or all of their care (Midwifery 2020, 2010). For women deemed to be at low **risk**, the midwife is likely to be the lead professional for their care. Women who are considered to have higher risks because of their own health and/or a previous or current pregnancy are seen by a consultant **obstetrician** in addition to or instead of a midwife. This model of care – differentiating women into low- and high-risk groups – has been criticised as reducing the choices open to women with higher risk pregnancies and as starting to offer a two-tier system of maternity care in the UK. The number of women whose pregnancies are categorised as high risk seems to be on the increase (Midwifery 2020, 2010).

Although this book is primarily aimed at normal midwifery practice and care, the underlying philosophy is that each woman and her pregnancy should be treated as unique, and that sharing of information and involvement in decision-making should be extended to all women, regardless of their pregnancy risk status. These concepts will be explored throughout this chapter as both the individual and the collective beliefs of midwives have an effect on pregnant women's experiences.

Defining midwifery

The official definition of a midwife comes from the International Confederation of Midwives (ICM, 2011). Before you read this definition, Activity 1.1 encourages you to try to work out your own midwifery priorities.

Activity 1.1   *Decision-making*

Try to write your own definition of a midwife.

Now access this website to read the ICM's full definition of a midwife:

www.internationalmidwives.org/Portals/5/2011/Definition%20of% 20the%20Midwife%20-%202011.pdf

How does this definition compare to yours? Probably you will have used many of the words in this internationally recognised document – for instance, competency, responsibility, accountable, partnership, normal.

See the suggested answer at the end of the chapter.

Now you have considered the definition of a midwife, what do you consider to be the most important aspects of this role? This chapter will set out the UK context of midwifery practice but take a moment to explore your own personal philosophy.

Activity 1.2   *Reflection*

What sort of a midwife do you want to become? Where have these ideas come from (if you know)? How will you remember this philosophy at the end of your training?

As this activity is based on your own reflection, there is no outline answer at the end of the chapter.

Just as the task above was personal to you, each woman's pregnancy and birth is personal and unique to her. But there are still standards and responsibilities that each midwife must achieve and uphold; these will be explored before we go on to consider other more complex concepts, such as normality and risk in midwifery practice.

In the UK the roles and responsibilities of a midwife are governed by the Nursing and Midwifery Council (NMC). Some of the most important documents that will shape your practice come from this source: for instance, the *Midwives rules and standards* (NMC, 2004a), *The code* (NMC 2008a) and the *Standards for pre-registration midwifery education* (NMC, 2009).

Activity 1.3   *Communication*

Take a look at the NMC website for midwifery-related content and documents:

www.nmc-uk.org/Nurses-and-midwives/Midwifery/Midwifery- Education-and-Practice

continued . . .

Discuss with a colleague on your course what you think of the content offered on this website. Consider the following: How easy is the site to navigate? Would you return to this site? If so, what for? What did you find particularly helpful?

There is no answer at the end of this chapter as each student will have their own views on the website.

It is worth accessing the NMC website a few times a year, as there are often consultations that are open to the public, students and qualified staff. If you participate in these surveys, you are contributing to both the nursing and the midwifery professions.

Although the NMC governs both professions, midwifery is not a subset of nursing: the two professions are very different. Nurses are often caring for patients who are sick, whereas in midwifery the woman is generally well. Pregnancy is a normal **physiological** process; it is not **pathological**, as with a disease. In nursing there is only one patient to care for, although the family is important to recovery (especially when nursing children). In midwifery there is a pregnant woman, her developing yet unborn baby and usually a partner, too, so family-centred care, information-sharing with all parties and decision-making are heightened. You do not need to be a nurse to be a midwife, yet some midwives are also or have previously been nurses. Most midwives now enter the profession by direct-entry routes, with a three-year preparation programme. They qualify as midwives with eligibility to the NMC register and a degree, and they can work anywhere in the world. The number of nurses in the UK is huge – there are fewer midwives: in 2008, 660,000 nurses and midwives were on the NMC register, of which 35,000 were midwives registered as eligible to work in the UK (**www.nmc-uk.org/Documents/ Statistical%20analysis%20of%20the%20register/NMC-Statistical-analysis-of-the-register-2007-2008.pdf**).

There are two publications/practices that set midwifery further apart from nursing, as nurses do not have either of these systems. One is the **statutory**/legal responsibility of midwives to have supervision (*Standards for the supervised practice of midwives* – NMC, 2007) and the other is the set of rules and standards that govern midwifery practice (*Midwives rules and standards* – NMC, 2004a).

Supervision

Just as midwives support pregnant women, supervisors of midwives support other midwives. Supervisors of midwives are experienced midwives who have undertaken extra training to support other practising midwives. The purpose of this supervision is to protect women and babies from poor practice but also to promote excellence in midwifery. Each midwife is supported by a named supervisor to ensure they are providing the right care to each woman, promoting normality and working in partnership with women; each midwife must meet their supervisor at least annually. Just as each midwife has a supervisor, each supervisor also has a supervisor above them, not as a system of hierarchy but as a system of continued collaboration to improve and maintain midwifery standards. The Local Supervising Authority (LSA) has a Midwifery Officer supervisor who reports directly to the NMC. As previously mentioned, the NMC is the professional regulator for the two professions and is currently the largest regulator in the UK. This framework aims to keep midwives safer and enhance their roles by providing support to improve and consolidate their practice in ever-changing contexts.

Midwives rules and standards

There are 16 rules in this publication, each detailing the responsibility of a midwife, with guidance to help each midwife understand the regulations. Rule 6 is the one that this chapter will focus on as it sets out the midwife's responsibility and sphere of practice (NMC, 2004a). *Midwives rules and standards* states that a midwife will provide midwifery care during the antenatal, intrapartum and postnatal periods and except in an emergency will not carry out any care they have not been trained for. The midwife is also responsible for recognising where there is a *deviation from the norm* (NMC, 2004a, p18). This means that a midwife must recognise what is normal and what is outside their sphere of practice. In order to undertake the following activity it might be useful to remind yourself of the *Midwives rules and standards* (which can be accessed at **www.nmc-uk.org/Publications/Standards**).

Activity 1.4   *Decision-making*

Consider whether the following are considered normal midwifery care.

- A woman is anxious about her pregnancy.
- A 32-week gestation pregnant woman's child has chickenpox.
- A woman requests an epidural in labour.
- A woman is 42 weeks and two days pregnant.

Discuss these with a fellow student and see if you come up with similar answers.

There are some sample answers at the end of this chapter.

This exercise might have highlighted to you how difficult it is to separate frequently occurring midwifery care with normal midwifery practice. It is also important to remember that the *Midwives rules and standards* govern our practice, but they do not say what we should do in each situation; this is something you have to learn through theory and practice, reading evidence and asking others – women and other midwives. There is not just one 'right' way in each aspect of midwifery, as each woman is unique and what matters to her might not matter to the next woman.

Normal midwifery care

We will first consider more broadly what care women can expect from a midwife. For most women, pregnancy and birth are normal physiological events. Pregnant women are usually healthy women in a perfectly natural state. Care of women during pregnancy, birth and the postnatal period in the UK is guided by documents compiled by the National Institute for Health and Clinical Excellence (NICE).

Who provides midwifery care?

The term *named midwife* was introduced by the *National service framework* (DH, 2004) as the midwife primarily responsible for an individual woman's care and named on the woman's **hand-held notes** (the documentation each woman has of her pregnancy) as the lead professional. At each visit the midwife records in the woman's hand-held notes the information exchanged, the observations performed and any maternal issues. The woman keeps her records and brings them to each visit. She knows who to contact in the first instance, as the midwife's name and contact details are clearly detailed on these notes. Should there be a problem in the pregnancy, the responsibility for ensuring this woman receives appropriate maternity care lies with this named midwife.

The importance of continuity in midwifery care is reinforced by other Department of Health documents such as *Maternity matters* (DH, 2007a), and we will return to this a little later. For women experiencing uncomplicated pregnancies the care is usually provided by the named midwife alone, a team of midwives or a model of shared care between the GP and midwifery services, and there is no need for women whose pregnancies are deemed low risk to visit an obstetrician. This is often referred to as **midwifery-led care** and is suitable for women who have uncomplicated pregnancies. The benefits include fewer hospital admissions during pregnancy and more vaginal births with no negative effect on neonatal outcome – that is, their babies are not at increased risk (Hatem et al., 2008). The relationship between midwifery-led care and improved pregnancy outcomes is complex; it could be attributed to the low-risk pregnancy, but in the review by Hatem et al. (2008) both low- and moderate-risk pregnancies were considered to benefit from this model of care.

Activity 1.5   *Reflection*

Consider the phrase *midwifery-led care*. What does it mean to you? Jot down your ideas.

Look at your notes and reflect upon the following.

*   How did you define midwifery-led care?
*   What do you know about this concept and how did this influence your ideas?
*   Did you consider your own birth experiences, those of family members, or your experiences of midwifery so far?

As this activity is based on your own reflection, there is no outline answer at the end of the chapter.

Midwifery-led care may mean valuing communication with women, seeing pregnancy and birth as normal or natural events and thus using less technology or interfering less than other models of care may. But midwifery is not only about letting nature take its course and not interfering; it is also about providing safe environments for women and their babies, and to do this the presence and absence of risk factors are identified.

The concept of risk within midwifery

Normal midwifery care is engulfed by the concept of risk; basically, every piece of information given by or gleaned from a woman is to identify whether her pregnancy is at greater or lesser risk. The information gleaned includes every aspect of the woman's life, from whether she gets enough sunlight and eats enough nutrients to what her body weight is, what sort of exercise she does and what her job is – and this is before we even begin to think about pregnancy risks. There is no middle ground on definitions of risk in UK midwifery: women either have low-risk pregnancies or high-risk pregnancies. In the Hatem et al. (2008) review of midwifery-led care, pregnancies were separated into low-, moderate- and high-risk pregnancies. In the NHS midwives are the lead carer for low-risk pregnancies only, although this notion shifts within independent midwifery practice. Remember, though, that this risk status is not necessarily fixed. This means that a woman can have a pregnancy deemed to be low risk at booking that becomes high risk due to raised blood pressure, for instance. On the other hand, a woman may have a pregnancy that is considered high risk because one of the **screening tests** suggests the **fetus** may have a congenital abnormality; this is unconfirmed following amniocentesis and the fetus is healthy, so her pregnancy is then considered low risk. However, this woman and her family may never feel reassured until the baby is born, and the anxiety felt during the period of not knowing may never leave them.

Although this book is fundamentally about normal – that is, low-risk – midwifery, remember that midwives care for all women. Table 1.1 sets out the factors that are considered to be of higher risk for pregnant women (this list is not exhaustive).

The list of risk factors on the table may seem daunting, but remember they are not all absolute risk factors. Consider the following examples to reassure yourselves. Even when fit and healthy, the woman who delays pregnancy until she is 40 years old has an increased risk of pregnancy associated problems; however, the likelihood is that everything will be fine for her and her baby. The absolute risk of delaying pregnancy is low; the relative risk is raised, but this does not mean that all will not be well. As another example, a woman who has had previous miscarriages is considered at greater risk; however, once the new pregnancy is established she is no less likely to have a complicated pregnancy than any other woman. Some of the risk factors listed in the table are rare, so you should try not to become too fixated on abnormal pregnancies. It is this risk status that some midwives – perhaps independent midwives more than others – question; they may see twin and breech presentations as normal for a particular woman, and within their sphere of practice. Reassuringly, the latest evidence from a national place of birth study showed that the majority of women were deemed low risk (Hollowell et al., 2011).

Low risk	Maternal social risk factors	Maternal health risk factors	Previous pregnancy risk factors	Current pregnancy risk factors
Age 15–39	Age below 14 or above 40	Endocrine conditions, diabetes	Recurrent miscarriage	Multiple pregnancy
Normal weight	Underweight: BMI less than 18; Obesity: BMI more than 35	Hypertension	**Pre-eclampsia**, eclampsia or HELLP syndrome	Grand multiparity
No other risk factors	Drug misuse, alcohol included	Cardiac disease	Blood group antibodies	Small for dates
	Vulnerable women, or those who lack social support	Epilepsy	Uterine surgery, *LSCS, cone biopsy	Bleeding, low **placenta**
		Psychiatric disorders	Bleeding; **APH or ***PPH	Malpresentation/ position including breech
		Severe asthma	Stillbirth or neonatal death	Pre-term labour
		HIV, hepatitis B	Small or large babies, less than 2.5 or more than 4.5 kg	Premature rupture of membranes
		Cancer	Fetus/baby with a congenital abnormality	Raised blood pressure
		Autoimmune disorders		Severe **anaemia**
		Haematological disease (****VTE)		Fetal anomaly detected

Table 1.1: Risk factors for pregnancy

Note: *LSCS = lower segment caesarean section; **APH = antepartum haemorrhage; ***PPH = post-partum haemorrhage; ****VTE = venous thromboembolism

Activity 1.6   *Evidence-based practice and research*

Access the birthplace cohort study at:

> **www.npeu.ox.ac.uk/birthplace/results**

> **www.npeu.ox.ac.uk/files/downloads/birthplace/Birthplace-Q-A.pdf**

Compare your experiences so far with the findings of this study. If you have not been out on placement yet, consider the birth experiences of your friends and families, and see if they are similar.

There are no answers at the end of this chapter because this activity is based on your own experiences. We hope, though, that this research will reassure you that a normal birth is not only possible but a reality for most women, regardless of what you have seen so far.

The quality of this research evidence, in combination with pre-existing research, will shape future maternity policy and practice. It may well increase the number of midwifery-led birthing units across the UK and promote these as the safest place for women with low-risk pregnancies to give birth. As other evidence has shown that both midwives and women in these environments have greater levels of satisfaction than those in other birthing units, this would seem to be a benefit for all society (Hatem et al., 2008). Another benefit for society is the new understanding arising from theories and research on coping in uncertain times (Bryar and Sinclair, 2011), which can be applied to midwifery practice.

Salutogenesis

The term **salutogenesis** is made up of two words, and it examines the origins (genesis) of health (salus). It was coined by a medical sociologist who studied how people manage stress and stay healthy. As much of this chapter – and, indeed, book – focuses on risk assessments, and these assessments can cause stress to women, the term has been adopted by midwifery researchers and writers recently (see, for example, Downe, 2008). The concept of salutogenesis explores how some individuals stay healthy when surrounded by stress yet others do not. The effects of stress according to Antonovsky (1996), the original author, can have three manifestations on individuals: pathogenic; neutral; or salutary. These three words mean that the effects of stress can have a bad (pathogenic) effect, no (neutral) effect or a beneficial (salutary) effect on people, depending on their coping strategies. The stress experienced has to make sense to the individual for a beneficial or salutogenic response to happen. This sense, which Antonvosky calls a sense of coherence, is achieved by people who have positive reactions to the experience in one of three ways: meaningful; manageable; or comprehensible. The way people cope with stress develops through their lives, and some people's ability to cope is greater than others.

While this theory looks at major life stress, pregnancy and birth can be seen as a stress too. Even in a low-risk pregnancy the decisions that women and their partners need to make can have huge implications. Immediately after the confirmation of the pregnancy come difficult choices –and if the pregnancy is unplanned, the woman and her partner may still be coming to terms with the idea of parenthood when these choices are offered. A woman and her partner will be asked to choose whether they should have screening tests and, if so, which ones; this leads to questions about what the possible outcomes of the screening tests are and what the chances are that a problem will not be detected by the screening. It is easy to see how this time of uncertainty – with decisions to make, concerns about whether the right decisions have been made, questions about whether 'my baby is OK' and other anxieties about the emotions and feelings both parents have – can cause stress to individuals.

As we have said, pregnancy and the effects of risk assessments may be stressful for some women and their partners. Looking at women from a midwifery model of care as opposed to a medical model of care could increase women's confidence and coping strategies during this time of stress and promote salutogenic or positive responses that promote well-being. As a midwife you will need to determine if the woman you are caring for is healthy and when she needs medical care. The differences between a midwifery model of care and a medical model of care can be compared to the differences between seeing birth as a normal physiological event and seeing birth as only normal in retrospect. Midwives promote maternal, fetal and family well-being; medics look for pathology, or things going wrong. The underpinning philosophy of midwife-led care is normality, continuity of care and being cared for by a known and trusted midwife during labour (Hatem et al., 2008).

Normality

We have already touched on normality – that the midwife is the lead practitioner in normal pregnancy. However, there are challenges to this concept. For instance, in a pregnancy deemed high risk, women often have fewer choices open to them, such as place of birth. It would not be wise to offer a woman a home birth if she is bleeding antenatally, but a midwife can promote normality even during the birthing process for this woman and her family. Simple aspects of her birth plan, listening to her own choice of music, reducing the ambient lighting for labour and being in a more upright position may enhance this woman's experience of birth, even in these stressful times. Of course, if the clinical picture becomes more serious, the lights may need to be raised and the music is unlikely to relax either of the prospective parents. The promotion of normal birth was only added to the ICM definition of a midwife in 2005, and this is the same year that the Royal College of Midwives (RCM) campaign for normal birth was launched. Perhaps these changes were in response to rising caesarean section rates globally, and to some extent they are a great idea; however, some women will not have natural vaginal births without intervention, and midwives need to support these women as much as any other, and cannot marginalise their experience. This is where knowing the woman can sometimes help, so we will look at continuity of care and carer next.

Continuity

According to Downe (2008) the term *continuity* is multi-layered. She offers several ways of interpreting the word: as a shared philosophy of care; as a streamlined approach to information; as the same person carrying out care; and as care in the same place. Continuity of care can mean that each woman gets the same care but this is delivered by different midwives even if the place of care is the same, such as a children's centre or room in a GP surgery. Continuity of care by the same midwife might offer the greatest rewards in terms of the relationship development between the woman and her midwife, but it seems that organisation of this interpretation of continuity is not always a priority for all maternity services. In labour, one-to-one support or care during birth has been shown to demonstrate increased satisfaction and improved outcomes for women, such as fewer caesarean sections, fewer induced or augmented labours, more normal births and more home births. This model of care has been prioritised in recent years, so fewer resources have been allocated to providing midwives for postnatal care. In a recent RCM audit of midwifery practice, most midwives did not provide continuity of care, especially not in the postnatal period (RCM, 2010).

Differing midwifery schemes or ways of working have also compounded the issue of continuity of carer. Caseload midwifery schemes are delivered by two or three midwives working together to care for a case of pregnant women. The midwives are responsible for the antenatal, intrapartum and postnatal care of the women within the case. The findings from research on this model of care provision have been positive, and both the women and the midwives have benefited from increased interactions and knowing each other. Other models such as team midwifery have also been evaluated, but in team midwifery up to six midwives work together, so this decreases the personal nature of the interactions between the women and midwives. Whichever model of care is provided where you work, the focus of care should be on providing women with individualised care that meets their requirements and promotes well-being for the family.

Individualised care

Individualised care means offering women care that meets their needs and wishes. You demonstrate respect for women if information is presented in an accessible way to them so they can make choices about their care. You will remember from earlier in the chapter that the evidence for care decisions, balancing the cost and effectiveness, is produced by NICE. This guidance, along with Trust policies, can sometimes seem to shape the care offered to women more than truly individualised care. Take, for instance, the number and schedule of antenatal visits women who are first-time mothers or already parents can expect. NICE (2008a) state that ten is the appropriate number of visits for first-time mothers and three fewer visits for subsequent pregnancies. This approach, it could be argued, is organisational-based care; the remedy to this is for the midwife to ensure that the content of the consultations is individualised. By going back to the *with woman* philosophy and seeing her as a whole person and not just another pregnant women, listening to her hopes and fears and unique experiences, the midwife can offer individualised care tailored to each woman. The relationship that then develops is individual to that midwife and woman, and if the resources are available in the area, other forms of support, such as drop-in clinics, parenting classes and other care can also be offered that each woman can choose to accept, if she wishes, in addition to the scheduled appointments.

Just as women have their own ways of knowing, midwives too have experiences, beliefs and knowledge about the world, relationships, women, pregnancy and birth that need to be explored. Discussion about how midwives join up their unique experiences and beliefs with the added dimension of knowledge and provide midwifery care will follow. The following theory is based on knowledge in nursing, but it is abstract enough to apply equally to midwifery practice. While much of this chapter has separated the philosophy of nursing from midwifery, this work is useful to analyse what knowledge is required by practising professionals and can thus be applied to midwives' knowledge as well as nurses'.

Patterns of knowledge

In 1978 Barbara Carper published her essay *Fundamental patterns of knowing in nursing* (Carper, 1978). Knowledge is divided into four patterns: empirics, ethics, esthetics (aesthetics) and personal knowledge. Empirical knowledge is the science – divided into laws and theories – that explains and describes phenomena. Ethics is about morals – what ought to be done as opposed to what is done. Aesthetics are specific as opposed to general components of an individual's care. They are what matter to that individual, and this is the aspect that has often been referred to as an art. Finally, personal knowledge is what the practitioner knows about the relationship of self to others – it is this that forms the basis of a therapeutic relationship with others. We can unpack the ways of knowing according to Carper by exploring a scenario.

Scenario

Jade is 39 weeks pregnant with her first baby. She is experiencing abdominal pain and her 'waters' have broken. On admission to hospital she is scared and needs reassurance. On examination she is not in labour, her **contractions** *are not regular and her cervix is not yet dilating.*

If we examine this scenario, the empirics or scientific knowledge is that the midwife knows Jade is likely to go into labour soon – most women will have a spontaneous onset of labour between 37 and 41 weeks gestation. Once the membranes have ruptured, most women go into labour within 24–48 hours; this has been scientifically proven (Walsh, 2007). The midwife could send Jade home now, but ethically she ought to support her, as we know she is in pain and might benefit from some breathing exercises or tools to cope with the pain, such as education about how the baby is born to help her understand what the pain is for. Aesthetically, although Jade is not in labour, what she needs that is pertinent to her is to be reassured, as she is scared. The midwife can do this by spending time with Jade, showing her around the birthing unit, reassuring her that being scared is normal and that she is managing well. Lastly, the midwife knows that the more time she spends with Jade now, the better Jade will be prepared for labour. The relationship between Jade and her midwife at this time is pivotal; it will shape her progress in labour.

A midwife who has an open view of the world and is intuitive to Jade's needs will provide a different form of care than one who believes Jade is not in labour and offers a more detached attitude.

At the beginning of your training you might be amazed at how a midwife knows what to do in each situation. This scenario might reassure you that being with the woman and not actually doing anything but listening, supporting and educating at this point is the best course of action. Breaking knowledge down into four patterns, as Carper has done, might help you to see what you need to know. Look at the *NMC Standards for pre-registration midwifery education* (NMC, 2009, p21), which are also broken down into four domains, and you will see that your education could have been shaped by Carper's theory. The four domains are: effective midwifery practice (empirics); professional and ethical practice (ethics); developing the individual midwife and others (personal knowledge); and achieving quality care through evaluation and research (aesthetics). While this theory might not feel helpful at the moment, it is hoped that over the course of your midwifery education, as you visit other theories – perhaps midwifery-specific ones – you will be better able to articulate your own philosophy of midwifery care and practice. The further reading section of this chapter offers some books and articles of theories relevant to midwifery.

The science of what happens in pregnancy and birth, the way women and their families are treated with ethical principles and individual care plans, and the interactions you will have with them all shape their experience. If, each time you meet a woman, you consider *How would I want my sister, friend or daughter treated?* and use this as a base to inform your communications with women, you will become a kind and empathetic midwife. Of course, this needs to be supported with science and knowledge of normal and abnormal anatomy and physiology, but this will come. First, we will consider ethics in greater detail.

Ethical principles

The ethical principles governing nursing and midwifery practice are written in the NMC *Code* (NMC, 2008a).

Activity 1.8　　　　　　　　　　　　　　　　　　　　　*Reflection*

Access the NMC website and look for *The code: standards of conduct, performance and ethics for nurses and midwives*. Have a read and think about the main messages being portrayed in this document. Do you understand what this document means to your practice?

This YouTube clip might enhance your understanding.

www.nmc-uk.org/Nurses-and-midwives/The-code/Launching-the-code/

The code is being rewritten in 2012, so you may need to check back for an updated version.

There are no suggested answers at the end of this chapter as this is based on your own understanding and reflections.

The NMC *Code* sets standards that nurses and midwives must abide by, for instance: always gain consent for treatments or tests so you are trusted; treat people with dignity and respect; advocate for them if they need someone on their side or are having difficulty putting their wishes across; and maintain their confidentiality and standards of care (NMC, 2008a).

One of the most influential textbooks that explores ethics in greater detail is *Principles of biomedical ethics* (Beauchamp and Childress, 2008); it is now in its sixth edition. This book explores four principles of ethics, but it also reminds the reader that the language we use may have a negative or positive effect on the women we care for.

Activity 1.9　　　　　　　　　　　　　　　　　　　*Critical thinking*

Make a list of midwifery words that are associated with positive and negative images.

Ask a colleague or your mentor to do this too, and compare and contrast the words and the effects that they have on you personally. You may find that your colleague or mentor has words on their list that they find unacceptable but that are not on your list. Discuss these differences especially.

As an example, think of the word *birth* as opposed to *delivery*. What do these two images conjure up for you?

There are no suggested answers at the end of this chapter as this is based on your own understanding and reflections.

Activity 1.10   *Critical thinking*

Access the ICM *International code of ethics for midwives.*

www.internationalmidwives.org/Portals/5/Code%20of%20Ethics%20 Long%20version-ENG.2003.doc

Ask yourself if it is still relevant today despite being adopted in 1993 (it was updated in 2003). Write down your thoughts on five statements that the code makes and then discuss them with a friend.

There are no sample answers at the end, but it seems like this code of ethics should still be applicable today. Read on for more about ethics.

Returning to the book by Beauchamp and Childress, the four ethical principles they explore are respect for **autonomy** and three principles of **beneficence**, **non-maleficence** and **justice**. These ethical considerations are, as you will see, rooted in midwifery models of care. If we examine each principle and relate it to midwifery, we can build up a fuller picture of normal midwifery practice. Some students want black-and-white answers to how or why we carry out care, but in an ever-changing world, there are no hard facts or truths about what must be done, and, as we have said, as each woman is an individual with her own values, each woman's needs will be different.

An example of respect for autonomy is when a midwife respects a decision made by a woman in her care, even if the decision is different from the one the midwife would make herself. If a woman chooses not to come for antenatal care, or continues to undertake risk-taking behaviours while pregnant – whether this is smoking, drinking or taking illicit drugs – as long as the midwife has informed her why antenatal care or a reduction in the risk-taking behaviours would benefit her and her fetus (and documented the interaction), the woman has the right to choose. The obligation of the midwife is to inform the woman of more optimal health choices but ultimately to respect her decision. The only deviation from this rule occurs if the woman has issues of mental capacity and is deemed, by a psychiatrist or court, unable to make a decision at that time. Informed consent can only occur if the woman and her family feel supported in their decisions.

The principle of beneficence involves acting in ways to promote well-being (or benefit) for others. We have already discussed salutogenesis, which is an example of a way of promoting well-being. Other examples of beneficence for midwifery include encouraging an obese woman to increase her daily activity and avoid 'eating for two' while ensuring that she understands what constitutes a healthy diet and answering a woman's question on topics such as vaginal birth after a previous caesarean section so she can weigh up and balance the possible benefits with the possible risks. Midwives should always act in the best interests of their clients.

The principle of non-maleficence, or not doing harm, is not easily understood in all areas of midwifery. Two examples illustrate the problem. It is known that the practices of routine episiotomies, artificial rupture of membranes and continuous **cardiotocograph** (CTG) can potentially harm the woman or her fetus and subject her to **iatrogenic** or hospital-induced harm. These and other practices should only be undertaken if there is a clinical indication, such as fetal distress or an abnormal heart rate upon **auscultation**. However, if a woman has severe pre-eclampsia at 26 weeks gestation and the only way she will recover from this multi-system disorder is to give birth, the doing of no harm to the woman is likely to cause harm to the fetus, since having the baby so early will be detrimental to its development.

The fourth principle, that of justice, refers to the obligation of treating others fairly. For Beauchamp and Childress it was about sharing what is inherently good in medicine with others, and about how justice was distributed. According to the NMC *Code* (NMC, 2008a), you must treat patients (or women) and colleagues fairly and may not discriminate between either group. You must not care differently for one woman than another. Consider, for instance, a woman who has not cared well for herself during pregnancy; she still deserves the best care that you can give. Just because one woman has a nicer house or an easier life does not mean that she should have more midwifery time.

Professionalism

The last concept to consider in this chapter is professionalism, which follows on from ethics. Your education will enable you to provide professional midwifery care. The concept of a professional has a shared meaning, regardless of the profession you enter, whether it is law, education or midwifery. The first shared meaning is that you know something – you have knowledge. As we have seen in the Carper definition above, knowledge in midwifery comes from many sources: for instance, sociology and psychology in addition to biological knowledge. You will also develop skills for practice; these include communication and maternal and fetal assessments and examinations. You will work to a high standard of professional ethics, including, but not only, the four principles discussed above and the NMC *Code*, rules and standards. You will be interested in pregnant women, their families and other midwives, and be part of and create a motivated environment for the profession's benefit.

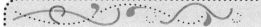

Chapter summary

This chapter has introduced normal midwifery practice. It has considered the opposing views of low- and high-risk pregnancies, and how midwives can incorporate philosophies of care that provide for women at both ends of the continuum of risk. Midwifery practice encompasses several forms of knowledge that can be compared to domains of practice within your own education programme. It has explored the ethical principles and those of continuity and normality to build up a whole spectrum of knowing in midwifery.

Activities: brief outline answers

Activity 1.1: Decision-making (page 6)

The midwife is recognised as a responsible and accountable professional who works in partnership with women to give the necessary support, care and advice during pregnancy, labour and the postpartum period, to conduct births on the midwife's own responsibility and to provide care for the newborn and the infant. This care includes preventative measures, the promotion of normal birth, the detection of complications in mother and child, the accessing of medical care or other appropriate assistance and the carrying out of emergency measures (ICM, 2011).

Activity 1.4: Decision-making (page 8)

Consider whether the following are considered normal midwifery care.

- A woman is anxious about her pregnancy: this depends on whether the woman is just pregnant and has just found out, whether she has a pre-existing history of anxiety or if something untoward has happened during this pregnancy. It could be considered normal for women to be anxious in the early stages of a first or an unplanned pregnancy (about how are they going to cope and whether everything will be OK). However, anxiety can also be a serious condition. The midwife will have to use all her skills to work out whether this is normal or not.
- A 32-week gestation pregnant woman's child has chickenpox: while this is not normal, it does happen on occasions. This woman and her fetus are probably fine; most women have immunity to chickenpox already from being infected as children. If the immune status is not known, women can be tested. At 32 weeks the consequences for the mother or baby of having chickenpox are minimal so you can reassure this woman; if she is not immune, there are treatments that can reduce transmission rates to the fetus.
- A woman requests an epidural in labour: while this can be considered normal as so many women choose epidural analgesia in labour, the RCM campaign for normal birth would not consider this a normal birth.
- A woman is 42 weeks and two days pregnant: while this may be normal for a woman with a menstrual cycle of 35 days or who has had previous prolonged pregnancies, it may be a cause for concern in another woman whose menstrual cycle is 26 days.

Further reading

The following texts are all useful for background reading.

Bryar, R and Sinclair, M (2011) *Theory for midwifery practice*, 2nd edition. Basingstoke: Palgrave Macmillan.

Downe, S (2008) *Normal childbirth, evidence and debate*, 2nd edition. London: Churchill Livingstone Elsevier.

Medforth, J, Battersby, S, Evans, M, Marsh, B and Walker, A (2006) *Oxford handbook of midwifery*. Oxford: Oxford University Press.

Walsh, D (2007) *Evidence-based care for normal labour and birth: a guide for midwives*. Oxford: Routledge.

Useful website

http://midwifethinking.com

Campaign for Normal Midwifery Birth: this blog is an interesting read; Rachel Reed is a midwife and educator based in Queensland, Australia.

Chapter 2
Communication and interpersonal skills in normal midwifery practice

Sam Chenery-Morris and Moira McLean

NMC Standards for Pre-registration Midwifery Education

This chapter will address the following competencies:

Domain: Effective midwifery practice

Communicate effectively with women and their families throughout the pre-conception, antenatal, intrapartum and postnatal periods. Communication will include:

- listening to women and helping them to identify their feelings and anxieties about their pregnancies, the birth and the related changes to themselves and their lives;
- enabling women to think through their feelings;
- enabling women to make informed choices about their health and health care;
- actively encouraging women to think about their own health and the health of their babies and families and how this can be improved;
- communicating with women through their pregnancy, labour and the period following birth.

Domain: Professional and ethical practice

Practise in accordance with *The code: standards of conduct, performance and ethics for nurses and midwives* (NMC, 2008a), within the limitations of the individual's own competence, knowledge and sphere of professional practice.

Practise in a way which respects, promotes and supports individuals' rights, interests, preferences, beliefs and cultures.

Maintain confidentiality of information.

Domain: Developing the individual midwife and others

Demonstrate effective working across professional boundaries and develop professional networks. This will include:

- effective collaboration and communication.

Domain: Achieving quality care through evaluation and research

Apply relevant knowledge to the midwife's own practice in structured ways which are capable of evaluation: This will include:

- gaining feedback from women and their families and appropriately applying this to practice.

NMC Essential Skills Clusters

This chapter will address the following ESCs:

The Essential Skills Clusters are separated into five key areas: communication; initial consultation between the woman and the midwife; normal labour and birth; initiation and continuance of breastfeeding; and medical products management. Communication is pivotal to all ESCs.

Chapter aims

After reading this chapter you will be able to:

*   understand terminology used in midwifery;
*   explore the impact of language used with women and the implications of this for the midwifery profession;
*   develop your ideas about how and what you are communicating with women;
*   recognise that it is not just the practical midwifery skills you need to practise but the *way* these skills are offered to women;
*   reflect upon and increase your communication strategies.

Introduction

This chapter will show you how communication is an essential skill. It is paramount in all midwifery care, whether communicating with the woman and her partner, another professional or colleagues. The chapter will also consider documentation as one way of communicating care. The importance of communication to all aspects of normal midwifery practice cannot be overstated. We will consider midwifery terminology, such as empowerment, and what types of language are appropriate in midwifery practice.

The chapter will help to prepare and develop you, the student, for professional practice, examining your role in the community and hospital environments, understanding your super-numerary status, your learning needs and your need to be an educator too. It will give you confidence to undertake clinical skills in practice as you become familiar with the language and the need for such assessment.

Clinical skills for midwifery will be covered. These will be expanded upon in each of the following antenatal, intrapartum and postnatal chapters, but the basics of maternal and fetal observations, abdominal palpation, vaginal examination and communication will be introduced in this chapter. Before we begin, use the following activity to try to recollect your thoughts the first time you heard 'midwifery speak'.

Activity 2.1   *Reflection*

Try to remember what you thought the first time you watched a pregnancy-related TV programme, such as *One Born Every Minute*. Did you understand the terminology used? Did you notice how the women and midwives communicated? What did you think was good and what did you think could be improved in this communication?

As this activity is based on your own experiences, there are no sample answers at the end of the chapter.

You may remember not understanding all the phrases or terminology used by the midwives on such programmes. Depending on where you are in your preparation programme, this may still be the case. Learning how to be a midwife and what all the complicated words mean may seem daunting. To break it down, let's start with what you have to demonstrate throughout your education.

Communication: an essential skill

You will notice that the list at the beginning of this chapter, detailing which domain of practice and essential skills you will be exploring, is longer than any other in this book. This is because communication is the essential skill listed first and in every one of the competencies you will need to succeed in becoming a midwife. The NMC standards (NMC, 2009) are separated into four domains of practice: effective midwifery practice; professional and ethical practice; developing the individual midwife and others; and achieving quality care through evaluation and research. These all require communication skills. It could be argued, therefore, that this is the most important chapter in this book. Many students think they have good communication skills before they begin their course, and while this may be true – you will obviously have communicated effectively during your interview – this skill is not static. It changes, develops and grows as you learn more about midwifery and develop your relationship with women, your peers, your mentor and the midwifery profession. There will always be another level you can take your communication skills to. This does not mean that you will speak in technical or complex ways, but that you will be able to listen, reflect, respond, empathise, motivate, educate and much more as you understand and practise these skills.

In Chapter 1 we looked at a theory of nursing examining the fundamental patterns of knowing (Carper, 1978) and explored how these four ways – empirics, ethics, personal knowledge and aesthetics – resonated with the four domains of midwifery practice (NMC, 2009). The following paragraphs explore in more detail how these fit in with communication and midwifery skills.

Empirics or empirical knowledge is described by Carper as the science – the laws and theories of science. So in effective midwifery practice this knowledge is communicated in how we talk to women about the physiological changes that are happening in their bodies. Your knowledge of signs and symptoms of pregnancy are communicated to a woman to reassure her all is well. This form of science is derived from biology – from the anatomy, physiology and pathology of the human body. So if you recognise a deviation from the normal physiological changes in pregnancy, you also need to be able to communicate this. The sciences also include sociology (how people live within society), psychology (how people think) and many other scientific laws and theories that inform midwifery practice and how we communicate well-being or otherwise to women and their families. Much of the scientific evidence that informs midwifery practice has been incorporated into evidence-based practice guidelines, so, for instance, because of scientific research we know the optimum number of antenatal appointments a woman needs and at what times they should occur in her pregnancy (NICE, 2008a). This forms one aspect of communicating with women.

Ethics – or professional and ethical practice – is informed by the NMC *Code* (NMC, 2008a). It is also shaped by the ethical principles we met in the previous chapter, such as non-maleficence, 'to do no harm', within the midwifery profession. So a midwife who practises without due thought, thus causing harm to the woman's birthing experience, is not upholding this principle. How we know what is likely to cause harm to a woman is by communicating with her, listening to her preferences, hearing her values and respecting these. If we offer her enough information, she can make a decision that is right for her and her family, and not based on someone else's beliefs. For Carper (1978), ethics is about morals, what ought to be done as opposed to what is done. So, as a student midwife, you don't only do what your mentor says or does, but you really consider how this woman would want this information to be relayed so she can make the best decision for herself.

Personal knowledge means knowing oneself. For the student midwife this might seem like a tall order. You came on the course to know about midwifery, but if you know yourself and develop this knowledge, you can use it to get to know others. It is an essential part of communication, as the ability or inability to be self-aware affects communication and relationship development. How well you know yourself informs the relationship you can develop with others, and it is this relationship that is considered therapeutic. As a student midwife, and then a registered midwife, you will have your own values, experiences, beliefs and knowledge about families, relationships and childbearing, whether you have experienced childbearing yourself or not. It is these values that can shape your communication both negatively and positively; recognising what it is that you believe in, and accepting that others may have different opinions is crucial in developing yourself and your communication skills with others.

Aesthetics is the art of midwifery; it is the practical knowledge the midwife experiences or feels. Aesthetics encompasses knowing the women in your care. It covers specific components of an individual's care as opposed to general components, so knowing what matters to that person and their birthing experience is the aspect that is most often referred to as an art. It is precisely this practical element that is sometimes hardest to evaluate – how you 'know' something. Practical knowledge might also encompass the skills that you need to demonstrate to achieve quality midwifery care. How to describe what one midwife lacks and how another has the ability or art of communication or a particular skill can be problematic, but many of us know what the art of quality midwifery looks and feels like even if it is hard to describe.

As Carper points out, all knowledge is subject to change and therefore even the empirical, scientific knowledge that is considered to be factual will change. Let's first see how language has changed in midwifery. It's not only what we say but also how we say it that matters (Leap, 2012). We must stop using words and phrases that have hidden or even not-so-hidden meanings.

Activity 2.2   *Critical thinking*

Consider the following words from Nicky Leap's article (2012, p18):

> Confinement; failure to progress; inadequate pelvis; incompetent cervix; failed homebirth; and referring to women as 'patients'

Use a dictionary to look up each of the terms above and see how the dictionary defines them. Then think of a more appropriate 'women and midwifery friendly' term that could be used instead.

Try this with a colleague, because two heads are usually better than one.

There are some suggested answers at the end of this chapter.

Now that we have thought about the power of language, let's look at communication strategies. Gibbon uses as an article title 'It's more than just talking' (Gibbon, 2010) in order to encompass the many interrelated aspects of communication skills. She explains how many of the most recent policy documents have improving communication strategies as their central message (DH, 2007b), improved communication can also save women's lives (Draycott et al., 2011). Gibbon (2010) offers strategies for improved communication, including reflecting, summarising, paraphrasing, hunching and checking, questioning and silences. So let's look at some of these techniques and see how we can incorporate them into caring for woman and their families.

Reflecting is a communication strategy that has two steps: first, you listen to what the woman has said; then you offer back her thoughts to show that you have understood them properly. The idea comes from a counselling technique (Rogers, 1986) and demonstrates, by using the woman's own words back to her, that you have accepted what she has said. Summarising is when you state the key issues to show the woman you understand what she has told you. Paraphrasing is when you repeat the woman's story back to her, in your own words. It, too, can reassure the woman that you understand her issue.

Hunching and checking involves the midwife responding to terms or issues a woman offers and trying to explore or understand them further. That is, the midwife has an idea – a hunch – about what the woman means when she says she feels something, but the midwife still checks that their understanding is the same as the woman's, to ensure they are communicating effectively. For instance, a woman might say she feels 'damp down below'; the midwife may not be sure whether the woman is describing increased vaginal discharge or spontaneous ruptured membranes; the midwife chooses the one she thinks fits the scenario most – has a hunch about the right interpretation – but then checks with the woman that they share the same interpretation of that phrase.

In communicating with women, it is more useful to ask open-ended questions than closed ones. To demonstrate the difference between the two try the following activity.

Activity 2.3   *Communication*

Ask a friend how they travelled to work today or how they are feeling by using the example closed and open questions below.

Open style: How did you get here today? How are you feeling today?

Closed style: Did you come to work by train? Are you sad today?

Think about the kinds of reactions and responses you received from these two styles of questioning.

There are some sample answers at the end of the chapter.

Having tried two very basic questioning styles, you can probably see that how we ask information from women either enables them to 'chat' and start to build a relationship or limits their responses. Open-ended questioning gives the woman a chance to take the lead, whereas closed questions mean the professional is leading with their agenda. In the short time you will have to get to know the women in your care, asking closed questions may seem like the best way to get the answers to make clinical decisions, yet this is not the case. The opportunity for the woman to be heard, to tell her story in the way she wants to and to know the listener is really there for her, is part of a therapeutic and trusting professional relationship. When you listen to a woman you can often link another open question into the ensuing conversation, which will help you to clarify the information you need. Examples of these types of questions include: Could you expand upon that a little more? Could you tell me more about what you are finding most difficult to deal with?

The last technique advocated by Gibbon is silences. For midwives this is sometimes essential as it allows the woman time to think about the question, reflect upon her situation, and gather her thoughts or compose herself, depending on the issue. For student midwives this is sometimes the hardest skill to master; knowing when to be silent is difficult to determine and can feel uncomfortable to begin with. All communication strategies require practice. Silence will be one of the non-verbal communication strategies you will be using. These strategies include: eye contact; smiling to reassure the woman; other facial expressions; your tone of voice; your posture; and even your appearance throughout the interaction.

But none of the strategies in the above paragraphs works on its own; each needs to be part of your interest in the woman and in her experience. The element that is missing from the communication techniques above and that holds them all together is the emotional connection with another person. The emotional component of care is unavoidable if we are to be there for the women we care for (Theodosius, 2008). Theodosius was studying nursing behaviours, but her theory is reiterated by others in the midwifery context (Hunter, 2004; Deery 2005). Both Hunter and Deery think that student midwives like you need to be introduced to emotional awareness during your education, so you are better equipped to deal with the challenges of practice. They suggest that using role play, drama, art and poetry in a supportive environment may help you to engage with your emotions and then you will be better able to connect with others.

We now need to take this a step further, to look at the stages of a woman's birth experience – antenatal, intrapartum and postnatal – to see what and how a midwife needs to communicate (Table 2.1).

As you can see, in Table 2.1 communication skills and midwifery skills have been intertwined. This is because it is often not just a matter of performing a skill that is important but also how this skill is communicated to women and their families. The range of skills included in the table

	Antenatal	**Intrapartum**	**Postnatal**
Pregnancy and birth knowledge	Physiological changes and symptoms that may be experienced by the woman that are normal, and those that require referral to another professional	Knowledge of birth used to communicate with women their progress in labour and reassure them	Return of the woman's body to non-pregnant state, recognising deviations from normal
Sharing information to facilitate informed choices	Screening tests – maternal and fetal, nutrition, smoking, alcohol, work-related hazards	Using the knowledge from the box above, facilitating conversations and enabling women to make decisions about mobility, pain relief if required and choices such as third-stage management	Reassurance in initiating and continuing breastfeeding; knowledge of the neonatal screening programme
Promoting physical and mental health	Assessing antenatal mental health and whether there are particular problems such as domestic violence. Antenatal preparation classes, place of birth discussions	Optimal fetal positioning, active birthing	Breastfeeding support, infant bonding
Midwifery skills	Blood pressure, urinalysis, abdominal measurement and palpation, **membrane sweeping**	As antenatal; maternal pulse and temperature, palpating uterine contractions, auscultating the fetal heart rate, vaginal examinations, management of labour and birth	Maternal and neonatal examinations and observations, including maternal blood pressure, temperature and pulse, neonatal examination, Apgar score,* temperature

Table 2.1: Skills and communications needed in normal midwifery practice

Note: * Apgar = Appearance, Pulse, Grimace, Activity, Respiratory effort (see Chapter 7 for details).

is too diverse to cover in detail within this chapter, so we will concentrate on three key skills: maternal blood pressure (BP); abdominal palpation, including auscultation of the fetal heart; and vaginal examination. Other skills, such as drug administration and examination of the newborn baby, will be covered in the later chapters. It's not necessarily how to perform the skills that you need to concentrate on – though many students do; it's how the *consequences* of undertaking each skill are communicated to women that is important, so they consent or decline the procedures with full understanding. To enhance this chapter, signposts to other more specific skills books are given in the further reading section.

Activity 2.4   *Evidence-based practice and research*

Find the Royal College of Midwives website and look under the student tab for the 'How To Guides'.

www.rcm.org.uk/college/your-career/students/

Read these through with a colleague and see whether your practice deviates from these articles, which cover manual and automated BP measurements, abdominal examination, hand washing and others.

There are no suggested answers at the end of this chapter as this activity is based on your own practice.

Now let us consider first one of the most frequently undertaken skills for midwifery – blood pressure measurement. Blood pressure measurements are offered throughout the pregnancy and birth experience: at the first booking appointment; at each appointment through the antenatal period; at admission to hospital, in labour and postnatally. It is a non-invasive procedure, meaning that the woman is not poked and prodded too much; the measurement is taken from the arm and usually the woman does not have to remove her clothes. However, it can occasionally be uncomfortable for the woman, especially if her blood pressure has been high or someone pumps the cuff up too tight or for too long. Even though this procedure is non-invasive and 'routine', you still need to ask each woman for permission to perform this measurement.

Concept summary: informed consent

To consent to care, a woman needs enough information on which to base her choice to accept or decline that care. The woman must also be deemed competent to consent, have the mental capacity to make the decision herself and enough information so her consent is fully informed. Ensuring this information is given in a non-judgemental way is part of your role and that of every midwife. Knowing how much information each woman needs is a problem faced by midwives every day.

Now that we have considered the concept of informed consent, we need to consider what information a woman needs in order to consent to a BP measurement. It's not just the action of taking the blood pressure measurement that is important in the woman's decision-making process; it's the implications if the measurement is found to be higher or lower than the normal parameters. The reason midwives take BP readings at every appointment is to recognise pre-eclampsia; thus, for the woman to give informed consent to this procedure, you need to tell her this. She may also need to know the normal parameters of BP measurement before she consents. Smoking, eating, talking and exercise immediately prior to a BP measurement can elevate the reading. If the BP is within normal range limits of 100–139 mmHg for the top (diastolic reading) and 60–89 mmHg for the lower (systolic reading) – 120/72, for instance – the woman will be reassured that all is well at that time. But she still needs to be alert to signs and symptoms of pre-eclampsia, such as headaches and visual disturbances, so she can self-refer if she is unwell. Now we consider how to undertake this skill.

Skill summary: recording blood pressure (see Figure 2.1)

Ask the woman you are caring for to sit or lie in a semi-recumbent position, depending on the environment and whether you are going to be undertaking another skill following this procedure, with her consent. Her arm should be at the level of her heart. The machine you use, a sphygmomanometer, has an inflatable cuff, which you place around the woman's upper arm and secure with the velcro, so when you pump the cuff up, it tightens to restrict the blood flow to her lower arm. You feel the woman's brachial pulse – the one in the inner aspect of her elbow – to see how high you need to pump the cuff; stop pumping when the pulse is no longer felt. Place your stethoscope over this pulse and listen for the sound of the blood flow to return as you slowly release the pressure from the cuff. The first sound, a tapping, gives you the systolic blood pressure measurement; you need to visually read this measurement in 2 mmHg increments as the dial on the manometer falls. As you continue to deflate the cuff, the sound of the blood flow will change; when the sound stops, look for the reading, which will give you your diastolic measurement.

Remove the cuff, and record the findings in the appropriate place, whether this is the woman's hand-held records or on her **partogram** or postnatal kardex, depending on when you are undertaking this skill.

You can see from the skill summary that you need to use two of your senses, hearing and sight, but you also need to use non-verbal observation skills to ensure that this woman is all right, and you could smile at her as well to reassure her during the procedure. You will perform this skill many times during your education period and once qualified as a midwife, as most women consent to BP measurements during their birthing journey.

You can begin to see that there is much more to consider than just performing a 'routine' observation. If we truly treat each woman as an individual, we need to ensure that the amount of information relayed to her meets her needs to consent to care. Now, the midwife also needs to

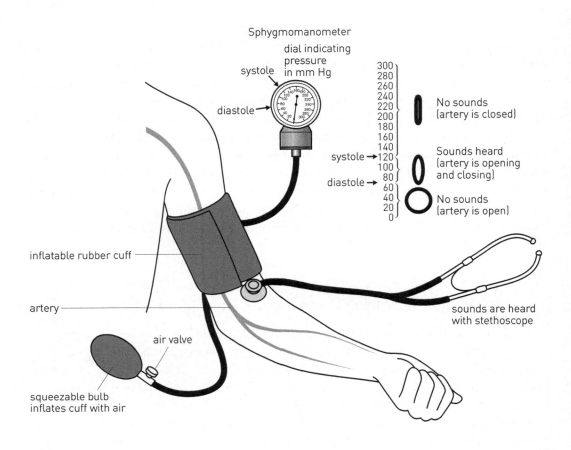

Sphygmomanometer

dial indicating
pressure
in mm Hg

systole

diastole

300
280
260
240
220
200
180
160
140
systole → 120
100
diastole → 80
60
40
20
0

No sounds
(artery is closed)

Sounds heard
(artery is opening
and closing)

No sounds
(artery is open)

inflatable rubber cuff

artery

sounds are heard
with stethoscope

air valve

squeezable bulb
inflates cuff with air

Figure 2.1:
Method for taking blood
pressure measurement

a) Technique

b) Consider environment, the
woman's comfort and informed
consent when taking blood
pressure

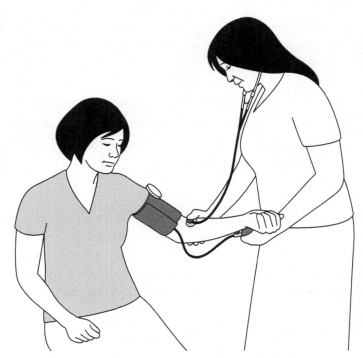

consider how she shares this information with the woman without causing excess anxiety. These are the sorts of questions that are barriers to informed consent in practice. But if the midwife does not offer all the information, the woman is making only half a decision. BP measurement is one example, and most women consent to this procedure as the reason for doing it is to identify a pregnancy-related disorder, and this identified care can be tailored to ensure both the mother's and the baby's needs are balanced to ensure as healthy an outcome as possible for both. But as we look at the rest of the childbearing process, you will see that the issues become more complex, in terms of both the information needed and the consequences of the choices women need to make.

Without enough information to make their own decisions women will not be empowered. Empowerment is encouraged by assisting women – through an intentional process of information sharing – with decision-making that reflects their values and enables women and their partners to be confident in their care choices and the actions that may arise from the choices. To explore this concept further and look at how midwives facilitate this, we will look at the three stages of the birth experience.

Antenatal communication and skills

During the woman's pregnancy, you need to listen to the way she initially communicates about her pregnancy news, to assess whether the woman is positive about this life-changing event. It is not just hearing the words that will alert you to her emotional response to pregnancy, but the way she uses non-verbal communication too. Let's examine what we mean here. Listening is a key aspect in communication skills; women frequently say that no one really listened to them, or tried to understand the reasons behind their emotions, hopes, fears or concerns (AIMS, 2012). Appointments can feel rushed, and you, as a new student, are concerned about practising your physical checks on the woman, learning how to take or perfect the blood pressure measurement or urinalysis. This inhibits your ability to concentrate on what the woman is actually saying – or not saying. Active listening is a skill and requires more of you than just listening to the woman's words. Up to 70 per cent of first impressions during communication are at a non-verbal level; as a student midwife, you will need to learn how to receive and interpret these non-verbal signs to better hear women (Mehrabian, 1971).

During the antenatal period the midwife is also using communication strategies to facilitate changes in behaviours that may be harmful to the developing fetus, such as smoking. In a study of the approaches of South African midwives to smoking cessation (Everett-Murphy et al., 2011), three types of communication styles were seen. These included: an authoritarian style where the midwife assumed the dominant expert approach and was angry and confrontational when women did not comply with their advice; a paternalistic 'I know best' approach where the midwife had little faith that their approach would alter the women's smoking behaviours; and an enthusiastic friend approach that embraced a woman-centred philosophy, consciously encouraging more interaction with the women, which enhanced the trusting midwife–women relationship.

Activity 2.5   *Evidence-based practice and research*

Imagine that you have a vice or behaviour that you wish to change. It could be smoking, writing your assignments at the last minute or taking only limited exercise. Now consider the three styles of communication described above: authoritarian, paternalistic and enthusiastic friend. Which of the approaches are you most likely to respond to? What do you see as the benefits and limitations of these communication strategies?

There are some sample answers at the end of this chapter.

The style of communication that is most applicable to midwifery is a woman-centred approach, which can be considered similar to the term 'professional friend' approach – knowing the balance between being detached and being over-involved, and also understanding that you are not social friends and that there are boundaries that you must not cross. The codes of professional behaviour are different from those of social behaviour, and as a student midwife you must uphold the rules of professional engagement, including confidentiality and maintaining a non-judgemental attitude, to ensure you uphold professional integrity.

As a midwife, you help facilitate a woman's education about all the screening tests she and her partner will be offered, not only to ensure her own health, but also the health and well-being of the developing fetus. The information offered will be one part of the process the woman and her partner will go through in deciding which tests they choose to accept or decline. To enable you to know what and how to communicate this knowledge, you need first to gather this information and digest it yourself. Then you need to listen to how your mentor communicates the information. You will probably first try relaying small chunks of information, and then larger parts of these consultations will become part of your role. Communication is not just repeating what your mentor says. As degree students you need to be able to critically analyse what information is required, to listen to the woman and her partner's responses to tailor the information to their needs, but also to recognise why a woman might be quiet, and deal with this too.

Screening tests are more difficult for women to consent to than blood pressure measurement for many reasons. First, the implications of **screening** are to detect a condition or disease. If the condition or disease is anaemia in the woman, the treatment – iron supplementation – is usually acceptable as the woman will feel better, with more energy, if their anaemia is treated. However, if the screening test detects a condition in the fetus, there may not be a treatment, and the parents-to-be then have bigger decisions to make, such as whether to continue with the pregnancy or not. The decision to accept or decline screening for fetal anomaly is therefore a much bigger decision than whether to accept BP measurement. As midwives we need to ensure women and their partners have enough information about all their care choices, not just the complex decisions, so they are truly informed.

Intrapartum communication and skills

The skills you will need in intrapartum care or labour include all of the above communication skills and some additional ones. For instance, in the antenatal period you usually communicate with women face-to-face, but this is not always the case in early labour. Although women can use the telephone at any time during their pregnancy to communicate their care needs and ask for advice and reassurance, it has become the first point of call in labour care (Green et al., 2011). This study by Green et al. (2011) recognises that telephone, as opposed to face-to-face communication, is a changing context of labour care and needs to be managed in a caring and sensitive manner; in particular, it is important that women are made to feel welcome to come into hospital. This philosophy of welcoming women to come into hospital in early labour might seem at odds with the idea of telephone assessment, which would suggest that, if all is well, the woman should remain at home for as long as possible. The skill of telephone communication is to enable women to feel they have control over the timing of coming into hospital; doing this may give them the confidence to stay at home for longer (Green et al., 2011). However, another study (Nolan and Smith, 2010) did not find the same results; these researchers found that the women they interviewed felt the need to have their labour validated by a health professional, which meant they wanted to go into hospital. The practice of advising women to stay at home in early labour may therefore be a professional as opposed to a woman-centred approach to care. The message to take from these two contrasting research studies is that one size does not fit all women, and we need to have a range of communication techniques to meet women's differing needs.

Whichever form of communication is employed in the hospital where you practise, what is certain is that women value the relationship they have with midwives throughout pregnancy and labour (Leap et al., 2010b). The communication between women and midwives, building trusting relationships, and encouraging and supporting each woman's ability to give birth had a positive effect on the woman's birth experience.

In the labour room, how midwives talk, and the surveillance method adopted, whether that is the **Pinard stethoscope**, Doppler hand-held **sonicaid** or **electronic fetal monitoring (EFM)**, have to be balanced to facilitate normal birth (Scammell, 2011). While in normal midwifery practice, which is the focus of this book, surveillance methods should not include EFM, the way a midwife is vigilant about monitoring the maternal and fetal well-being can sometimes communicate certain less 'normal' understandings of birth and could be perceived by women and their partners as 'danger'. Balancing the benefits of assessing the maternal and fetal well-being and the maintenance of a sense of calm is obviously a skill. Let's look at the skills of assessing a woman admitted in labour to see how we communicate well-being.

Skill summary: abdominal examination of a pregnant woman

This is a key skill and something you will learn early in your training and develop and refine throughout professional practice.

Before the examination

Understand what you aim to achieve by the examination. In the antenatal period, from 24 weeks, the aim of the examination is to measure the fundas height only: in early labour it is usually to determine the position of the fetus. Consent prior to this or any examination is important. Encourage the woman to empty her bladder and adopt a comfortable position. Make sure that you have washed your hands and that they are warm with short nails. Ensure that the woman will be warm and comfortable with privacy and dignity maintained: you expose her abdomen for the shortest time and always ask for permission before uncovering her.

Equipment

You will need a tape measure to measure the **symphysis-fundal height**, a Pinard stethoscope or sonicaid and the woman's hand-held records.

Observation

Look at size, shape and contour of the woman's abdomen. You may be able to see fetal movements, rashes and lines (linea) or stretch marks (striae gravidarum).

Palpation (undertaken from 36 weeks only)

The palpation has three elements: fundal, lateral and pelvic. To begin with, the top of the uterus, the **fundus**, is palpated to see if a fetal pole – a head or buttocks – can be felt. If either of these parts of the fetus can be palpated, the lie is usually longitudinal. The symphysis-fundal height is then measured (see the 25-week antenatal appointment in Chapter 4 for details). Lateral palpation follows; this is where you use your hands to feel the sides of the uterus and fetus underneath to see which position the fetus is in (see Figure 2.2). The pelvic palpation determines whether the presenting part (PP), most frequently the fetal head, is engaged in the pelvis.

In labour, following this abdominal examination, the fetal heart is auscultated. This is not a requirement of antenatal examinations unless the woman specifically asks (NICE, 2008a). Having found the position of the fetus from the abdominal palpation, you will know where to place the Pinard stethoscope, aiming to hear the fetal heart through its back (see Figure 2.3).

To ensure that it is the fetal heart that you are listening to, you next need to differentiate it from the maternal pulse. Take the maternal pulse rate (see Figure 2.4), record it, and check that it is not the same as the fetal heart rate you are listening to – if it is the same, you may be listening to maternal rather than fetal sounds. Position the Pinard stethoscope and listen carefully; if the sound is muffled, try moving the Pinard. Once the fetal heart is heard, listen for one full minute.

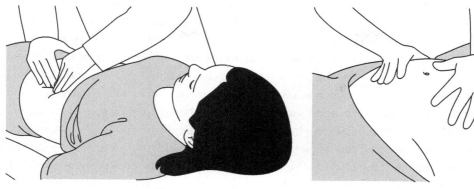
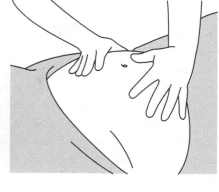

Figure 2.2: Abdominal palpation: a) early in pregnancy   *b) lateral hand position*

Figure 2.3:
Auscultating the fetal heart
with a Pinard stethoscope

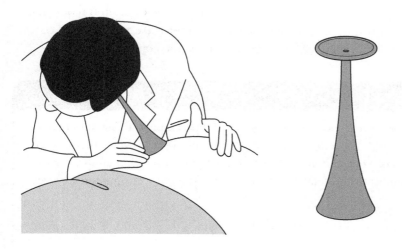

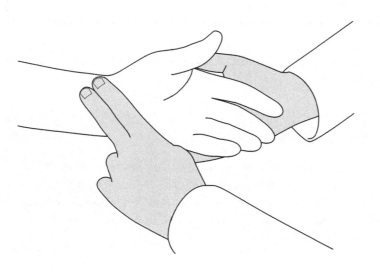

Figure 2.4:
Taking the maternal pulse

While the above skill summary assumes you are using a Pinard stethoscope, in reality most midwives now use technological means to listen to the fetal heart, and 'sonicaid' is the generic term used to describe the electronic hand-held machine. The sonicaid (sometimes called a Doppler, because of the wave it measures) uses **ultrasound** to detect the motion of the fetal heart valves or walls and converts this information into a sound that is heard and also usually displayed as a number on the digital readout. While some midwives and women prefer the sonicaid because of the audible sound, as opposed to the Pinard stethoscope when only one person, the midwife, is able to hear the fetal heart, there are disadvantages to its use. Artefact (an undesired technological error) can be picked up by the ultrasound – for example, the maternal heart rate – and added to the fetal heat rate, giving a digital display of a tachycardia; for this reason the acuity of *listening* is recommended rather than relying on the digital display. The maternal pulse should be palpated to ensure differentiation as with the Pinard method. Whichever method is used, it is essential that records of findings are kept (NMC, 2004b).

If we reconsider informed consent as one of the most important communication requirements of midwifery care, especially when women are in labour, we can undertake an activity to see what and how we need to ensure that women have enough information to consent to procedures.

Activity 2.6 — *Decision-making*

Imagine you are in spontaneous labour after an uneventful pregnancy. Think about all the observations, activities and procedures a midwife might 'do' to you, such as BP measurement, palpation of your abdomen to determine the fetal position and strength of your contractions, listening to the fetal heart rate and a vaginal examination to assess progress in labour.

Which of these procedures would you wish to have explained to you (and, if appropriate, to your partner)? Why?

There are some suggested answers at the end of this chapter.

Now that you have considered the procedures a woman is asked to consent to in labour, we will look at the skill of vaginal examinations.

Skill summary: Vaginal examination

This examination needs more preparation than many because of the intimate nature of the examination. As the woman's midwife, you must ensure that the rationale for the examination is explained and documented in the notes before you begin. The woman needs to understand what is involved, what she may expect to feel and how long it may take. For her to consent, she needs all of this information.

Encourage the woman to empty her bladder prior to examination and ensure that she is in a comfortable position – usually a semi-recumbent position – taking care to avoid a reduction in the maternal blood pressure caused by the weight of the pregnant uterus on the blood vessels that return to the heart (supine hypotension syndrome). An abdominal examination, including auscultation of the fetal heart, must always be carried out prior to a vaginal examination.

Reassure the woman that you will discontinue the examination at her request at any point. There are many principles you will need to consider and maintain while undertaking this examination, including the woman's privacy and dignity, infection control and good communication skills.

Observe the vulva for any discharge, fluid draining or unusual features, for example, warts, varicosities, oedema, scars or piercings. Apply water-based lubricant to gloved forefinger and middle finger and insert fingers into vagina gently. As you advance your competency of this skill you will begin to notice subtle differences in the tone of the pelvic floor, moisture and temperature of the vagina.

Identify the cervix (this may be all you will be able to achieve for many vaginal examinations); once you have accomplished this, you will be able to identify other points such as the cervical position, consistency, **effacement** and **dilatation**. Note the application of the cervix to the presenting part.

Feel for membranes and the consistency. Are they bulging or smooth?

Identify the presenting part; you will have clues from your abdominal palpation to help you here. Feel for sutures and fontanelles to determine the position of the head and its relationship to the pelvis. Feel for **moulding** or **caput succedaneum**. After the examination, listen to the fetal heart rate again and record all your findings on the partogram.

Following the examination, give the woman a paper towel to dry herself, help her reposition into a more comfortable position and share the findings of the examination with her, explaining how this relates to her plan of care in labour. Take care with the language used in explaining your findings; for example, try to avoid minimising words such as using *you are only*, as it's not the woman who is 'only' anything but her cervix, and saying in a positive way *Your cervix is getting thinner and ready to dilate* is better than saying *You are only in the early stages of labour*.

Now that you have considered the vaginal examination, the skill most students find the hardest, we need to consider what else needs to be communicated to a woman in labour. Birth choices make positive and negative experiences for women and you will find more about communicating with labouring women in Chapter 5.

We will now consider the last phase of the birth experience, postnatal care.

Postpartum communication and skills

Unfortunately, attitudes of staff are frequently cited as indicators of poor satisfaction in the postnatal period (Beake et al., 2010). In this study women felt their needs for information were unmet and that the level of support for breastfeeding was poor. Staff should be aware of how they interact with women, and this interaction makes the difference as to whether care is viewed as positive or negative. Consider the following scenario as an example of how care may be viewed.

Scenario

Two women, Helen and Sarah, both want to breastfeed their babies. Helen had a vaginal birth and is well; she is able to care for all her baby's needs but requires support with breastfeeding. Sarah had an **emergency caesarean section**; *she is tearful that the birth was not as she planned. She is in pain and needs help each time the baby moves in his cot, in addition to breastfeeding support. By the end of your shift Helen has rung for help only three times and is confident about breastfeeding her baby. Sarah is still tearful, has rung at least 20 times for help and is no more confident than she was at the beginning of the shift. Consider what you could have done differently.*

In the case study above, perhaps Sarah needed some spontaneous contact from you, to show her you cared. By reaching out to women we can gain more than we do if we respond only when they call. You may not have needed to say anything differently, but communication is about the messages we give women, and spontaneously approaching Sarah would have said more than many words could have. This concept of *presence* or being *with*, as opposed to doing anything practical for Sarah or other women in your care, can be used throughout the birthing experience.

Strategies you can use to improve your communication that are fundamental to the philosophy of midwifery include making sure the woman and partner are asked for permission each time their baby is touched or examined by staff. Hold the belief that effective communication, including warmth and a genuine interest in the woman and her experiences, are the hallmarks of connecting and relationship building throughout a family's experience.

So to draw all the above together, it's not just what midwives say or where they say it that matters in communication; it's how they work together that affects care. While midwives need to work together, we need to work to the highest possible standard of communication. Occasionally, the 'culture' in which midwives work negatively affects the communication strategies. If we do not stand up for what we believe to be right and go along with others, in what has been called a *herd instinct*, we let the profession down (Gould, 2011). One of the barriers to practising and improving your communication techniques is the socialisation process you are going through. You want to be *seen* as a midwife, and this means you want to talk and behave like your mentors. This professional socialisation can sometimes have a negative effect on your development. Social pressure from qualified staff and other students can enforce behaviours that do not always put the woman and her family first. The need to *fit in* by meeting the expectations of those you work with, especially those in authority, can hamper your communication with women. There may be times when you have to stand up for the woman in your care, which may be at odds with your wanting to be part of the group and fit in.

It is not just student midwives who find that communication issues affect the care they can give. Pollock (2011) describes how many factors – for example, gender, professionalism, medicalisation of birth and power relationships – still contribute to poor outcomes for childbearing women. The communication strategies (discursive practices) were hampered by previously established hierarchies and power relationships, which meant that the best possible communication between practitioners was not always achieved.

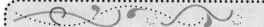

Chapter summary

This chapter has explained and examined the fundamentals of communication and some of the skills that you will need to learn through your midwifery education. It is expected that each time you read this chapter you will see how you could improve another aspect of your communication skills. Initially, you will emulate your mentor's style of communication, but as your knowledge and confidence develop you will try your own way. Just as new words come into the English language and other words are used less frequently, your initial style of communication will be replaced by a more professional and woman-centred one as you develop.

Activities: brief outline answers

Activity 2.2: Critical thinking (page 25)

'Confinement' suggests that one is imprisoned or confined.

While traditionally, women rested at home or in hospital – and this was described by the phrase 'lying-in', this term now sounds very dated and is no longer used.

'Failure to progress' has connotations of failure to achieve. For this reason it is better to use the term 'slow progress' or 'long latent phase'.

'Inadequate pelvis' is another negative-sounding term. There are three factors that need to be right for birth: the power of the contraction, the shape of the pelvis, and the movement of the passenger (fetus). Measuring the pelvis is difficult so this term should not be used. A combination of events rather than just one issue usually prevents vaginal birth.

'Incompetent' or 'failed' are both negative terms meaning not able to complete or do as expected. Instead of using negative terms, try to give women reasons why their experiences may not have been as anticipated.

Activity 2.3: Communication (page 26)

The open style of questioning probably elicited more of a conversation between you, the questioner, and the person answering, as it gave the person answering more opportunity to use their own words and feelings.

The closed-style questions often only require a 'yes' or 'no' answer; there is limited opportunity to start a conversation. By asking if someone is sad or any other emotion, you can project an emotion on to them that they were not previously experiencing, and this can then mask their real emotions. However, if you said, *From the tone of your voice or your limited responses I wondered if you were OK*, this might enable the respondent to say they were sad, or worried, or talk about another emotion they might be experiencing.

Activity 2.5: Evidence-based practice and research (page 32)

The enthusiastic friend approach, supporting and encouraging you, is most likely to work. The authoritarian and paternalistic approaches are not part of a partnership model.

Activity 2.6: Decision-making (page 36)

As you are physically being touched as each procedure is carried out, you will want the opportunity to consent to all these procedures, no matter how 'routine' they may be. Each activity is a screening tool in a way and as such has a consequence. For example, if your midwife finds that the fetus is in the breech presentation, this may limit your birth choices. If the fetal heart is found to be outside the normal parameters, this may necessitate a conversation about electronic fetal monitoring. While in low-risk women each of these examples are unlikely, it is up to your midwife to ensure that you, as the woman, consent to each of these procedures once you understand the implications of each of them.

Further reading

Fraser, D and Cooper, M (eds) (2009) *Myles' textbook for midwives*, 15th edition. London: Churchill Livingstone.

Hunter, B and Deery, R (2009) *Emotions in midwifery and reproduction*. Basingstoke: Palgrave Macmillan.

Johnson, R and Taylor, W (2010) *Skills for midwifery practice*, 3rd edition. London: Churchill Livingstone.

Kirkham, M (2004) *Informed choice in maternity care*. Basingstoke: Palgrave Macmillan.

Medforth, J, Battersby, S, Evans, M, Marsh, B and Walker, A (2006) *Oxford handbook of midwifery*. Oxford: Oxford University Press.

Raynor, M and England, C (2010) *Psychology for midwives: pregnancy, childbirth and puerperium*. Maidenhead: Open University Press

Useful websites

http://webarchive.nationalarchives.gov.uk/20090104012205/healthcarecommission. org.uk/homepage.cfm
www.cqc.org.uk/_db/_documents/Towards_better_births_200807221338.pdf

The Healthcare Commission website and reports make interesting reading, which we can use to alter how we care and communicate for women to improve their experiences.

www.nct.org.uk/professional

The National Childbirth Trust is a valuable resource and has a section for professionals that you might like to access to improve your communication strategies.

Chapter 3
The initial antenatal appointment and care

Sam Chenery-Morris

NMC Standards for Pre-registration Midwifery Education

This chapter will address the following competencies:

Domain: Effective midwifery practice
Communicate effectively with women and their families throughout the pre-conception, antenatal, intrapartum and postnatal periods. Communication will include:

- listening to women and helping them to identify their feelings and anxieties about their pregnancies, the birth and the related changes to themselves and their lives;
- actively encouraging women to think about their own health and the health of their babies and families, and how this can be improved.

Provide seamless care and, where appropriate, interventions, in partnership with women and other care providers during the antenatal period which:

- are appropriate for women's assessed needs, context and culture;
- promote their continuing health and well-being;
- are evidence based;
- are consistent with the management of risk;
- draw upon the skills of others to optimise health outcomes and resource use.

NMC Essential Skills Clusters

This chapter will address the following ESCs:

Cluster: Communication
Women can trust/expect a newly registered midwife to:

3. enable women to make choices about their care by informing women of the choices available to them and providing evidence-based information about benefits and risks of options so that women can make a fully informed decision.

continued . . .

Cluster: Initial consultation between the woman and the midwife

Women can trust/expect a newly registered midwife to:

1. be confident in sharing information about common antenatal screening tests;
2. complete an initial consultation accurately ensuring women are at the centre of care.

Chapter aims

After reading this chapter you will be able to:

- conduct an initial booking interview with a woman;
- discuss lifestyle choices with women;
- understand the concept of risk assessment;
- offer women choices, such as choice of place of birth, model of care and screening choices.

Introduction

The purpose of antenatal care depends upon the point of view of those involved. A midwife's role is to record the normal and reassure the woman. In this context, the purpose of antenatal care is to confirm that, despite minor symptoms of pregnancy such as nausea or backache, the woman is well and her pregnancy progressing normally. The midwife is also responsible for recognising deviations from normality, both in the mother (such as raised blood pressure), or in the growing fetus (such as small for dates fundal height), and referring to another health care professional, as appropriate. The midwife is also seen as the woman's professional friend. An obstetrician, on the other hand, might consider the aim of antenatal care to be maternal and fetal surveillance (e.g. blood tests to exclude maternal infections or anaemia and fetal screening). The obstetrician might consider pregnancy normal after the birth (if everything has gone well), whereas the midwife might consider it normal during the pregnancy, unless complications arise. A pregnant woman and her partner might see the aims of antenatal care as being supported by their midwife, having their anxieties listened to and being given information.

The relationship between the woman and her midwife, or midwifery team, is pivotal; the woman needs to feel relaxed enough to ask questions, yet sufficiently well informed to make autonomous decisions. The only way for this interaction to work is to allow time for the relationship to develop. In today's society, where workloads are measured and resources scarce, midwives have to build relationships faster than ever. The volume of information to be communicated to the woman in your care, from screening tests to dietary advice, is massive, and when you add to this maternal and fetal observations and an opportunity for the woman to discuss her issues, you can easily see how some women may not feel cared for. As a student midwife you need to learn from your mentors how to conduct antenatal appointments that balance all the requirements of the woman, her family and your employer as well as your own personal ethics. The initial meeting is especially important, as this is where the relationship between the woman and her midwife begins, and first impressions do count.

This chapter looks at the first trimester of pregnancy, focusing on the care you need to provide, balancing the information needs of the woman and her family with the observations you should perform. Relevant anatomy and physiology will be summarised so that you can see how it relates to and underpins the care you are providing; however, this book does not comprehensively cover the basic anatomy and physiology, so you should revise this before reading the chapter (see suggested texts in the further reading section on page 64).

Activity 3.1   *Critical thinking*

Take a look at how these two websites present information on the first trimester of pregnancy:

    **www.bbc.co.uk/health/physical_health/pregnancy/pregnancy_
    trimester1_info.shtml**

    www.nct.org.uk/pregnancy/first-trimester

Think about which website is more appealing to pregnant women and why. What information do they give? How straightforward is it to navigate through that information? Is it presented in an easy-to-read way?

Ask a fellow student to do the same and share your thoughts.

As this activity is based on your own reflection, there is no outline answer at the end of the chapter.

The first trimester is a period of great change in a pregnant woman's life. Not only are she and her partner adapting to their news, but her body is altering greatly, too. Women are often hungry for information about the pregnancy and developing fetus: all of the websites and resources used in this book are from reputable sources and suitable for sharing with women if they ask.

The antenatal booking interview

The midwife may be the first professional the woman sees when she is pregnant, or she may make an appointment with her GP first and then see her named midwife for a booking appointment. The booking interview is the first introduction between the maternity services, usually the midwife, and the woman.

Although midwives are able to provide pre-conceptual care, in reality, women rarely seek this resource. Women of childbearing age with certain medical conditions such as diabetes or epilepsy are likely to be offered pre-conceptual care by their medical consultant because their pregnancies are likely to be complicated by their conditions, but for most women the first time they meet their midwife will be at the booking interview.

Concept summary: the first trimester

The first trimester of pregnancy starts with the first day of the last menstrual period and lasts 13 weeks. **Ovulation** (the release of the egg from the ovary) has occurred, and if sperm are available, **fertilisation** (of the egg or ovum and sperm) will occur in the **fallopian tubes** and the **implantation** of the dividing cells comprising the egg and sperm in the lining of the uterus follows. It is during this time, usually around the first missed period (**amenorrhea**), that women begin to consider they might be pregnant. It can be a very exciting time for many women; for others it is an anxious time. There are signs and symptoms of pregnancy that a woman may experience, such as nausea (feeling sick), breast sensitivity, frequency of **micturition** (passing urine) and fatigue (tiredness). The developing cells are called an **embryo** initially and a fetus at ten weeks gestation, eight weeks after fertilisation. The **gestation period** is 40 weeks in total, 38 weeks from conception.

Activity 3.2   *Evidence-based practice and research*

To enhance your learning within this chapter, refresh your knowledge of the anatomy and physiology of the first trimester of pregnancy: both the woman's physiological changes and embryology. Look at the photos of human embryo development at **http://embryo. soad.umich.edu/** and cross-refer to an anatomy and physiology textbook.

There are no answers at the end of this chapter as this is a self-learning activity.

The booking appointment is likely to take place between 6 and 12 weeks gestation. It is a longer appointment than subsequent antenatal appointments, so that all relevant information about the woman's medical, obstetric and family history can be gathered. Other information is offered by the midwife to the woman and her partner, to enable them to make informed decisions on lifestyle choices such as smoking and alcohol consumption and screening choices. The appointment details and choices offered to women will be covered in separate sections in more detail below.

In the past a lot of irrelevant data was obtained from women, such as whether they were married and what form of contraception they had been using.

Activity 3.3   *Critical thinking*

Try to think about why each question you and your midwife ask women during booking interviews is required, and consider how relevant this information is to their current pregnancies. If you have not been out in practice yet, look at the Scottish national maternity records and see how many questions women are asked.

continued . . .

**www.healthcareimprovementscotland.org/his/idoc.ashx?docid=467
e846b-6649-4e2d-a125-5657452bf7b1&version=-1**

Try to consider this activity from the point of view of the midwife as well as that of the woman. What might it be useful to know about a woman and her pregnancy, and why? Are there any questions that might be asked but are irrelevant? You could compare the Scottish maternity record to your own Trust notes.

As this activity is based on reflection and your own personal experiences, there is no outline answer at the end of the chapter.

During the booking interview, you and your mentor will also consider your own and the woman's communication skills, body language and mood to build up an overall picture of this pregnancy, to confirm normality and as part of the overall assessment.

Recording antenatal care

The health care professional, namely the midwife or GP, will document any care given and maternal or fetal observations within the woman's hand-held records. The woman is responsible for bringing this documentation to each appointment. Depending on whether this is the woman's first or subsequent pregnancy, a schedule of appointments will be offered to each woman. This usually equates to ten visits for a first pregnancy (also called a **primigravida**) and seven for women who have had babies before (called **multigravida**) (NICE, 2008a). Although the term primigravida (first time pregnant) and **nulliparous** (never previously given birth) are often used in practice interchangeably, there are differences between the two words and they mean different things. Parous refers to giving birth at least once, whereas gravid refers to the pregnancy within the uterus. The nulliparous woman may have been pregnant before – she may have had a miscarriage or a termination of pregnancy – but she has never given birth before, whereas the primigravid woman has never been pregnant before. As it is not necessary to enquire whether women have had previous terminations of pregnancy, although many will confide in their midwife, the correct term to use is nulliparous for all first-time mothers. Remember that some women who have had a miscarriage may not like being called primigravida (first-time pregnant) as this is not their first pregnancy. Similarly, women who have had terminations do not need reminding of this.

Women should be informed about the schedule of appointments in early pregnancy. Most women stick to the recommended schedule, but drop-in clinics may also be offered in some areas where women are able to see a midwife without an appointment on a specific day and place and between specific times. The details of the drop-in clinics will be recorded in the woman's hand-held records should she require an unscheduled appointment, feel more anxious than usual or need extra support.

Conducting a booking appointment

Around the UK there are variations in where the booking interview occurs. Sometimes the booking interview is conducted in the woman's home; some areas use a clinic, such as an antenatal clinic in a hospital; other areas use a GP surgery or room in a local children's centre. The activity below explores which location may be best and for whom.

Activity 3.4   *Critical thinking*

Consider the pros and cons of the place where the booking interview takes place. Think about which location is usually used in your area of practice. Is it the GP surgery, the women's home or a children's centre? Try to consider the environment and impact of this appointment on the woman and the midwife.

There are some thoughts at the end of this chapter.

Now that you have considered the place for the booking interview, let's consider the optimal timing of the first contact. Booking interviews used to be undertaken within the first 12 weeks of pregnancy; now this initial interview is scheduled sooner, ideally by ten weeks, to allow women and their partners time to consider screening choices. In a recent survey, 54 per cent of women were seen by seven weeks of pregnancy and a further 41 per cent by 12 weeks (DH, 2010). Wherever the booking interview is undertaken, it is essential that the woman is made to feel comfortable as there is a great deal of information to be gathered and shared with the midwife at this meeting. The section below covers the history, lifestyle advice, weight, nutritional needs, clinical observations, screening choices and communication skills the midwife needs to know and impart.

What questions to ask

You will be required to undertake a maternal history; initially, you will watch your mentor, but as your course, knowledge and confidence progress, you will need to undertake this history on your own. Details such as the woman's age, events of previous pregnancies, medical history and occupation will all be explored. This information is used to determine her risk during this pregnancy. For instance, in relation to age, women at both ends of the reproductive spectrum (young mothers and women aged 35 or over) are at increased risk of pre-eclampsia, low birth weight babies, fetal abnormalities and caesarean section births. Although you cannot alter the mother's age or her risk factors, you can be aware of them and vigilant to deviations from the normal.

Details of previous births, including previous babies' birth weights and recoveries following her pregnancies, are all considered. If the woman has had three uneventful pregnancies and births, it can be assumed that this pregnancy will also be uneventful; however, if the woman experienced a bleed after her last birth, this might increase the risk or chance of this happening again, depending on the cause of the bleed. The medical history questions are looking at whether the woman has any known disabilities or disorders that may be exacerbated by the pregnancy, such as kidney disease. Details of the woman's occupation are needed to determine any occupational hazards for the pregnancy; any advice given to reduce hazards will be recorded.

The following activity will help you to assess how effectively you are communicating.

Activity 3.5   *Evidence-based practice and research*

NHS Quality Improvement Scotland has devised best practice statements, including taking a maternal history. Access this resource via a search engine and use the audit tool to reflect upon whether you and your mentor are using the best available evidence to take a maternal history.

As this answer relies on your own experiences, there is no outline answer at the end of the chapter.

You can go on to ask the woman and her partner how they feel about the pregnancy. Many conceptions within the UK are unplanned, so take care not to assume that all women will be delighted with their news, although of course many are. Emotions during the first trimester can fluctuate between positive and negatives, such as pleasure, dismay, ambivalence, tearfulness and increased or decreased sexual libido. All of these emotions are normal; however, you must take care to identify a woman's deteriorating mental health. The document *Antenatal and postnatal mental health guidance* (NICE, 2007a) offers midwives advice on how to predict and detect antenatal and postnatal mental health issues. At the woman's first appointment, her midwife should enquire about past or present mental illness and treatment, and ask the following questions to identify possible depression.

1. During the past month, have you often been bothered by feeling down, depressed or hopeless?
2. During the past month, have you often been bothered by having little interest or pleasure in doing things?

If the answer to either of these is 'yes', the midwife needs to ask the following question too.

3. Is this something you feel you need or want help with?

You may worry about asking sensitive questions about a woman's mental health, but depression impacts on the whole family. Research suggests that both women and midwives find screening for depression acceptable; if the woman feels comfortable with the screening process, she is more likely to answer honestly (Brealey et al., 2010).

What the midwife does at the booking interview

Blood tests

Maternal blood tests are taken with consent for a variety of purposes. Initially, the woman's blood group – A, B, AB or O – is determined, and then whether the blood is **rhesus positive** or **rhesus negative**. Both rhesus positive and negative are perfectly normal; the problems occur when the mother is rhesus negative and the fetus is rhesus positive. If fetal and maternal blood mixes during the pregnancy or birth the subsequent pregnancy may be affected and the fetus not develop normally – it may develop haemolytic disease of the newborn. A simple treatment is preventative anti-D, a blood product, which prevents problems with the developing fetus in the subsequent pregnancy. Women who are rhesus negative will be offered further antibody testing during their pregnancy and also **prophylactic anti-D** (a preventative medicine should mixing of the two bloods occur). For more information on prophylactic anti-D and rhesus isoimmunisation, see the further reading section at the end of this chapter. Other red cell antibodies are also determined from the initial bloods, and should there be any abnormality the woman will be informed by her midwife at the next appointment.

The blood is also examined for **haemoglobinopathies**, recessively inherited conditions of the red blood cells such as **sickle cell anaemia** or **thalassaemia**. Screening for anaemia is also undertaken; this is a measurement of the level of **haemoglobin** within the maternal blood. A reduction in the usual amounts of haemoglobin is easily treated with a diet rich in iron and sometimes medication. (This is covered in more detail in the book on high-risk pregnancy also in this series.)

The blood tests also give information about infections, such as whether the woman has acquired immunity to rubella or contracted HIV, hepatitis B virus or syphilis. All these infections can have serious consequences for the developing fetus. Some cannot be treated, and termination of pregnancy may be offered as an option. Women must be sure they want to consent to screening tests, so their implications and the consequences must be explored. Women and their partners should ensure they understand the condition that is being screened for, what their views on this condition are and how they might proceed once a diagnosis has been made. No one should undertake a test without having all the information needed to make a decision that is right for them; it is your role, as a midwife, to explore these issues with expectant parents. Research suggests that parents would like information on screening early in pregnancy and that midwives lack knowledge about screening (Skirton and Barr, 2010). As professionals, it is our responsibility to keep up to date and educate the clients in our care. For more information on screening for infectious diseases go to **http://infectiousdiseases.screening.nhs.uk/public**.

Women under the age of 25 are offered screening for chlamydia, a sexually transmitted infection that is often asymptomatic and prevalent among young people. If detected, antibiotics can treat this infection, and partners can be treated too, to prevent reinfection. Further details of this screening programme can be found in the useful websites section at the end of this chapter.

Discussing lifestyle advice

You need to ask sensitive questions around lifestyle issues, such as smoking, alcohol consumption and recreational drug use, and whether the woman is a victim of domestic violence. All of these lifestyle issues can have implications for both the mother and the developing fetus, and appropriate advice and information about support services in the area can be given to a woman if she is affected by these issues.

Broaching subjects such as smoking, alcohol consumption and domestic violence can be difficult. There is no one right way of asking these sensitive questions. The following examples can be explored by you and your mentor, and tried out with women, until you find a balance between asking for the information and how you ask. Remember that as a midwife you may use all your senses to assess a woman's health, including smelling smoke or alcohol on a woman's breath or clothing.

Activity 3.6 — Communication

Consider the different ways you can ask about lifestyle choices. One way of asking these sensitive questions is to be direct and ask *How many cigarettes per day do you smoke?* If the woman does not smoke, she will say so. Women who do smoke might be more likely to answer a direct question than a two-part *Do you smoke?* that then needs following up with *How many per day?*

The alternative way to ask the question would be to say, *Do you mind if I ask whether you smoke?* This way might allow more women to say that they do mind the question being asked and prefer not to answer.

One way midwives can broach the alcohol question is to ask *How many units of alcohol have you consumed in the last week?* and then follow this question up with *And the last month?* to give a fuller picture of the woman's drinking habits.

In relation to domestic violence the following question might be helpful: *Do you feel safe at home?*

Think about how *you* would prefer to be asked these questions and which you feel is most appropriate and why.

As this is based on your own reflection, there are no outline answers at the end of the chapter.

Now that you have considered how you communicate these issues to women, consider why we need to. Smoking in pregnancy is associated with low birth weight babies and pre-term labour, and can be seen as one of the reasons for stillbirth. It has also been associated with some birth defects (Hackshaw et al., 2011). Two of the most harmful substances inhaled while smoking are nicotine and carbon monoxide. These substances pass through the placenta to the developing fetus and jointly reduce the amount of oxygen the fetus receives.

Activity 3.7 — Evidence-based practice and research

Take a critical look at the website **http://smokefree.nhs.uk/smoking-and-pregnancy/**

Explore the 'Just the Facts' section and see how research on smoking in pregnancy and the effects smoking has on the fetus are communicated to the public. Reflect on this communication.

---

continued . . .

- Is it powerful?
- Do you understand the information?
- Does it help you to explore smoking cessation with women?

As this activity is based on your own reflections, there are no outline answers at the end of this chapter.

Now think about how a midwife may help to support a woman and her partner to stop smoking in pregnancy. Some community midwives have carbon monoxide detectors that show women how much carbon monoxide they are breathing out. This can be used to help women to reduce or quit smoking (NICE, 2010b). There are also smoking cessation teams around the UK to which women can be referred. Some are opt-out services, which mean that a woman will be automatically referred if she smokes, unless she says specifically that she is not interested in quitting smoking.

Alcohol consumption in early pregnancy can cause major damage to the developing organs and nervous system of the embryo. If a pregnant woman continues to drink heavily during the pregnancy, her baby can be affected by **fetal alcohol syndrome**. Counting how many cigarettes a woman smokes may be easier than counting the number of units of alcohol she consumes.

Activity 3.8   *Evidence-based practice and research*

Look at resources about responsible drinking on the internet, such as **www.drink aware.co.uk**, to increase your knowledge of alcoholic units. Then read the evidence about alcohol intake in pregnancy:

www.drinkaware.co.uk/facts/factsheets/pregnancy-and-alcohol

Think about how we, as midwives, communicate this information to women.

As this activity is based on your own reflections, there is no outline answer at the end of the chapter; however guidance on drinking limits in pregnancy follows.

The safe and acceptable limit of alcohol consumption in pregnancy is not in excess of one to two units once or twice a week, but preferably no alcohol should be consumed (NICE, 2008a). Because the effects of alcohol consumption are variable, it is difficult to say absolutely that no effect will manifest in the fetus. Therefore, in the first three months of pregnancy especially, while most of the development of the embryo is taking place, it is recommended that no alcohol is consumed.

Women who use recreational drugs may be offered help by a specialist service such as a specialist substance abuse midwife. Ask your mentor where the local services are, look at the notice boards in the GP surgeries, clinics or children's centres to find out about support services in your area or use an internet search engine for national organisations.

Remember that you must be non-judgemental in your care. The reason for your questions is to inform women of the risks involved and to offer advice and support to reduce these behaviours for optimal maternal and fetal health. Not all women may want this advice, however, and you must respect this.

Domestic violence affects one in six women at some point in their lives, and around 30 per cent of domestic violence starts or worsens during pregnancy. The midwife's role is therefore to identify women at risk of this abuse and offer them support. Evidence shows that the more often women are asked about domestic violence, the greater the likelihood of disclosure. Research into domestic violence (Keeling and Mason, 2011) has suggested that women may be receptive to disclosing domestic violence at different points during their pregnancy and postnatal period.

Activity 3.9   *Evidence-based practice and research*

The RCM position paper on domestic violence explains how and why midwives should ask women about their experiences. Read this position paper, which can be found at:

www.standingtogether.org.uk/fileadmin/user_upload/standingUpload /Maternity/RCM_Position_Paper_No_19a.pdf

Then consider how you have heard questions about domestic violence asked.

- How did you feel?
- How do you think women receive this question? Consider their body language when this question is asked.
- How can this important question be asked so that it is better received by women?

As this activity is based on your own reflections, there is no outline answer at the end of this chapter.

Now that we have considered sensitive lifestyle questions, we have one more issue – weight – to consider.

Body weight

Body weight – at both extremes – is an important indicator of risk in maternity care; those who are severely underweight or overweight require extra support and surveillance. Obesity has become one of the most often occurring risk factors in pregnancy. As the nation becomes more obese you will encounter more pregnant women who are obese. Obesity is defined as a Body Mass Index (BMI) of 30 kg/m^2, whereas underweight is categorised as a BMI below 18.5 kg/m^2. A BMI of 18.5–25 is considered healthy, and a BMI above 25 is classified as overweight.

Concept summary: calculating the BMI

First you need to weigh the woman and measure her height.

Then divide the woman's weight in kilograms by the square of her height in metres (i.e. kg/m^2).

For instance, a 72 kg woman who measures 1.72 m will have a BMI of $72/(1.72 \times 1.72) = 24.3$ – a healthy weight. If, however, the woman weighs 94 kg at the same height, her BMI will be $94/(1.72 \times 1.72) = 31.8$, which is classified as obese.

Obesity especially increases the chances of problems in pregnancy, for both the mother and the fetus. For instance, obese women are more likely to have high blood pressure, pre-eclampsia (see the book in this series on high-risk pregnancy care), fetal anomalies and diabetes, and are more likely to need a caesarean section. Babies born to obese mothers are more likely to be admitted to a neonatal unit following birth than those of women with a lower BMI.

If a woman is found to be obese, dietary advice may be offered; for more information on what advice to give, read the NICE guidance (NICE, 2010c). Of course, all women should be offered advice about healthy eating in pregnancy. It does not follow that just because a woman has a BMI of 22 she understands or consumes a nutritious diet – she may eat few vegetables, for instance. The following activity is aimed at increasing your knowledge and evidence base of a healthy diet in pregnancy, for all women.

Activity 3.10   *Evidence-based practice and research*

Explore this website:

www.nhs.uk/Planners/pregnancycareplanner/pages/Eating.aspx

You will find there all the information you need on a healthy diet and food advice in pregnancy. Reflect upon your prior knowledge and jot down limitations in your knowledge, so you can improve your communications with women.

Another interesting and informative read is the publication by the Royal College of Obstetricians and Gynaecologists (RCOG) and the Centre for Maternal and Child Enquiries (CMACE) on planning care for women who are obese and pregnant (CMACE and RCOG, 2010). Sadly, the number of obese women who die in the childbearing period is higher than the number of women of normal weight who die in the childbearing period. Read some of the above guidance online or listen to your mentor to hear how they offer advice and support to women who are obese, then consider how you would care for Diane, who you will meet in the scenario below.

This activity is personal to you, so there is no outline answer at the end of this chapter

After undertaking this activity you should be better able to communicate a healthy diet to all women, not just women whose weight is at either end of the ideal spectrum.

Scenario

Imagine you are caring for Diane, who is 25. She is concerned about gaining too much weight during her pregnancy. The gestation period is ten weeks and she has a BMI of 30, which is considered to be on the border between overweight and obese. As her midwife, how do you broach this sensitive subject with Diane and what information does she need to know about weight management during her pregnancy?

Although it is difficult to talk about weight management with women, as a midwife you should ensure that all women in your care know what a balanced diet entails. Talk to Diane about optimal food and drinks to eat, and ensure she knows which foods to avoid during pregnancy. Explain that she does not need to 'eat for two' and that small changes, such as increasing her activity by walking 15 minutes each day, will help her maintain her weight during this pregnancy. Guidance (NICE, 2010a) suggests midwives should explain that a BMI of 30 or more is considered to be a risk during pregnancy; you can access this information online and read it for yourself. Diane can be referred to a dietician during her pregnancy to help her maintain her weight and to support her to reduce her weight after the birth of her baby.

As her midwife, try to remember to ask Diane about her weight management and exercise at antenatal appointments to support and encourage her and to show you acknowledge the concerns she mentioned during her first appointment. You could also try to read up on health psychology to improve your understanding of what motivates people to change their behaviour.

Now you have considered weight in pregnancy we will look at other nutritional needs, some of which are covered in Activity 3.10.

Nutrition and supplements

The midwife needs to ensure that the woman knows about food supplementation – you will need to access the NICE antenatal guidance (2008a) for more information on this. Folic acid supplementation of 400 micrograms per day is recommended pre-conceptually until 12 weeks of pregnancy for all women to reduce the risk of having a baby with a neural tube defect such as anencephaly or spina bifida (NICE 2008a). A higher dose of folic acid is recommended for women who are obese. It is in the first few weeks after conception when this supplement is most important as the neural tube is developing; refresh your knowledge on embryology by referring to an anatomy textbook such as Stables and Rankin (2005).

Vitamin D is suggested for some women, such as those who are not exposed to naturally occurring vitamin D in sunlight because they are predominantly covered when outside, those who have diet low in meat, fish or eggs and those with a BMI of 30 kg/m^2 or more.

Other dietary advice includes food safety, avoiding listeriosis, toxoplasmosis, high vitamin A consumption and caffeine consumption. Listeriosis is a bacterium found in some foods, such as mould-ripened cheeses (Stilton and Brie, for instance) and pâté; and you should advise the woman to avoid these. Ready-cooked meals should be thoroughly reheated to destroy any potential bacteria. Toxoplasmosis is a parasitic infection found in raw meats, and cat and sheep faeces. Hand hygiene should be strictly maintained when touching raw meats, and you should advise the woman to avoid eating raw cured meats such as Parma ham and to eat well-cooked meats. You should advise women to take care when handling cat litter trays and, when gardening, to wear gloves and wash hands thoroughly. Women should avoid lambing sheep because of the risk of contracting diseases carried in animals' blood. Vitamin A consumption above 700 micrograms is considered to be unsafe. Women should avoid eating liver and liver products as these are high in vitamin A. Caffeine intake should also be moderated in pregnancy: four mugs of instant coffee or three smaller cups of filter coffee contain 300 mg of caffeine, and this is the recommended maximum; remember that tea, chocolate and cola products also contain caffeine. All of this information is documented in greater detail in the NICE (2008a) guidance available to read online or in print.

Clinical observations

Other clinical observations taken at this time are the woman's blood pressure (BP) and a urine test for signs of **proteinuria** (protein in the urine). At this point you should revise the normal physiological effects of pregnancy on a woman's cardiovascular and renal systems to understand why these are such important observations to undertake; see Chapter 13 of *Myles' textbook for midwives* (Fraser and Cooper, 2009). These measurements are recorded and act as a reference for the woman's baseline observations during her pregnancy.

A rise in the blood pressure or proteinuria may indicate pre-eclampsia (a medical condition of pregnancy that can be harmful for the mother and require early delivery of the fetus). A single diastolic BP of 110 mmHg (if you need to remind yourself of normal blood pressure readings, refer back to Chapter 2) or two consecutive systolic readings of 90 mmHg at a four-hour interval with or without proteinuria need further surveillance, usually an appointment with the obstetrician. The obstetrician may prescribe medication to lower the BP and regular BP checks, perhaps twice per week – this is covered in detail in the book on high-risk pregnancies in this series.

The first urine sample is usually sent to the laboratory to test for **asymptomatic bacteriuria** – bacteria in the urine – which may increase the woman's chance of pre-term labour. Asymptomatic means the woman has no symptoms of the bacteria being present, and is therefore unaware of having this infection. The bacteria can be treated easily by antibiotics, and this will reduce the chances of the woman going into pre-term labour, which is before 37 completed weeks of pregnancy. The midwife's role here is to detect and treat an abnormality that may cause upset and harm to the mother and her baby.

Each time urine is tested, glucosuria – glucose in the urine – may also be detected. This may indicate that a woman is consuming too many high-sugar meals or drinks, or it may indicate a more serious complication of pregnancy, gestational diabetes, a topic that is covered in the book in this series on high-risk pregnancies. If the glucosuria is due to dietary intake, the midwife must educate the woman about healthier foods and drinks for pregnancy; refer back to Activity 3.10 if you need reminding about this.

Risk assessment

Understanding the concept of risk

The maternal history taking and all antenatal care identify whether a woman is at increased risk during this pregnancy. The concept of risk is explored by Robinson et al. (2011) who argue that a trusting relationship between the patient/client and provider reduces the incidence of risk over-estimation. This is where the pregnant woman feels the burden of risk even if the chance of it occurring is low.

Risk of pre-existing maternal diseases such as cardiac disease or pregnancy-related disorders such as gestational diabetes, as well as previous pregnancy events that can increase the risk in this pregnancy, can all be identified in the maternal history taking. Additional care, such as appointments with an obstetrician, can then be planned. Women whose pregnancies are considered to be high risk will have a consultant obstetrician as the lead professional for their care. This is known as consultant-led care and will be covered elsewhere in this series. Women who fall into this category may have renal, cardiac or endocrine disease, blood or immune disorders, epilepsy or cancer, use Class 1 recreational drugs, have HIV, a complicated obstetric history such as previous caesarean section, bleeding in pregnancy or high blood pressure, or obesity that may increase the risk to their lives or those of their fetuses (NICE, 2008a). Remember, though, that most women have uneventful pregnancies and that birth is a normal physiological process.

Concept summary: risk

The concept of risk is pervasive in midwifery. This means it is everywhere, from defining a woman's pregnancy as low risk and suitable for midwifery care as opposed to high risk and needing consultant-led care (also referred to as obstetric-led care) to screening and the associated risk of having a baby affected with some condition.

A wide range of factors may influence the way women and their partners perceive risk. These include:

- previous personal experience;
- their own physical and/or mental health;
- experience of illness among family members;
- obstetric history, where there have been any problems in previous pregnancies;
- cultural or religious values;
- personal attitudes to, and understanding of, risk, fate and inheritance of genetic diseases;
- age;
- controllability of risk and ability to cope with uncertainty;

Risk can be portrayed in many ways, as Activity 3.11 suggests.

Activity 3.11   *Communication*

Think about the following sentences and consider how these could be altered to reduce the power of the language used.

- Obese women are more likely to have complications in pregnancy.
- It is not dangerous to have your baby at home.
- The chance of having a baby with Down's syndrome is high.
- The probability of bleeding after birth is low.

Restructure these sentences to make them more positive.

An answer to this activity is given at the end of the chapter.

Communicating risk

Risk can be communicated in many ways, and how you communicate risk to women is important. Think about who communicates risk to women and their partners, and how this might affect their pregnancy experience. Women and their partners will use their previous experiences to subjectively appraise risk; midwives can use language to reframe the sentence so the concept of risk is more objectively understood by women and their partners.

Within the UK there is no definition of moderate risk pregnancies. Risk can alter during the course of a pregnancy; for example, an antenatal scan of a woman classified as being at low risk might detect a low-lying placenta necessitating another, later scan. Depending on the findings at the second scan, this pregnancy would either continue to be classified as low risk or would be re-classified as high risk and care transferred to an obstetrician.

Offering choices

Now that you have considered risk, remember that continuity of care is important to women (DH, 2010). This is not the same as continuity of carer, where the same person (probably the same community midwife) cares for the same woman each time she visits. Continuity of care means that all the health care professionals involved in her care offer the same information and choices. Where possible, a limited number of midwives working in a small team should provide the care rather than a series of different midwives meeting the woman at each scheduled appointment. Women who are seen by the same midwife at each appointment are more likely to say they were always treated with respect, kindness and given choices about their care (DH, 2007b). Women should be offered choices about who provides their care (and where).

Screening choices and diagnostic tests

In addition to the clinical examination and information exchange offered above, you will have to address another important issue with women, that of screening choices and **diagnostic tests**.

Many women might think that a blood test would be diagnostic, that is, it would give you a definite answer: 'yes', you have this condition, or 'no', you do not. Many of the tests undertaken in midwifery, however, are screening tests, that is to say, they indicate your level of risk of having a particular condition rather than stating definitely whether the condition is present. The midwife needs to ensure the woman and her partner understand the risks, benefits and limitations of all the screening tests they are offered (NICE, 2008a), and that they both have time to consider whether the tests are something they would like to pursue. The NHS UK screening choices booklet, which you can find online (**http://cpd.screening.nhs.uk/timeline**), has a timeline of a pregnancy that includes the timing of these tests to help women make decisions about whether to have any or all of them. The number of screening tests, the times they are offered, and their risks and limitations follow. If you are still unclear after reading this, use the additional learning resources at the end of the chapter to build on your knowledge. In the meantime, consider the concept summary below to ensure that you understand which tests offered to women and their partners are screening tests and which are diagnostic tests.

Concept summary: diagnostic tests and screening tests

The difference between a diagnostic test and a screening test is a subtle but important concept to grasp. A diagnostic test states whether the person being tested *has* the specific disorder or not; a screening test can only *suggest* that the person being tested are at greater or less risk of having a specific disease or condition. Screening is a process of identifying apparently healthy people who may be at increased risk. They can be offered information, further tests and appropriate treatment to reduce their risk and/or any complications arising from the disease or condition. Tests offered during pregnancy can be broken down into both diagnostic and screening tests, both for the mother and the developing fetus.

Now that you have considered the concept, let's look at the specific tests offered during the booking appointment.

Test results and choices

There are a number of screening tests that you will offer for assessing the well-being of the fetus. Some parents prefer to know, so that if there is a likelihood of giving birth to a baby with additional needs, they can prepare for this; others would choose to terminate the pregnancy in these circumstances. Consenting to screening is not only about agreeing to have a blood test; it is also about considering your options and continuing with diagnostic testing if a high risk is found.

Before women agree to these tests, you should discuss with them the implications and consequences of screening, such as the rate of false positives – where the woman has a high-risk result but their baby turns out to be healthy – and the rate of false negatives – where the woman has a low-risk result and is not offered any further follow-up, but their baby turns out to have the condition. The UK National Screening committee benchmark is a detection rate greater than

90 per cent of affected pregnancies, with a false positive rate of less than 2 per cent. This means, for example, that 10 per cent of babies affected by Down's syndrome will not be detected by the screening test, and out of 100 women whose screening test result was high risk, two women will have had all the worry but an unaffected pregnancy.

These screening tests are detailed below after an activity that helps you to think about communication skills when discussing screening choices.

Activity 3.12   *Communication*

As Emma's midwife, you offer her and her partner the opportunity for fetal screening. She says, *Oh yes, that's routine isn't it? I had it last time: it was fine.*

How do you respond?

There are some thoughts and a sample answer at the end of the chapter.

If you have completed the above activity, you will probably have realised that although Emma and her partner have had screening before, they still need to be reminded of what tests are available in their area now. Screening tests change over time, so the tests they previously consented to may not be the same. You may have asked Emma and her partner what they remember about the screening tests, and then you can build on their previous knowledge to ensure it is up to date and that they have the right information to consent this time.

A woman is offered an ultrasound to determine the gestational age between 10 weeks and 13 weeks and 6 days. Some women will be entirely sure of their last menstrual period dates and may decline this ultrasound as they know how many weeks pregnant they are; others may be unsure of their dates or curious to see their 'baby'. For optimal accuracy, screening tests rely on exact gestational ages, so women who are unsure of their last menstrual period are encouraged to have this ultrasound. If the fetus is between 11 weeks and 13 weeks and 6 days, the combined Down's syndrome test may be undertaken at this time (this test may also detect less common genetic abnormalities such as trisomy 13, or 18, or neural tube defects), as long as the woman understands what it is and the consequences of this form of screening. For example, for every 100 women screened for Down's syndrome, one pregnancy will be affected; the woman and her partner will be offered a diagnostic test, such as amniocentesis, to determine whether their fetus is affected. There is no cure for Down's syndrome, however. If it is detected, the options offered to a woman and her partner are a planned birth in a hospital with facilities for any emergency treatment that might be needed, or a termination of the pregnancy.

This test combines the **nuchal translucency measurement** (a measure of the fluid at the nape of the neck of the 'baby'), with two measurements in the maternal blood (**beta-human chorionic gonadotrophin** and pregnancy-associated plasma protein-A). A computer analyses the measurements along with the women's age and ethnicity to determine her risk of having a fetus affected by a chromosomal abnormality or an open neural tube defect. A risk result of 1:150 or greater will be considered high risk, whereas a risk of 1:2000 is considered low risk.

If the nuchal translucency is not measured at the optimal timing, either because fetal positioning or raised maternal BMI mean the ultrasonographer is unable to take a sufficiently good picture of the fetal neck, or if the woman books her pregnancy after 13 weeks gestation, then another slightly less accurate test is offered. This is called the **triple** or **quadruple screening test** and is offered in the second trimester (see page 68).

Consider the following activity in relation to screening choices.

Activity 3.13   *Decision-making*

Put the following tests into either a diagnostic or screening category.

*   Fetal: chorionic villus sampling (CVS), amniocentesis, nuchal translucency scan, fetal anomaly scan.
*   Maternal: chlamydia, rubella antibodies, anaemia, blood group, syphilis.

There is a sample answer at the end of the chapter.

One of the most important roles you will have as a midwife is to communicate information to women and their partners, so they can make an informed decision about accepting or declining any tests. If the parents-to-be do not have enough information to make an informed decision, they may accept the tests without considering the consequences of screening, such as what would they do if their baby is affected by a condition. It is paramount that you encourage women and their partners to think through all tests offered to ensure they make the decision that is right for them and do not just accept something because it is offered. The NICE guidance (NICE, 2008a) suggests that antenatal screening choices should be offered to women in a place where discussion can take place and suggest a group setting before the booking appointment. This may be difficult to organise because of the time frame, and also may be difficult to manage, as each individual will have a different perspective and value on life and the subsequent choices screening may offer. At present you will probably be offering women opportunities to discuss screening choices individually. Table 3.1 is useful for ensuring that women and their partners consider all the screening tests offered in pregnancy.

Where is antenatal care offered?

Antenatal appointments should be offered within the local community so women can access them more easily. Children's centres have become more popular for antenatal care; they are within the local community and offer a range of services that women may like to continue with after their baby is born, from baby massage classes to music and postnatal exercise classes. If women see other women accessing these classes, they may be more likely to participate.

Information giving and place of birth

In addition to all of the above, which probably seems a lot already, you are expected to give information to women on how their baby develops during pregnancy; look at the summary within

Please use this form to make a record of your choices about what tests you want to have (antenatal screening choices).

Test	Yes, I am interested in having this test.	No, I am not interested in having this test.	I don't know. I would like more information.
Early pregnancy ultrasound scan			
Screening for HIV			
Screening for hepatitis B			
Screening for syphilis			
Screening for rubella			
Screening for blood group and antibodies			
Screening for sickle cell anaemia and thalassaemia			
Screening for Down's syndrome			
Fetal anomaly ultrasound scan			

Table 3.1: Your antenatal screening choices

Source: **www.screeningservices.org.uk/asw/public/screen_tests/screen_tests.asp**

this chapter and also at the titles on anatomy and physiology for pregnancy in the further reading section. A Department of Health booklet, *The pregnancy guide*, is given to all first-time mothers as a reference to support the information given verbally by the midwife (DH, 2009). You should also discuss place of birth and the options available for the mother to choose from; however, this choice is only tentative, as events during the antenatal period may restrict a woman's choices. Previous medical and obstetric history is also a factor, and women who have complications will not have all the choices open to them either. Common places of birth are home birth, midwifery-led units and consultant-led units. See Chapter 1 for more details of these. The following case study asks you to consider place of birth with Jill.

Case study: place of birth

Jill requests a home birth. She has had six previous births. Her first pregnancy was induced at 42 weeks gestation, and after 48 hours she gave birth to a 3.3 kg baby but had a postnatal bleed also called a postpartum haemorrhage (PPH) of 500 mls. The second and subsequent labours have been uneventful but progressively more rapid. Jill is concerned about travelling to hospital this time as she barely made it in time for her last birth.

*The midwife is concerned that Jill's previous birth experience and bleed might reduce her chances of having a home birth. Her history of a previous PPH predisposes her to another PPH, as does her grand multip (having had more than five babies before) status; however, the last five births have been uneventful. The midwife has said that she will document Jill's wishes and try to support her decision. As Jill's pregnancy is deemed high risk, her midwife offers Jill an appointment to discuss her care with her consultant. The midwife also discusses her anxieties with her supervisor of midwives. A plan is agreed upon. Misoprostol (a drug that stops postpartum bleeding, should the need arise) is prescribed by the consultant; Jill collects this from the pharmacy and stores it in her refrigerator as a precaution, should she bleed again. She agrees to be **cannulated**, which is to have a tube inserted into one of the veins of her lower arm in case fluids or further drugs are required. If all maternal and fetal observations are within normal limits, she will stay at home for as long as she is comfortable.*

The midwife acted as an advocate for Jill, by being honest about her concerns but facilitating Jill's wishes on this occasion. On balance, there were fewer risks for Jill if she took precautions for a home birth prior to labour than if she went into spontaneous labour at home and was not able to make it to the hospital in time because of a rapid delivery.

As an advocate for women, you, as their midwife, should also advise women on the maternity benefits they may be entitled to. There are resources such as the 'Directgov' website and 'A parent's guide to money' website listed in the further reading section. Dental care is free for all pregnant women and begins as soon as they know they are pregnant.

This completes the booking and first trimester appointments and meetings. To see how much information and knowledge you have retained already, try the activity below.

Activity 3.14   *Reflection*

Reflect upon the first time you were involved in a booking interview; if you have not yet been out in practice, think about the information written in this chapter so far. Write down your initial thoughts.

What forms of communication did the midwife use? For example, listening, eye contact, smiling, open posture? Did you understand what the midwife was saying to the woman (or all that was written in this chapter if you haven't yet been out on a placement)? Did you have an opportunity to look at any information leaflets? How did you feel after the interview? Now consider how the woman may have felt.

There are some thoughts at the end of the chapter.

There was a lot of information in this chapter, as demonstrated by the reflection activities. To consolidate this learning it is important to set this in context and think about the pregnancy in more detail. To finish this chapter, think about the major changes in the anatomy and physiology of the woman and developing fetus during the first trimester.

Chapter summary

This chapter has covered the initial consultation between a pregnant woman and her midwife. There is a great deal of information that needs to be received from the woman by the midwife and offered by the midwife to the woman. This developing relationship needs to be tailored to the woman's needs. Establishing the woman's understanding and promoting a healthy pregnancy, including lifestyle issues surrounding diet, smoking and alcohol consumption, are aspects of the midwife's role. Another feature of the midwife's role is recognising when a woman and her partner may need further support and information in making decisions about accepting or declining screening tests. Balancing these two facets of midwifery care – promoting normality and screening for risk – is a skill that takes time to learn. This chapter has discussed the antenatal care options available and implications for practice, so you can develop and enhance the initial antenatal care offered to women.

Activities: brief outline answers

Activity 3.4: Critical thinking (page 46)

Some midwives feel women are more comfortable in their own homes; others feel it is unnecessary to visit the women as they are fit and well. A home booking appointment used to be an opportunity to assess the home if the woman requested a home birth. Fewer women now consider a home birth, and inspecting a woman's home is no longer deemed necessary.

Confidentiality is sometimes an issue if the community midwife is well known in the local area; if women want to wait before they tell their neighbours their news, some women may prefer to come to a more anonymous clinic than to have the midwife's car parked outside their house. Alternatively, the clinic may be difficult to access for some women.

Another factor is a financial one: a midwife can see more women if she is based in a clinic with the women coming to her than travelling to each of their houses, especially if the community is in a rural location. This may be the more cost-effective method, but it does not allow for women to have a choice.

Activity 3.11: Communication (page 56)

These are more positive ways of addressing the same topics.
- Limiting excessive weight gain during this pregnancy will optimise your pregnancy and own health.
- Home birth is a safe option for most women.
- Out of 100 women with the same test result, 99 will have a healthy baby.
- A rare complication is bleeding following birth.

Activity 3.12: Communication (page 58)

It is not acceptable to accept on face value that a woman and her partner have all the knowledge they require to make an informed decision about screening choice. Even if they say, *Oh, yes I remember that from last time*, it is your responsibility to ascertain how much they remember and fill in the gaps in their knowledge or update them on current changes.

Begin by asking them to tell you about what was on offer last time; this helps you to decide how much more information they know or how confident they are that they have all the knowledge they need. Do this in a non-threatening way such as *Tell me what you remember about last time*. If they then say that they cannot, in fact, remember much, you know you need to give them all the information again. Some couples, though, will remember every agonising decision because they had a high-risk result or someone close to them did or they researched their original decision comprehensively. For these couples the communication of new or changed policies only may be required.

Communicating is an essential skill. You are required to have knowledge of the main NHS-managed screening programmes. You are also expected to facilitate informed choices regarding antenatal screening tests to ensure women fully understand the purpose of all the tests before they are taken. Therefore, it is your responsibility to inform Emma and her partner that it is not a routine procedure; they must think about the consequences of consenting to this test. Just because her previous screening was uneventful does not mean that this pregnancy will also be considered low risk. Once Emma and her partner consent to the test, they may have other decisions to make if the result is high risk, such as whether to agree to a diagnostic test. They need to consider how this news and possible future decisions will impact upon this pregnancy and their family. Take time to ensure that Emma understands the consequences of screening decisions. Your personal values and attitudes – that is, whether you think screening should or should not be undertaken – should not cloud the consultation, but you need to ensure that Emma and her partner know that this is a choice they are making and not a routine procedure.

Activity 3.13: Decision-making (page 59)

The following are diagnostic tests that are able to diagnose certain conditions.

1. With chorionic villus sampling, a sample of placental tissue is removed vaginally and examined for **chromosomal make-up** to determine if the fetus is affected by various genetic conditions. It says that this fetus has this particular genetic make-up and therefore this condition.
2. Amniocentesis is similar to CVS, but the test is offered later in pregnancy. The amniotic fluid, as opposed to the placental tissue, is examined to determine the chromosomal make-up of the fetus; again, this diagnoses genetic conditions.
3. Chlamydia, rubella and syphilis are infections, and tests determine for definite whether the woman has these infections or not.
4. The blood group test states whether the women has one of four blood groups: A, B, O and AB. There is no uncertainty here.

The following test is a screening test.

- The anaemia test will determine if the woman's haemoglobin level is low; it will not diagnose why, and further tests may be required to find out the cause.

There are two tests that may be both diagnostic and screening tests.

- Nuchal translucency is offered as a screening test, but it can be diagnostic of Down's syndrome if the measurement is excessive.
- The fetal anomaly scan (more commonly just called ultrasound scan) is offered as a screening test to all women, but it may diagnose cardiac abnormalities or other structural problems in the fetus.

Activity 3.14: Reflection (page 61)

Often when students first go out into practice, especially after their first booking interview, they feel overwhelmed by the amount of information they have heard. The students worry they will never be able to understand all the information offered, let alone remember what to say. Remember this feeling, as it may be how women are also feeling. You can use this experience to reflect upon how the midwife delivers the information, whether they are kind, offering the woman and her partner time to ask questions and suggesting ways the family-to-be can process these decisions. Referring back to the leaflets you offer and suggesting that the woman write notes on them if anything is unclear or she would like further support/discussion on any points is a good way to tailor care to individual needs. It may also help you learn and question why certain tests are offered and can help your development too.

Further reading

Stables, D and Rankin, J (2005). *Physiology in childbearing with anatomy and related biosciences*. London: Elsevier.

A more in-depth anatomy and physiology book about changes to the woman during pregnancy and embryonic development to complement your learning.

The following articles also give more information about maternal blood testing and rhesus isoimmunisation during pregnancy.

Crowther, S (2010) Blood tests for investigating maternal wellbeing (2). Testing for anaemia in pregnancy. *The Practising Midwife*, 13(10): 48–52.

Gunn, J (2010) Blood tests for investigating maternal wellbeing (3). Blood group and red blood cell antibody screening. *The Practising Midwife*, 13(11): 46–49.

Hall, J (2010) Midwifery basics: Blood tests for investigating maternal wellbeing. *The Practising Midwife*, 13(9): 40–42.

Useful websites

www.arc-uk.org/

The website of Antenatal Results and Choices, a national charity, has an easy to navigate website explaining the rationale for the blood and screening tests offered to pregnant women. The resources are for women and professionals.

www.nctpregnancyandbabycare.com/

Another charity, the National Childbirth Trust also has an excellent website with easy-to-follow sections and information on all aspects of pregnancy and baby care.

www.chlamydiascreening.nhs.uk/

www.chlamydiascreening.nhs.uk/ps/index.html

For women under 25 another screening programme is offered; for more information visit the National Chlamydia screening programme. The site has information provided in different ways for professionals and the under 25s.

www.direct.gov.uk

www.moneyadviceservice.org.uk/parents/

These are two useful advice websites.

Chapter 4
Ongoing antenatal care

Sam Chenery-Morris

NMC Standards for Pre-registration Midwifery Education

This chapter will address the following competencies:

Domain: Effective midwifery practice

Determine and provide programmes of care and support for women which:

- are appropriate to the needs, contexts, culture and choices of women, babies and their families;
- are made in partnership with women;
- are ethical;
- are based on best evidence and clinical judgement;
- involve other healthcare professionals when this will improve health outcomes.

This will include consideration of:

- plans for birth;
- place of birth;
- plans for feeding babies;
- needs for postnatal support;
- preparation for parenthood needs.

Complete, store and retain records of practice which:

- are accurate, legible and continuous;
- detail the reasoning behind any actions taken;
- contain the information necessary for the record's purpose.

Records will include:

- biographical details of women and babies;
- assessments made, outcomes of assessments and action taken as a result;
- outcomes of decisions with women and advice offered;
- any drugs administered;
- action plans and commentary on their evaluation.

NMC Essential Skills Clusters

This chapter will address the following ESC:

Cluster: Communication

Women can trust/expect a newly registered midwife to:

1. be attentive and share information that is clear, accurate and meaningful at a level which women, their partners and family can understand;
4. ensure that consent will be sought from the woman prior to care being given and that the rights of women are respected;
7. provide care that is delivered in a warm, sensitive and compassionate way.

Chapter aims

After reading this chapter you will be able to:

* offer women ongoing antenatal care;
* understand the reasons behind the various assessments made during this period;
* identify women in need of additional support;
* understand the importance of communication in your relationship with women in your care and reflect on how much you can learn by listening to them..

Introduction

This chapter follows on from the care set out in Chapter 3. It assumes that you, the midwife, have met the woman and undertaken her booking appointment; however, a few women may not have had this opportunity yet. For women who 'book' late – that is, after 12–13 weeks gestation – the initial appointment and ongoing care may happen simultaneously.

This chapter will focus on the two remaining trimesters of pregnancy: the second trimester from 14 to 27 weeks gestation and the third trimester from 28 to 40 weeks. Although midwives do not necessarily think in trimesters – they are more likely to think in weeks – women and the books they read often do, so this arrangement offers the opportunity for you to combine the two approaches.

The relationship between the woman and you, her midwife, continues to develop at each contact point, and a warm, caring and compassionate attitude to care for all women will help this.

The second trimester of pregnancy (weeks 14–27)

The second trimester of pregnancy starts at week 14 and finishes at week 27. During this time women often feel at their healthiest, as the initial early symptoms of nausea and fatigue have usually disappeared, and the growing fetus has not yet become heavy enough to restrict their movement. During this period, the fetus doubles in length (from 120 mm at 13 weeks to 260 mm at 27 weeks), while its weight increases by a factor of ten (from 110 grams to 1150 grams). Fetal movements are first felt by the mother between 17 and 20 weeks. Towards the end of the second trimester the fetus is considered viable, which means that it has a chance of survival if it is born after 24 weeks gestation.

Activity 4.1   *Critical thinking*

Take another look at these two websites and reflect upon the different ways they present information about the second trimester of pregnancy:

> **www.bbc.co.uk/health/physical_health/pregnancy/pregnancy_trimester2_info.shtml**

> **www.nct.org.uk/pregnancy/14weeks**

Why do you think one website offers a week-by-week account of the second trimester, while the other offers advice about aspects of the pregnancy? Which do you find most informative and why? Does either website refer to the midwife?

As this activity is based on your own reflection, there is no outline answer at the end of the chapter.

Having used these websites to think about the woman's perspective, let's now think about the midwife's role.

The midwife's role during the second trimester

Your role in the second trimester of a woman's pregnancy is to continue to support her, inform her of the next phase of her pregnancy and continue to undertake the necessary observations to confirm that all is progressing well with her health and that of her developing fetus. During this period, you should be able to develop your relationship with her, as you are likely to meet the woman on several occasions, depending on the model of midwifery care offered where you work (see Chapter 1 to remind yourself about this). Midwives will see nulliparous women (who have never given birth before) on at least three occasions (at 16, 25 and 28 weeks gestation) but the low-risk multiparous woman only twice routinely (16 and 28 weeks) (NICE, 2008a).

Nulliparous woman are seen more frequently antenatally because they are at greater risk of developing pre-eclampsia. They may also develop pre-eclampsia earlier in the pregnancy than multiparous women, so they are seen at 25 weeks when early signs and symptoms of pre-eclampsia may develop. Another reason for the additional appointment is to offer nulliparous women extra support at this time of great transition from a single person or couple to a family. Yet another reason is that in an age where cost analysis drives care choices, it has not proved cost-effective for multiparous women to receive the same number of antenatal appointments in this trimester (or the next) as nulliparous women (Sandall et al., 2010). The resourcing of the appointments outweighs the chance of finding a deviation from the normal, so they are not deemed necessary.

During the second trimester all women will also be offered an antenatal ultrasound to screen for fetal abnormalities; this will be explored in greater detail later in the chapter.

Second trimester screening

If the combined screening test (see Chapter 3) was not undertaken during the first trimester, the triple or quadruple screening test needs to be offered between 15 and 20 weeks. We have already stated that the combined screening test is the most accurate as it has a 90 per cent detection rate and false negatives of only 2 per cent. However, in some circumstances – for example, if a woman has not met her midwife before 14 weeks gestation, or if it has not been possible to record the nuchal translucency measurement – the woman and her partner will be offered the triple or the quadruple screening test, depending on which test is offered by the local Trust. These tests have less accurate detection rates than the combined test – 75 per cent rather than 90 per cent – so 25 per cent of babies affected by Down's syndrome will not be picked up by these screening tests. The triple or quadruple screening tests use a maternal blood test to measure protein and pregnancy hormones – either three or four, depending on the test – to determine the chance of the fetus being affected by Down's syndrome. Table 4.1 sets out the various screening tests and their characteristics.

Gestation	Test	Sensitivity	Markers
11–13+6 weeks	Combined – blood test and ultrasound	90% detection rate; false negatives 2%	Nuchal translucency, determined by ultrasound; 2 serum markers
15–20 weeks	Triple – serum screening, blood test only, measures three blood chemicals	75% detection rate	3 serum markers
15–20 weeks	Quadruple – serum screening, blood test only, measures four blood chemicals	75% detection rate	4 serum markers

Table 4.1: Screening tests

If the screening tests have all been accepted and undertaken, you should review the results with the woman to ensure she fully understands them and their implications. A risk of 1:1000 is considered low risk and should be communicated to the woman as such by rephrasing the numbers and saying that for every thousand women screened, one will have a baby with Down's syndrome, whereas 999 will not be affected by this condition. The cut-off point is 1:150, so women whose risk is calculated to be greater than 1:150 for screening tests – for example, with a risk of 1:10, 1:49 or 1:149 – will be offered a further diagnostic test. Remember, though, that even 1:149 means that of 149 women screened, 148 will not have a baby affected by this condition, that is, there is a 99.25 per cent chance the baby will not be affected and a 0.75 per cent chance the baby will have Down's syndrome. Table 4.2 might help you understand these numbers.

These discussions and results need to be recorded in the woman's hand-held notes, for example 'Results discussed with . . .', using the woman's name here to make it more personal to her.

Advice on the fetal anomaly scan, or ultrasound for structural fetal anomalies, also needs to be given; this usually occurs between 18 weeks and 20 weeks and 6 days. This scan is different from the first dating scan in that it is scheduled to detect abnormalities, as the fetus is large enough for the ultrasonographer to visualise the major organs of the heart and brain, for instance. The previous (first) dating scan merely measures the growth of the fetus to estimate a date of delivery; some major structural anomalies may have been visualised, but that is not the purpose of the scan. Not only can the ultrasonographer detect structural anomalies during the 20-week scan, but they are also able to detect 'soft markers'. Soft markers may be suggestive of a fetal anomaly, but they are not indicative. As science and ultrasound technologies improve, the significance of soft markers changed: once, shapes in the brain were seen as a soft marker – now they are considered normal. The decision as to whether to inform the parent of unusual images on ultrasound, therefore, is complex. This is where technology and women's

Risk	As a %	Reframed
1:16. High risk	6.25% chance of affected fetus; 93.75% chance of unaffected fetus	For every 16 pregnancies, 15 will be unaffected by Down's syndrome
1:100. High risk	1% chance of affected fetus; 99% chance of unaffected fetus	99 pregnancies out of 100 will be unaffected by Down's syndrome
1:149. High risk	0.75% chance of affected fetus; 99.25% chance of unaffected fetus	148 women in this group will have a pregnancy unaffected by Down's syndrome
1:1000. Low risk	0.01% chance of affected fetus; 99.9% chance of unaffected fetus	For every 1000 women, 999 will have a baby unaffected by Down's syndrome

Table 4.2: Reframing the risk

perceptions of technology can often cause anxiety, and is the reason why the processes of obtaining informed consent and counselling prior to ultrasound scan are so important and must be adhered to. In a study of women's knowledge on ultrasound (Cash et al., 2010), the women had mixed views about being informed of soft markers: half the women wanted to know, 20 per cent wanted to know only if significant and a further 20 per cent wanted to know only if discussed previously, suggesting that prior to any screening test, all possible outcomes should be explained to parents-to-be.

If during this second (20-week) scan the placenta is found to be lying low in the uterus (the usual place is the upper anterior aspect or fundus of the uterus), women will be offered another ultrasound scan during the third trimester, at 32 weeks, to check on the placental site. During the third trimester the lower segment of the uterus elongates and the placenta, which is attached to the lower segment, moves up and away from the cervix, which is desirable. If the placenta remains low-lying, it may obstruct labour; delivery will require extra vigilance and it may be necessary to perform a caesarean section. For more on this, read the book in this series on high-risk pregnancy.

The 16-week appointment

The first scheduled midwifery appointment in the second trimester is at 16 weeks. During every appointment you should allow time for the woman to ask questions and for her to talk about her pregnancy as well as for carrying out the formal checks. Remember that the relationship between you, the midwife, and the woman needs to be established and develop. Communication is an essential skill, and this is demonstrated by listening and body language, as well as giving and receiving information (see Chapter 2 for more detail).

The maternal blood tests that were taken at the previous appointment (see Chapter 3) need to be reviewed at the 16-week appointment, and considerations made for further appointments depending on the results. For instance, if the woman is rhesus negative, she needs to be told about the anti-D prophylaxis programme (see page 48, or read NICE, 2008d) offered to all women, so she can decide whether to consent to this injection. If the woman's haemoglobin level was low initially, further tests may be indicated, to detect low folic acid levels, or you may discuss her diet in greater detail to increase her knowledge and consumption of foods rich in naturally occurring iron, such as whole grains (wholemeal bread and cereals), green leafy vegetables (broccoli and cabbage), red meat (beef and lamb) and pulses (beans or lentils) as well as reducing tea and coffee consumption, which inhibit iron absorption. As a woman is now more likely to feel like altering their diet than in early pregnancy when they may have been affected by nausea, it might be an opportune time to reiterate the basis of a good diet in pregnancy and beyond. For more food advice in pregnancy visit: **www.nhs.uk/planners/pregnancycareplanner/pages/ eating.aspx**.

The maternal observations are repeated at the 16-week appointment, and blood pressure testing and urine testing for proteinuria are undertaken (see Table 4.3 for an example of recorded observations and actions taken). Remember that these are important measurements as they may detect abnormal rises in blood pressure. Remember that during the second trimester it is usual for the blood pressure to reduce. The presence of proteinuria may be indicative of urinary tract

Gestation	BP mm/Hg	Urinalysis	SFH*	Care decision	Rationale
16 weeks	110/70	Nil detected	N/a	Routine care	Normal observations
25 weeks	130/80	Nil detected	22 cm	Continue with routine care	Normal observations
28 weeks	140/90	Nil detected	25 cm	Routine care but be vigilant	Fetal growth evident, BP borderline
31 weeks	140/90	Trace protein	27 cm	Refer to obstetrician, ask about headaches, epigastric pain and oedema	Two 90 mmHg BP measurements trace of protein and decreased fetal growth all indicate obstetric review – send to hospital

Table 4.3: Maternal observations

* SFH = symphysis-fundal height

infection at any gestation or a symptom of pre-eclampsia from 20 weeks gestation. If you did not revise the cardiovascular and renal system when you read Chapter 3, consider revising it now to enhance your anatomy and physiology (look at one of the recommended anatomy and physiology books in the further reading section).

If the BP is above 160 mmHg on two occasions, medication may be considered by the obstetrician, and the woman needs to be seen in the hospital that day for an obstetric review and follow-up appointments arranged. All women should be informed that symptoms of pre-eclampsia such as severe headache, blurred vision, epigastric pain (pain under the ribs) and oedema (swelling, usually of the lower legs) need investigating; they should seek urgent medical attention if they experience these symptoms (NICE, 2008a).

The 25-week appointment

At 25 weeks only nulliparous women are seen – this is one of their extra antenatal appointments. The appointment has two main purposes.

• To screen for pre-eclampsia (which is more prevalent in nulliparous women).
• To offer extra midwifery support for the transition to parenthood.

You will need to ask the woman how she is feeling – her emotions as well as her pregnancy symptoms. Some women will talk about the equipment they may be looking at, such as cots and prams; others will be relieved they are feeling better. Listen to the woman's conversation with you and think about whether she is really OK or whether there may be some underlying issue that she is not telling you. Hearing what is said and what is unsaid is a challenging skill to learn. Listen to your mentor and see how she gives women the opportunity to talk during the antenatal appointments. It is during these conversations that individual additional needs may be assessed and support offered by you or another agency, such as a social worker or health visitor (refer back to Chapter 2 for more on communication skills).

The antenatal observations at 25 weeks include measuring BP and urine for proteinuria, as before, but it is at this gestation and onwards that the symphysis-fundal height (SFH) is measured at all appointments.

Concept summary: symphysis-fundal height (SFH)

Symphysis-fundal height (SFH) is used instead of abdominal palpation. Abdominal palpation is where a midwife feels through the maternal abdomen to determine how the fetus is positioned within the uterus and determines the fetal growth by using landmarks on the maternal abdomen, such as the umbilicus to measure the estimated height of the fundus (top of the uterus). SFH is measured with a tape measure, in centimetres, from the fundus to the pubic bone. This measurement is then plotted on a graph and should correspond (within 1–3 cm either side) to the gestation. Thus, at 25 weeks a normal SFH measurement would be from 22 to 28 cm, depending on the woman. Variations from this can indicate a larger- or smaller-for-dates fetus, or too much (polyhydramnios) or too little (oligohydramnios) liquid (liquor) within the uterus.

There is considerable variation in the accuracy of detecting small- or large-for-gestational-age fetuses using fundal height measurements (Sparks et al., 2011). Measurements for obese women are less reliable; measurements for multiparous women are more reliable. The accuracy of this measurement in detecting large-for-gestational-age fetuses is improved in women aged over 35 years and in Caucasian women but reduced in other ethnicities. In another study (Hargreaves et al., 2011) the detection of small or large fetuses by fundal measurement was not sensitive enough, and only 20 per cent of affected fetuses were detected clinically by this method.

Poor fetal growth is associated with perinatal morbidity and mortality; thus, measuring SFH at intervals (at antenatal appointments) and plotting these measurements on a graph can alert the midwife to poor fetal growth, in which case the midwife will refer the woman to the hospital for an ultrasound scan and to see an obstetrician to plan ongoing care (NMC, 2008a).

At these appointments the midwife should also ask the mother about fetal movements – this is considered to be a more effective method of assessing fetal well-being than listening to (auscultation of) the fetal heart during routine antenatal appointments because the mother can sit quietly and feel for fetal movements every day and be the expert in the movements of her 'baby', whereas the midwife can only confirm the fetal well-being at infrequent points during the pregnancy. It is not possible to rely on technology for all assessments of fetal well-being, and a mother's perception of her 'baby' must be considered a valid source of knowledge.

If the woman notices reduced fetal movements after 24 weeks gestation, she may be asked to attend a maternity assessment unit or central delivery suite for fetal assessment. Auscultation of the fetal heart may be performed in conjunction with perhaps an ultrasound scan or cardiotoco-graph (CTG) trace as the pregnancy progresses. However, for uneventful pregnancies asking the mother to count routine fetal movements, that is, counting each day, is deemed unnecessary; so too is antenatal auscultation of the fetal heart rate by the midwife, unless the woman requests it (NICE, 2008a). Consider the following scenario and activity to explore why.

Scenario: fetal heart rate

During an antenatal appointment a nulliparous women, Karina, asks you, the midwife, to listen to the fetal heart rate as she would like to hear it. She is 25 weeks pregnant and has felt the baby move more frequently lately. She is accompanied by her sister who recently had a baby and heard her fetus's heart rate at her antenatal appointments.

Activity 4.2   *Communication*

Read the scenario above and consider for a minute what you might do here and why.

Consider how you would communicate best practice of assuring fetal well-being to Karina and her sister.

There are some thoughts at the end of the chapter.

In this activity you will have acknowledged Karina's request, offered her and her sister education and respected her newly informed decision. All of these skills are required by you, as the midwife, during each consultation with women. Now consider the next scenario.

Scenario: emotions

Jade, a nulliparous 19-year-old woman, tells you she is having difficulty sleeping and is crying more frequently than usual. She is now 25 weeks pregnant. You have met Jade before and know that she, her boyfriend and her mother, who previously accompanied Jade to appointments, were excited about her pregnancy. This is the first appointment of the afternoon of a busy clinic; you want to listen to Jade's concerns but are aware of competing priorities for your time. Consider how you might manage this scenario.

On this occasion you decide to sit and chat with Jade. You ask her when this sleeplessness started and what else is on her mind. You enquire about domestic violence and are alert to other social factors, such as the fact that her

continued . . .

> *boyfriend has just moved into her family home and they have little money between them, which may have affected her mood. She tells you that everything is fine, her relationship with her partner and mother are good, and she is still happy about the pregnancy, but she feels the weight of responsibility of becoming a mother is keeping her awake. You reassure her that this is normal and suggest she talks to her partner and mum about her feelings. You ask her if she would like to reschedule another appointment for next week at the end of the clinic or inform her of the drop-in clinic you run, to allow more time for Jade to talk if she needs to, so you can undertake her antenatal observations and see how she is feeling one week later. You document the discussions in Jade's hand-held record and the need for a further appointment to follow this up and undertake the necessary measurements.*

During this scenario, you needed more time than you were able to give Jade, so you listened to her instead of undertaking the routine observations. By offering Jade another visit you will ensure that she does not miss routine care, but at the time you thought listening to her concerns was more important than the scheduled care. This is women-centred care at its best; although it adds another appointment to the following clinic, it also allows you to follow up on Jade's feelings in a timely manner. Had you not listened, her feelings might have escalated and she could have been more distressed at the next appointment.

Antenatal education classes

During the second trimester, usually at 25 weeks for nulliparous women, it is important to mention antenatal education classes and breastfeeding workshops, so women can think about whether antenatal education is appropriate for them. Although the antenatal education classes are typically not offered until the third trimester of pregnancy, around 34 weeks gestation, there are regional variations, and sometimes high volumes of pregnant women in one area may necessitate women being offered these classes slightly earlier than usual to meet the local demand. Historically, antenatal education classes were offered as a series of classes, one two-hour session per week, often in the evening for both women and their partners to attend. Nowadays, differing patterns may be offered depending on the local Trust, the demographics of its catchment area and the needs of the population. For instance, there may be all-day Saturday classes, six hours of intense education for women and their partners, afternoon classes for women only, classes delivered in Portuguese or Hindi, and classes for teenagers or single women. Some classes are delivered by outside agencies, such as the National Childbirth Trust, either for a fee or free of charge to all women. Ask your mentor and look at local notice boards to ascertain what services are offered in your local areas.

The third trimester of pregnancy (weeks 28–40)

Now we will consider the third trimester of pregnancy and the ongoing midwifery care that is offered during this period.

Activity 4.3   *Reflection*

Take another look at these two websites and reflect upon how they present information on the third trimester of pregnancy.

> **www.bbc.co.uk/health/physical_health/pregnancy/pregnancy_trimest er3_info.shtml**

> **www.nct.org.uk/pregnancy/29weeks**

One website seems to offer advice on things that are considered high risk: premature birth, high blood pressure and non-engaged heads. What do you think about the quality of information offered here?

Although it mentions back pain, the other website is encouraging women to think about the birth and parenthood. Reflect on these two approaches. Which is more realistic from your experience?

As this activity is based on your own reflection, there is no outline answer at the end of the chapter.

Now you have reviewed the websites, let's think about the third trimester and the midwife's role.

The third trimester of pregnancy starts at 28 weeks gestation and ends with the birth. Normally, birth can occur from 37 completed weeks of pregnancy to 41 or 42 weeks. Typically, pregnancy lasts 40 weeks. During this time symptoms of pregnancy such as heartburn, reduced appetite, constipation and backache may occur due to the size and weight of the fetus within the uterus disturbing the usual physiology of the woman. Refer to your anatomy and physiology textbooks, starting with Fraser and Cooper (2009), perhaps, if you are a first-year student, moving on to more complex books, such as Stables and Rankin (2005), as your knowledge develops. This will help you to understand why women experience these symptoms; to enhance your knowledge, we suggest you pay particular attention to the gastrointestinal and skeletal systems. It may be advisable also to look up fetal development at this stage. The additional reading will help you understand the midwife's role during this period.

The midwife's role during the third trimester

Antenatal appointments become more frequent during the third trimester, with over half the schedule of care being offered in this period – at 28, 31, 34, 36, 38, 40 and 41 weeks. Much of the care undertaken earlier in the pregnancy is repeated at each visit, such as measuring the maternal BP and urine testing for proteinuria, and enquiring about maternal well-being and fetal movements. In addition to these checks you will be measuring the symphysis-fundal height (SFH) from now on (see page 72).

The 28-week appointment

At 28 weeks you will undertake the usual BP and urinalysis for proteinuria. You will measure the symphysis-fundal height as before and plot this on a growth chart, as well as enquiring about fetal movements and maternal well-being, with questions such as *How are you feeling today?* Remember significant conversations from previous appointments and follow them up, or read the woman's antenatal notes if you have not met her previously or if she saw another midwife last time, to enable you to follow up on recorded conversations earlier in the pregnancy. This demonstrates a woman-centred philosophy of care and shows the woman that you are responding to her needs and well-being. Remember that offering women the opportunity to talk may be what they need in order to disclose their worries. By performing just the tasks of a midwife, you will be meeting only half the woman's needs and half the care you are required to carry out as a midwife, regardless of how busy the clinic is.

A second screening for anaemia and atypical blood cells is offered (the first one was undertaken during the booking interview – see page 43). This involves a blood test along with investigations for anaemia; if the haemoglobin level is below 10.5 g/100 ml, iron supplementation is also considered here. Women who are rhesus negative are offered anti-D prophylaxis (NICE, 2008d) (refer back to pages 47–8 to consolidate your learning).

Breastfeeding workshops should be offered to all women at this point, although women who have breastfed successfully before may not require them. Breastfeeding workshops are typically two-hour classes of information about breastfeeding offered by specially trained midwives or others, within either the hospital or the local community. Sometimes classes are tailored to women only, sometimes for their partners, too. Topics generally include the benefits for the mother and baby of breastfeeding, techniques to support effective positioning, latching on, and the prevention of common problems. Information on hand expression of breast milk and storing milk are often included. Benefits of the classes include meeting mothers-to-be who may choose to breastfeed, providing women (and their partners) with information and confidence to breastfeed, pre-empting common breastfeeding challenges and offering solutions for successful breastfeeding. If you have not attended a breastfeeding workshop yourself, ask your mentor if you can arrange to participate in one; also find out what services are offered to support women intending to breastfeed in your local area (for more information go to: **www.babyfriendly.org.uk**).

The 31-week appointment

At 31 weeks, nulliparous women have another appointment that parous women are not routinely offered. This again measures BP, proteinuria, SFH and fetal movements. Reviews and discussions about the results of the blood tests from three weeks ago are also recorded in the woman's hand-held records.

The 34-week appointment

At 34 weeks gestation all women are seen. The multiparous women have their blood results reviewed, discussed and recorded. All rhesus negative women are offered the second of the prophylactic anti-D injections. Every woman has her BP measured, urine checked for proteinuria, SFH measured and recorded, and fetal movements enquired about.

You should/will be giving to each woman specific information in this appointment on preparation for labour, birth plans, and recognising and coping with the onset of labour. This will either be on a one-to-one basis or during a group antenatal class.

Antenatal classes

Antenatal education aims to enable women to be more actively involved in their labour, for instance by exploring the mechanisms of labour so that women can understand what is happening to their bodies and make informed choices that may affect their progress in labour. Encouraging women to maintain a more upright posture or labouring in water, the bath or shower may reduce or delay the need tor pharmacological analgesia and facilitate a physiological birth. By informing women and their partners and showing them how to cope with contractions, they may be able to make more active choices in labour or understand more fully why their labour deviates from the normal. It also helps parents to meet the challenges of caring for a newborn baby as labour is only one aspect of the journey.

Antenatal education classes offer information on caring for the new baby as well as on labour, on **vitamin K prophylaxis** (a preventative medicine that helps the blood to clot and reduces the chance of the baby developing haemorrhagic disorders of the newborn), newborn screening choices, maternal postnatal care and awareness of altered moods in the postnatal period.

Classes are sometimes offered each week over four to six weeks or as a whole day, often at the weekend for birth partners to attend too or as shorter refresher classes for women who have given birth before. For further information on antenatal classes, look at the NCT website (**www.nct.org.uk**).

The 36-week appointment

At 36 weeks the usual checks, BP, proteinuria and SFH are undertaken as well as determining fetal position. This additional skill used to be routine; in fact, you may still be regularly performing abdominal palpation on all women, although SFH seems to have superseded this now. You can read more about abdominal palpation in Chapter 2 on page 34, but Figure 4.1 below shows palpation in late pregnancy.

The correct method of abdominal palpation requires the use of three individual positions that together build up a picture of the fetal lie, attitude, presentation, position and engagement; these are the fundal palpation, lateral palpation and pelvic palpation.

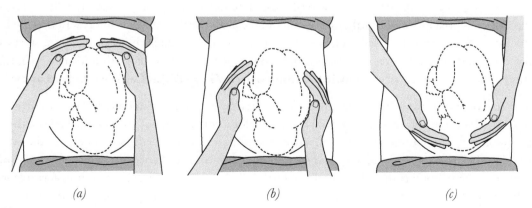

(a)   *(b)*   *(c)*

Figure 4.1: Abdominal palpation: (a) fundal palpation; (b) lateral palpation; (c) pelvic palpation

Determining the fetal position is a hard skill to master and often not correctly identified. It is only of clinical significance in the last few weeks of pregnancy, which is why it is no longer deemed necessary to perform an abdominal palpation until 36 weeks gestation. It can be uncomfortable for some women, especially the pelvic palpation, so the fewer times women are palpated the better.

Activity 4.4   *Reflection*

You are concerned about your clinical skills, especially abdominal palpation skills. It is your first placement in the community, and only a few women seem to be 36 weeks gestation or over. You wonder how you will ever have enough opportunity to develop this skill.

Consider what you have learned already in university; refer back to your notes or textbook and think about when you might need to perform an abdominal palpation to increase your skill and confidence in performing this skill.

There are some answers at the end of the chapter.

After considering how you will increase your clinical skill, we need to think about why this examination is performed. Clinically, abdominal palpation is performed to confirm that the fetus is in a position favourable for a vaginal birth. If a deviation from the norm is detected, the midwife will refer the woman for an obstetric review and possible confirmation of clinical findings with technological ones, such as ultrasound.

The most commonly identified position that needs consideration for birth is the breech presentation. If the fetus is in a breech position, women with no risk factors will be offered an **external cephalic version (ECV)** by their obstetrician, to turn their 'baby' from breech to a more favourable cephalic position for birth. Vaginal breech birth is considered riskier than cephalic birth, so women are offered ECV or caesarean sections, although there seems to be a revival of women choosing vaginal breech births, and more research is needed to offer women the best available evidence and advice.

At 36 weeks women are often offered a 'birth talk'. This is where the midwife individually explores the woman's preferences for birth; this is sometimes called a birth plan chat. Information, often in the form of leaflets, can be left with women to remind them of their choices for labour, such as the informed choice leaflets on position in labour and birth, place of birth and non-epidural strategies for pain relief (see: **www.infochoice.org/ic/ic.nsf/RevLeaflets?OpenForm**).

The role of the 36-week birth talk has been explored by Kemp and Sandall (2010), who suggest that the philosophy of caseloading, which is caring for a small group of women throughout their pregnancy, is inseparable from the effectiveness of the 36-week birth talk. They say that the positive effects of the 36-week visit and the subsequent birth experience are due to the model of midwifery care, not just the addition of the birth talk. While the 36-week talk is transferrable to other models of midwifery care, the positive effects in this study may be more to do with the relationship between women and midwives than the intervention alone.

The 38-week appointment

At 38 weeks, after the BP, proteinuria and SFH measurements are recorded, discussions about ongoing birth preferences and prolonged pregnancy may ensue. This refers to the options women may choose from if their pregnancy exceeds 41 weeks gestation. The three main options are membrane sweeping, induction of labour and expectant management. Women will be given information on membrane sweeping (a digital examination and stimulation of the cervix and attached membranes) offered at 41 weeks if spontaneous labour has not occurred. Membrane sweeping has only recently become routinely offered to women. It stimulates the cervix, and labour might begin spontaneously. There are few side effects – the most obvious one is that the examination is uncomfortable, but if it prevents induction of labour, it is considered worth the examination. Induction of labour usually commences at term +10; expectant management means 'to wait and see'. Few women choose this option but if they do after 42 completed weeks of pregnancy, they may be offered CTGs twice per week to monitor the fetus.

The 40-week appointment

Only nulliparous women are seen again at 40 weeks. All the usual measurements are undertaken – BP, urinalysis and SFH as well as abdominal presentation – and management of prolonged pregnancy may be discussed again.

The 41-week appointment

At 41 weeks all women who are still pregnant are seen and offered a membrane sweep and induction of labour (NICE, 2008c), as well as the usual care: BP, urine testing and SFH measurements. The risks of inducing a postdate pregnancy has to be communicated to women, so they and their partners can decide if this is something they wish to embark upon. Compared to spontaneous labour, nulliparous women whose pregnancies are induced tend to have more interventions and caesarean sections, and their babies have lower Apgar scores (Selo-Ojeme et al., 2011). Guidelines developed by five countries (Italy, UK, USA, Norway and Finland) remind practitioners that women experiencing postdate pregnancies have two routes they may choose: either induction or expectant management after 41 weeks (Mandruzzato et al., 2010). If the woman chooses the expectant management approach, she will be supported in her decision to allow spontaneous labour to ensue, and regular fetal and maternal well-being checks will continue.

Case study 1

Roxanne is a nulliparous woman; she has no medical conditions and was fit and healthy prior to this pregnancy. She has all her scheduled care with her midwife as her pregnancy is considered to be low risk. She is still pregnant six days after her due date, and she is uncomfortable. She sees her midwife, who performs a membrane sweep, and Roxanne starts contracting later that evening. She gives birth to a healthy boy the following lunchtime. Mother, father and baby are all well and happy.

Consider the two cases and think about how, you as a midwife, use different skills in each case. Both women have antenatal care, but their needs are very different, just as their birth experiences are, too – more of that in the next chapter.

The two cases demonstrate that every woman is individual, and so is her experience of pregnancy and the care she receives. Although the care for each visit is standard, to the woman it is anything but standard – it is a unique opportunity to talk to a professional about an extraordinary life event. Although the pregnancy may progress within normal parameters, remember that this experience is unique for each woman. Try to get to know each woman a little more each time you meet, so you build up your relationship with her and her partner. This is as important as the observations and record keeping.

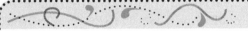

Chapter summary

This chapter introduced the schedule of antenatal care during the second and third trimesters with the tests and checks a midwife must discuss with the woman at each visit. The philosophy of woman-centred care – that is, valuing the woman and listening to her questions, anxieties or feelings – must not be overshadowed by the surveillance of the pregnancy. The woman should be supported by her midwife, and this takes time. A relationship between the woman and midwife should develop over the antenatal period so women will feel they have all the information necessary to make the right decisions for them regarding screening choices, place of birth and infant-feeding intention during their pregnancy.

Activities: brief outline answers

Activity 4.2: Communication (page 73)

First, as a midwife you might acknowledge that Karina's sister had the opportunity to listen to the fetal heart rate of her 'baby' and that you *can* listen to Karina's 'baby' as well. However, it is not necessary to listen to a fetal heart rate at each antenatal appointment and the mother is in a better position to discern fetal well-being than a midwife. Ask Karina when the 'baby' most noticeably moves, for example, what time of day it is and what Karina is doing at the time – it may be in the evening or when she gets into bed. Reassure Karina that feeling fetal movements is important and that she is doing well by noticing the pattern. The fact that her fetus is active is a positive sign and one she has noticed herself. Tell Karina and her sister that you can listen to the fetal heart rate but it is only a reliable indicator of fetal well-being in that moment. If the fetus moves, it is reassuring; if its pattern of movement alters, it may be less reassuring, and Karina is the best person to notice this. Ask Karina if she would still like to hear the fetal heart rate. If she says 'yes' respond to her request. After this discussion, she may decide that she does not need to hear the heart rate.

Activity 4.4: Reflection (page 78)

There will be plenty of opportunities for you to practise your abdominal palpations. These are likely to be at each antenatal visit subsequent to the 36-week appointment, during each antenatal admission, prior to induction of labour, before each vaginal examination in labour and at each change of care in labour. There is therefore no need to perform abdominal examinations on women prior to 36 weeks in order to practise your skills, as it is not clinically indicated here.

Further reading

All of these items are essential documents that support your care decisions. During the course of your training it is a good idea to read these so you can provide contemporary antenatal care.

NICE (2008) *Antenatal care: routine care for the healthy pregnant woman.* London: RCOG Press.

NICE (2008) *Induction of labour.* London: NICE.

NICE (2008) *Pregnancy (rhesus negative women): routine anti-D.* London: NICE.

The following is a selection of anatomy and physiology books to complement this chapter; they will give you the underpinning knowledge of what happens in pregnancy on which to base your care.

Fraser, D and Cooper M (2009) *Myles' textbook for midwives*, 15th edition. London: Churchill Livingstone.

Stables, D and Rankin, J (2005) *Physiology in childbearing with anatomy and related biosciences.* London: Elsevier.

The following book is a supplementary resource to antenatal care and may help consolidate some of this chapter and your learning.

Baston, H and Hall, J (2009) *Midwifery essentials: antenatal*, Volume 2. London: Elsevier.

Useful websites

www.dh.gov.uk/en/Publicationsandstatistics/Publications/PublicationsPolicyAndGuidance/DH_107302

The Department of Health Pregnancy Book includes not only the schedule of care and physiology of pregnancy for women, but also their rights and benefits; as such this is a particularly useful reference for midwives.

http://cpd.screening.nhs.uk/annb_elearning_module

Although you have to register to undertake these NHS screening e-learning modules, they are free of charge and a valuable resource for any health care professional.

www.cks.nhs.uk/pre_conception_advice_and_management/management/quick_answers/scenario_advice_for_all_women

NHS Clinical Knowledge Summaries is a great web-based resource that offers recaps and in-depth evidence on a wide range of clinical scenarios.

Chapter 5
Midwifery care in normal labour

Moira McLean

NMC Standards for Pre-registration Midwifery Education

This chapter will address the following competencies:

Domain: Effective midwifery practice
- Communicate effectively with women and assess and monitor women holistically throughout the intrapartum period using a range of assessment methods and reaching valid reliable and comprehensive conclusions.
- Care for and support women during labour and monitor the condition of the fetus, supporting spontaneous births.

NMC Essential Skills Clusters

This chapter will address the following ESCs:

Cluster: Normal labour and birth
Women can trust/expect a newly registered midwife to:

1. work in partnership with women to facilitate a birth environment that supports their needs;
2. be attentive to the comfort needs of women before, during and after the birth;
3. determine the onset of labour;
4. determine the well-being of the women and their unborn babies;
5. measure, assess and facilitate the progress of normal labour;
6. support the women and their partners in the birth of their babies;
7. facilitate the mother and baby to remain together.

Chapter aims

After reading this chapter you will be able to:

- understand the effects on labour of the birth environment and your demeanour as a midwife;

- understand labour and birth as a continual process that is not only physiological but emotional, social and spiritual;
- explain the principles of care throughout the labour process.

Introduction

This chapter looks at the role of the midwife in normal labour. It looks at the importance of the place of birth and discusses how the woman and her partner can be best supported to achieve normal birth. The phases of labour are described and the role of the midwife examined, paying particular attention to how midwives can fulfil women's needs for comfort and support during and after birth, at the same time as providing safe and effective professional care.

Place of birth

'Place of birth' is a much debated topic. Pregnancy and birth are a special episode in a woman's life and it is important that she makes a choice that is right for her and her family. In theory, a woman will be offered explicit choices about where to have her baby based on safety alone (Enkin et al., 2000; DH, 2007a). Currently in the UK, however, a majority of women give birth in obstetric units, with only about 2.8 per cent giving birth at home, around 3 per cent in midwifery-led units and just under 2 per cent in a free-standing midwifery unit (Redshaw et al., 2011). It remains to be seen whether this recently published birthplace study, with its emphasis on the safety of 'out of hospital' settings, will make any difference to where the vast majority of women will choose to have their babies. The choices currently available are:

- hospital;
- **birth centre alongside a consultant unit**;
- a **free-standing birth centre**;
- the woman's own home
  (Walsh, 2012)

Activity 5.1 — *Reflection*

Look again at the list above. What do you think the advantages and disadvantages (from the woman's point of view) might be for each of these options?

Consider what may influence women's choices about place of birth. What do you think is the midwife's role in ensuring women and their families are informed about the choices they have?

---

continued . . .

Now look at the following websites which may help you think about possible answers to these questions:

www.nct.org.uk/birth/faqs-home-birth

www.nct.org.uk/birth/choosing-where-have-your-baby

In order to understand a little about the differences of each of these environments for birth, take a look at:

www.nhs.uk/conditions/pregnancy-and-baby/pages/where-can-i-give-birth.aspx (some short video clips about home birth and hospital birth can also be accessed from this page)

www.healthtalkonline.org/Pregnancy_children/Pregnancy/Topic/1716/

Some thoughts on this activity are given at the end of the chapter.

Birth environment

The right birth environment is being increasingly recognised for the important role it plays in a woman's chances of having a normal birth. There is now clear evidence, supported by NICE (2007b), that reinforces the need for birth environments that support a woman's sense of control and increase her comfort. In some areas, new, smaller birthing units provide a relaxed, intimate atmosphere and give a real alternative to hospital or home births; to see inside one of these look at: **www.expressandstar.com/news/2012/01/03/inside-sandwells-new-birthing-unit/**.

Whatever the birth location, it needs to be one in which the woman has freedom to move and the ability to choose and control her level of comfort and ease. It is unlikely that facilities alone, or the lack of them, are the only considerations for women and the outcomes of their births. It seems probable that in settings where the facilities meet parents' needs, the attitudes and support from midwives and other staff may also differ. Women's expectations influence both what happens during labour and how they feel about their experience. Researchers suggest that positive expectations are associated with positive experiences and that women's satisfaction is strongly related to a sense of being in control and, in particular, being able to control panic (Green et al., 1998). It seems that controlling anxiety and panic are more important than reducing pain, because many women can tolerate pain provided they do not feel in a panic. Thus, a combination of low expectations, poor facilities, limited staff support and a sense of panic puts women at a disadvantage. This may increase their need for pharmacological pain relief and other interventions, reducing their opportunity for a straightforward vaginal birth and increasing the chance that they will have an **emergency caesarean section**. Improving the physical environment, increasing women's expectations and confidence through antenatal support and preparation, and increasing their sense of being supported and in control during labour could make a significant difference to the number of women who achieve the kind of birth they want, decreasing the need for emergency surgery.

During labour, women need to feel safe and secure, be protected from disturbances and adverse stimulation, and be able to let their body work most effectively. Labour rooms that are hard and cold, too hot, or open to uninvited visitors do not facilitate straightforward birth. Nor do environments that leave women and their partners feeling isolated or unsupported. Relaxing surroundings, deep baths, soft pillows, comfortable sofas and pleasant views may make all the difference, helping women to tune into their body's needs (NCT, 2006).

Women report finding encouragement and praise motivating. Practical suggestions (for example, about positions to adopt in labour), trusting the woman's instinct, valuing what she is trying to do, reassuring, being friendly, kind and chatty, and giving firm guidance when appropriate can all be helpful. Explaining what is happening, being a constant presence and not leaving the woman, seeming confident and in control of the situation but also involving the woman's partner are also highly valued. The woman should feel safe enough to let go (Anderson, 2010) and to express herself freely.

Activity 5.2 — *Evidence-based practice and research*

Go to the following websites:

www.midwiferytoday.com/enews/enews0317.asp

www.sarahbuckley.com/pain-in-labour-your-hormones-are-your-helpers

Take some time to read about the stress hormones and reflect about what effect these may have on a woman and how she may feel. Consider how this may affect her labour.

Now read:

Foureur, M (2008) Creating birth space to enable undisturbed birth, in Fahy, K , Foureur, M and Hastie, C (eds) *Birth territory and midwifery guardianship: theory for practice, education and research*. Edinburgh: Butterworth Heinemann.

As this activity involves your own research, there is no outline answer at the end of the chapter.

What is 'normal birth'?

The description of normal birth as *without induction, without the use of instruments, not by caesarean section and without general, spinal or epidural anaesthetic before or during delivery* (DH, 2006) is the definition often used to collect statistical data. The Royal College of Midwives defines components of normal birth as birth that follows an uncomplicated pregnancy and is spontaneous in onset between 37 and 42 weeks where the birth occurs within 24 hours of commencement of labour. This recognises birth as a unique and dynamic process where the fetal and maternal physiologies interact symbiotically and there is minimal trauma to either mother or baby (Bates, 1997). Care for a 'normal birth' can be provided either at home or in a birth centre by a midwife, though it is also possible in a hospital setting (Dodwell and Newburn, 2010).

It is also known that some factors help to facilitate straightforward birth without evidence of additional risks. These factors include: one-to-one support (Hodnett et al., 2011); immersion in water (Cluett et al., 2004; Alfirevic and Gould, 2006); low-risk women planning for a home birth; care from known midwives; and the employment of consultant midwives focusing on normality.

Activity 5.3   *Reflection*

Read Beech, BA and Phipps, B (2008) Normal birth: women's stories, in Downe, S (ed.) *Normal childbirth: evidence and debate*, 2nd edition. Edinburgh: Churchill Livingstone: 67–79.

Reflect on the voices of the women in this chapter and what appears to be of value to them. Consider how you might include some of this in your own practice.

As this activity depends on your own responses to the text there is no outline answer at the end of the chapter.

The World Health Organization (WHO, 1996) identifies four key practices that promote and support normal birth, and Lamaze International (2012) has identified two more.

1. Allowing labour to start on its own.
2. Freedom of movement in labour.
3. Continuous labour support.
4. Spontaneous pushing in non-supine position.
5. No separation of mother and baby.
6. No routine intervention.

Initiation of labour

While what starts labour is still not fully understood, it is believed to be a combination of inter-related factors, and labour may be experienced differently by different women and by the same woman in different pregnancies.

Activity 5.4   *Evidence-based practice and research*

Go to the following website:

http://mothering.com/pregnancy-birth/ecstatic-birth-the-hormonal-blueprint-of-labor

What do you learn about the role of the following hormones?

- Prostaglandin.
- Progesterone.
- Oxytocin.

---

continued . . .

- Oestrogen.
- Corticotrophin-releasing factor.

Visit the website below and complete the activity:

http://quizlet.com/7679452/initiation-of-labor-flash-cards/

As this activity involves your own research, there is no outline answer at the end of the chapter.

Stages or phases of labour

Labour is the process by which the fetus, placenta and membranes are born. Traditionally, labour has been divided into three stages; however, physiologically the process is a continuum and each phase is unique to each woman. Downe and McCourt (2008) use the term *unique normality* rather than descriptions of the stages of labour, but the concept of stages of labour and assessment of progress is deeply embedded in our birth culture and practice. With most women currently giving birth in consultant units within a medical framework of care, this is unlikely to change dramatically.

While the three-stage model may be helpful for students, you need to remember that the individual woman is at the core of all you do.

The first stage of labour

The first stage of labour involves regular and coordinated uterine contractions accompanied by cervical dilatation. There are three phases to this stage: **latent**, **active** and **transitional**.

While birth is an extremely complex physiological process, three main things occur.

1. Dilatation of the cervix.
2. Rotation of the fetus through the pelvis.
3. Descent of the fetus through the pelvis.

This is not a step-by-step process – it's all happening at the same time, and at different rates. So while the cervix is dilating the fetus is also rotating and descending. Dilatation is a gradual process that occurs because the muscle fibres in the fundus retract and shorten with contractions, pulling the cervix open (Coad, 2005). This does not require the pressure of a presenting part; however, the head can influence the shape of the cervix as it dilates up around it.

The fetus enters the pelvis through the **brim**. Usually in a transverse position, as it descends into the **pelvic cavity** the head will be **asynclitic**. This is because the angle of the pelvis requires the baby to enter at an angle. Once in the cavity the fetus has room to rotate into a good position for the outlet, which is usually an **occipito anterior** (OA) **position**. Rotation is aided by the shape of the pelvic floor and often by pushing by the mother.

The definition of 'established labour' includes regular rhythmic contractions with at least three occurring every 10 minutes, lasting for 45 seconds and accompanied by progressive dilatation of the cervix. However, women's contraction patterns are as unique as their bodies. Assessing the progression of the 'first stage of labour' also relies on knowing what the cervix is doing. Vaginal examination remains an element of 'routine' care, and in many units the timing of assessments is usually four-hourly. Some hospitals no longer have a policy of routine vaginal examinations in labour, perhaps reflecting concerns about the practice (Crowther, 2000). A vaginal examination only reveals what the cervix is doing at the time of the examination – it cannot provide information about what the cervix was doing before, or what it will do in the future. There should always be sound rationale for carrying out a vaginal examination.

Activity 5.5   *Critical thinking*

Lucy is four days past term in her first pregnancy. She has called the delivery unit twice with contractions and backache over the past two days. She has now had a show and the contractions are every ten minutes. She is very excited, and her family are all telling her different things, especially that she ought to go into the birthing unit where she has chosen to have her baby. The baby is moving well, and Lucy would like to wait till her partner Lawrence comes home in two hours' time.

Using the information above, consider what information you might give to Lucy over the phone when she next rings.

An outline answer to this activity is given at the end of the chapter.

Assessing progress in labour

There are a number of ways of 'measuring' progress in labour, including assessment of contractions, of the descent and position of the fetal head by abdominal palpation and of cervical dilatation by vaginal examination (VE). Attention to changes in a woman's behaviour and anatomical changes are additional tools the midwife can use to try to avoid disturbing labour rhythms and reduce invasive interventions. For example, the midwife can watch for the **purple line** (Shepherd et al., 2010), or the **Rhombus of Michaelis** (Simpkin and Ancheta, 2011), observing the way the woman's legs get progressively colder from ankle to the knee as labour progresses (Davies, 2011b).

Abdominal examination and uterine activity

Palpation of the uterus to assess the lie and progressive descent of the fetus can help to establish progress. Contractions can be palpated by gently laying a hand on the fundus of the uterus. Between contractions the fundus should feel soft and relaxed and, as a contraction establishes, the fundus starts to feel hard. The onset of a contraction may be palpated before the woman feels that it is a contraction. Normal labour is characterised by uterine contractions that are involuntary and intermittent with increasing frequency and duration. Intensity and frequency are measured from the start of one contraction to the start of the next. Normally, the number of contractions in a ten-minute period is counted. Up to five contractions in ten minutes are normal. This allows adequate relaxation of the uterus between contractions, enabling the placental bed to be perfused with blood and oxygen. The duration of contractions is assessed as the time from the start to the end of the contraction, with early labour contractions lasting 20 to 30 seconds, and active labour contractions 60 to 90 seconds. The resting time is noted, as is the resting tone in which the uterus relaxes between contractions.

Vaginal examination

Vaginal examination remains a contentious issue. It is most frequently used as a means of assessing progress in normal labour, and it remains a key skill for the midwife to learn and to apply intelligently. Technology may also elicit information and in the future may offer an alternative. Guidelines from the Royal College of Midwives suggest that VEs should be carried out by the same midwife throughout labour to reduce inter-observer variability and inaccuracy (RCM, 2008).

The examination should always be carried out with sensitivity, maintaining privacy and dignity, and always with consent; communication and feedback are important aspects, too.

The importance of maintaining hand hygiene cannot be overstressed – the chapter by Johnson and Taylor on the principles of infection control hand hygiene in *Skills for midwifery practice* (as listed in the further reading list on page 113) is essential reading.

Case study

Paula, who is having her second baby, is contracting regularly every three minutes and gives a history of having passed a mucoid show several hours ago. She arrives at the birth centre and by visual appearance appears to be in established labour. After all other assessments have been carried out (maternal and fetal observations, urinalysis, palpation of contractions for length strength and frequency), Sandra the midwife discusses whether or not Paula would like vaginal assessment. Paula is coping with each contraction and has got herself into a comfortable position kneeling over a birthing ball. She declines the offer of vaginal examination. Sandra nods in support and continues to offer support and gentle encouragement to Paula who, 50 minutes later, births her baby spontaneously in the all-fours position. A few hours later, while Sandra is helping Paula into the shower, Paula tells Sandra that her last birth experience has left her with a real fear of vaginal examinations. She feels so much better not having had to have one.

Support in labour

Continuous support in labour is an effective and inexpensive means of improving maternity care. Hodnett et al. (2011) found that women allocated to continuous support were more likely to have normal births and less likely to require intrapartum analgesia or report dissatisfaction in labour. In addition, the labours were shorter and less likely to involve caesarean section, instrumental childbirth, regional analgesia or babies with a low five-minute Apgar score. Continuous support was most effective when provided by someone (such as a doula) who was not part of either the hospital staff or the woman's social network. Continuous support during labour has clinically meaningful benefits such as a reduced need for pain relief and increased normal birth rates. It causes no known harm and can therefore be recommended (Walsh, 2012).

Emotional support includes continuous presence, reassurance and praise, information about labour progress and advice on coping techniques, comfort measures (comforting touch, massage, warm baths/showers, promoting adequate fluid intake and output), and **advocacy**. The labour supporter is also able to anticipate the expected behaviours of the woman in labour, such as tiredness, anxiety, concern, crying, screaming and/or the woman's feelings of not being able to cope (Bruggemann et al., 2007). Women have said that supporters should: focus on normality; decrease their fear; increase their trust and confidence in their ability to give birth; listen, respect and accept their ideals; provide spiritual, emotional and physical care; and provide clear information on which to base their decisions (Edwards, 2000).

Assessment of women's well-being in labour

Well-being is an important consideration for women in normal labour. While many of the physical observations discussed below are important, the midwife should also assess how the woman is feeling about the labour and what kind of support she wants. If the woman has made a birth plan, this should be discussed with her and acknowledged throughout her labour and birth. Where aspects of the birth plan cannot be implemented, this should be discussed with the woman (who should be kept fully informed) and a compromise reached if at all possible. A general assessment of well-being, including the woman's emotional and behavioural response, should be made.

Physical observations such as blood pressure (BP), pulse, temperature, respiration and urinalysis should be recorded (see Table 5.1). Most maternity units currently carry out a **modified early obstetric warning score (MEOWS)** at the outset of labour and repeat this four-hourly. In addition to this, observations of vaginal loss and the colour of the liquor, if present, should be made. Appropriate action should be taken on any deviation from the normal parameters, and this may include medical referral. A partogram (see Figure 5.1) should be used to record all findings, as it is an effective means of exchanging information about labour progress between caregivers where continuity of carer cannot be given. While individual units have developed their own variations of partograms, many have included action lines, which allow the midwife to recognise promptly any deviation from what is being used as a guide to progress in labour. See the further reading section on page 113 for more information on using the partogram.

Observation/ Examination	Frequency	Rationale	Action
Temperature	4 hourly	To identify pyrexia >37.6°C	If temperature is raised on more than two occasions, refer to medical staff
Pulse	1 hourly	To identify infection, haemorrhage and establish the difference between fetal heart rate and maternal pulse	If tachycardia present on two occasions, refer to medical staff
Blood pressure	4 hourly	To identify pre-eclampsia, haemorrhage	If raised in range 140/90 mm/Hg on 2 occasions 30 mins apart or a single reading of systolic 150/110 mm/Hg, contact medical staff.
Bladder emptying and urinalysis	2–4 hourly	To reduce damage to bladder from the presenting part and make room for descent of head; to identify normal micturition, underlying bacteraemia, proteinuria and/or infection and ketoacidosis	If unable to pass urine encourage ambulatory positions, privacy and dignity; in the absence of rupture of membranes, urinalysis shows 3+ protein on two separate tests, contact medical staff; if bladder palpable and woman unable to spontaneously void urine, consider intermittent catheterisation prior to onset of second stage labour
Bowel movement	On admission	To identify constipation, which may prevent progress in labour	Discuss last bowel movement and bowel habits through pregnancy; offer enema if constipated/concerned
Abdominal palpation	On admission and then before every vaginal	To confirm that the fundus is equal to weeks gestation, long lie, cephalic presentation,	If fundus is greater or less than dates suggest or suspected breech presentation, contact medical staff

Table 5.1: Observations in normal labour, all of which should be documented following local policy and NMC standards for record keeping (NMC, 2004b; NICE, 2007b)

Observation/ Examination	Frequency	Rationale	Action
	examination	position of the fetus and descent of presenting part.	
Contractions	On admission and at a minimum hourly during first stage labour	To confirm frequency, strength, tone and any changes	If frequency of contractions are more than 7:10 – suspect hyperstimulation; if contractions are less than 3:10, ensure labour is established; if labour has progressed and contractions reduce in frequency tone and strength, then suspect maternal acidosis and encourage fluids, isotonic drinks and easily digested foods. If problem persists, contact delivery suite consultant obstetrician.
Fetal heart auscultation	On admission, before any vaginal examination; every 15 mins first stage labour; at least every 5 mins or after each contraction second stage	To identify fetal well-being and identify abnormal features and/ or fetal distress	If any fetal heart rate abnormality is detected, use NICE fetal heart rate guidelines assessment and if first stage of labour, consider period of electronic fetal monitoring and contact medical staff (NICE, 2007b); if fetal heart rate abnormality during second stage of labour, ask for medical assistance from neonatal team to attend and medical support if suspected maternal problem.
Vaginal examination	On admission, as requested by woman and in the absence of	To assess: cervix position; texture of cervix; application of cervix to presenting part (PP); dilatation of cervix; membranes present/absent;	Vaginal examinations are useful to determine malposition, failure to progress in labour and to identify any anticipated birth problems (see Rimmer, 2009). If there is delay in first stage of labour due to above factors, ask for advice. If delay

Parameter	Timing		
other signs of progress in labour		fetal position; position of PP in relation to maternal pelvis; presence of caput/moulding; presence of abnormal features such as cord/placenta; to confirm full dilatation of cervix	or problems such as shoulder dystocia during second stage of labour; ask for assistance, perform immediate manoeuvres, with support from medical staff
Diet/fluid intake	On admission and throughout labour	To confirm that appetite is normal and no evidence of illness. H2 receptor antagonist drugs such as Ranitidine should not be used	Women should be offered light diet and continue with fluids through first stage of labour; this helps to prevent acidosis and dehydration.
Behaviour	On admission and throughout labour	To observe normal features of labour; any adverse behaviour concerns should alert the midwife and advice sought	Some women find labour more difficult to cope with than others; 1:1 support from the midwife will help to promote best outcomes and identify problems early. Some cultures expect women to be very noisy during labour – the midwife should be aware and supportive of this. If, however, a woman is struggling to cope, the midwife should offer support and, if this does not help, arrange transfer from a midwifery-led unit or home to a consultant unit.

Table 5.1: Continued

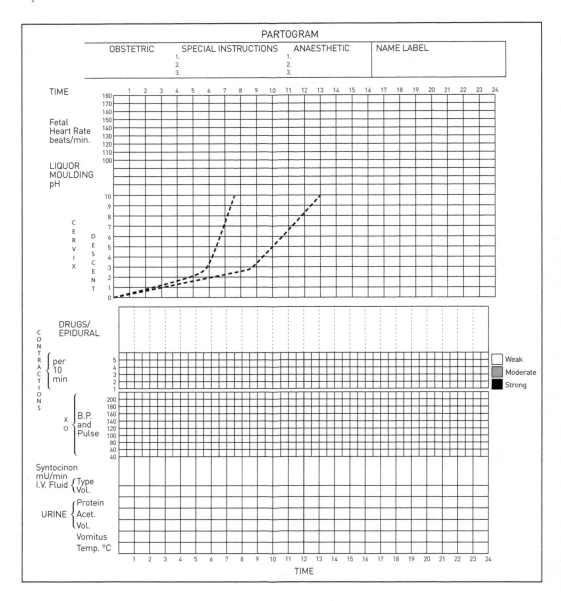

Figure 5.1: Partogram example

Assessment of fetal well-being in labour

A significant aspect of midwifery care during labour is the regular auscultation of the fetal heart rate sounds and uterine activity patterns, and the contemporaneous documentation within the health care record. While various methods are employed to do this, ranging from auscultation using a Pinard stethoscope or sonicaid/Doppler to more complex electronic monitoring, in normal labour the evidence is clear that intermittent auscultation is safe and that routine use of electronic fetal monitoring has not been shown to improve outcomes and is associated with operative birth increase (Alfirevic et al., 2006). Despite this, many women who are recognised as having normal pregnancies and are planning to birth in hospital are 'processed', and part of this is to have an admission episode of electronic fetal monitoring or cardiotocography (CTG) (Rattray et al., 2011). However, the admission CTG is a poor predictor of adverse outcomes, is not preventative of abnormalities and does not improve neonatal outcomes (Blix et al., 2005; Devane et al., 2012).

Activity 5.6 — *Evidence-based practice and research*

Read the chapter 'Fetal heart rate monitoring in labour' in Walsh, D (2012) *Evidence and skills for normal labour and birth*. London: Routledge. Then write down three issues that impact on the use of technology in normal pregnancies.

Now listen to the podcast at **www.cochrane.org/podcasts/issue-1-3-january-march-2012/cardiotocography-versus-intermittent-auscultation-fetal-heart-** for a review of the most recent evidence.

An outline answer to this activity is given at the end of the chapter.

Intermittent auscultation

Intermittent auscultation (IA) involves listening to and documenting the fetal heart rate at predetermined intervals during labour either by a Pinard stethoscope or a hand-held Doppler device (Leslie and Arulkumaran, 2011).

The National Institute for Clinical Excellence guideline on intrapartum care (NICE, 2007b) advises auscultation for the duration of one minute after a contraction at 15-minute intervals in the first stage of labour and five-minute intervals in the second stage. The importance of listening after a contraction is to detect prolonged, atypical variable and late decelerations, which are associated with poor fetal outcome. Abnormalities identified through IA or changes in the woman's well-being should prompt discussion with the mother and consideration of continuous monitoring; this may also involve a transfer of planned place of birth.

Activity 5.7 — *Evidence-based practice and research*

To be able to utilise intermittent auscultation of fetal well-being effectively and appropriately there needs to be some basic understanding of the control and physiology of the fetal heart rate and how oxygen and carbon dioxide transfer occurs in the fetus.

To help you answer the following questions, read the chapter on 'The fetus' by I Serci in Fraser, D and Cooper, M (eds) (2009) *Myles' textbook for midwives*, London: Churchill Livingstone.

1. What does the transfer of oxygen and carbon dioxide between the maternal and fetal circulations depend on?

---

continued . . .

2. In the placenta oxygen and carbon dioxide are exchanged via diffusion; this occurs quickly and is facilitated by the differential between the higher O_2 pressure in the maternal blood and the lower pressure in fetal capillaries. The fetus survives with less pressure of oxygen (PO_2) relative to adult values – why?
3. What are the differences in fetal haemoglobin that enable oxygen transfer more readily?

An outline answer to this activity is given at the end of the chapter.

Intermittent auscultation in labour

Using a Pinard stethoscope the fetal heart rate tones can be listened to and counted (using bone conduction). The Pinard stethoscope should be held flat against the maternal abdomen by gentle pressure provided by the practitioner's head. Auscultation requires extremely focused listening. Accuracy is increased with longer listening times and listening for a minimum of 60 seconds is recommended practice (NICE, 2007b). The Pinard stethoscope allows for fetal heart rate, baseline rhythm and changes to the baseline to be heard (Feinstein et al., 2000).

Instead of providing audible heart rate sounds, sonicaid or Doppler devices convert detected fetal heart rate movement into an auditory signal. Deflected ultrasound waves detect motion of the fetal heart rate valves or walls, and the Doppler converts the information received into a sound that is heard as a representation of the cardiac cycle (Mainstone, 2004).

Activity 5.8 — *Teamwork*

With two or three fellow students, discuss the following questions.

* Which method of auscultation of fetal heart rate is recognised as being most beneficial for low-risk women in labour?
* What sounds may be heard on auscultation?
* How can the practitioner differentiate between the sounds heard?
* When listening with either a Pinard or sonicaid what is the minimum length of time that you should listen?

To be able to accurately hear and understand what you are listening to, you should be familiar with the recognised definitions of key parameters of normality. Look up the definitions for the following terms in the glossary and discuss them with your fellow students.

* **Baseline rate**, including normal baseline rate.
* **Baseline variability**, including normal baseline variability.
* **Accelerations**.
* **Decelerations**.

continued . . . ••

A normal fetal heart rate should have a baseline between 110 and 160 beats per minute (bpm). It should have variability of greater than 5 bpm and have accelerations present and no decelerations.

An overview of your possible discussions can be found at the end of the chapter.

Working with pain in labour

The 'working with pain' ethos includes the belief that there are long-term benefits to promoting normal birth in terms of women's experiences and lives, and that pain plays an important role in the physiology of this process. In contrast, the 'pain relief' ethos is characterised by the belief that no woman needs to suffer the pain of labour and it is a kindness to alleviate it by a variety of pharmacological methods of pain relief (Walsh, 2012).Women are offered a 'pain relief menu', including the pros and cons of each method to enable them to make an 'informed choice'. Women may also interpret this as an implied message that it is not possible to get through labour without resorting to pain relief. Many health professionals also promote the use of pain relief because they feel disturbed by the noise and behaviour of women labouring naturally (England and Horowitz, 2007; Leap et al., 2010a).

Activity 5.9	*Reflection*

As a student you will be exposed to a variety of philosophies. Take some time to reflect on what influences your personal beliefs.

Read the following scenarios and consider what may affect women and the choices they make during childbirth. You may want to consider some of the points discussed earlier in this chapter and elsewhere in this book.

Scenario 1

Carrie is having her second baby in hospital on the delivery unit and has been labouring for three hours. It is two years since her first labour, which was a long, slow induced labour. This time, labour started spontaneously and the contractions are already every three minutes. Carrie had a vaginal assessment at her request as she was considering an epidural for pain relief, feeling that she just wouldn't be able to cope. Her cervix is already 8 cm dilated, the baby is in an optimum position and the membranes are intact. She is surprised but still feels that she won't be able to manage without the help of an epidural.

continued . . .

Scenario 2

Louise is having her first baby, and after labouring for five hours is now in the birth pool at home, her contractions are regular, and she has her eyes closed and is listening to gentle music. Her labour is progressing well and, prior to getting in the pool, her cervix was 5 cm dilated. She is confident that water is all she will need and has attended aquanatal classes.

How do you respond to each of these scenarios?

As this activity is based on your own reflection, there is no outline answer at the end of the chapter.

As labour progresses women should be encouraged to trust their instincts about what pain relief options and support might help and suit them. Depending on the environment for birth, various choices are available.

Women and midwives can work together using a variety of tools and techniques, including: using different positions; using movement such as swaying, walking, dancing and circling hips; focusing on breathing out very slowly; panting or blowing; vocalising (making sounds, e.g. singing, moaning, humming); using distraction such as keeping busy, watching TV, listening to music; using water by getting in a warm bath or a shower; using a birth TENS (transcutaneous electronic nerve stimulation) machine; and using relaxation techniques.

Some of these options, such as distraction, are most useful in early labour, while others, such as warm water, movement and focusing on breathing, can be invaluable all the way through.

The philosophy of this type of care has the underpinning belief that pain has a physiological purpose related to appropriate hormonal release, but it can also indicate emotional distress. Learning to discriminate between these is a key role of the midwife. Spending time with labouring women in a variety of situations can help to develop this skill. Developing trust and rapport are essential to this, and is discussed in part in Chapter 2 on communication skills. Learning to reflect on each experience can also develop this skill, but, as stated earlier, emotional distress can be caused by many past experiences and triggers, and not simply by the pain of labour. Clearly, this is a complex and challenging area.

Case study

Denise is having her first baby and is fit and well. She enjoys all types of exercise and is keen to avoid any interventions in her labour but particularly pharmacological pain relief. Helen, her midwife, suggests that using water may be an idea for her to explore. Helen explains that water has many benefits: it has analgesic properties and it will enable her to move more easily and maintain relaxation. She also tells Denise that all the midwives in the birthing unit she has chosen are trained in its use and that over 70 per cent of women use water for pain relief, some choosing to get out of the pool for birth, and others remaining in the water. Helen gives Denise some leaflets and website addresses to look at, and tells her about a local workshop on using water for pregnancy and birth that she might like to attend.

Positions for labour and birth

Women in labour often instinctively need to remain upright, move around and adopt a range of positions, thereby facilitating their labour and, for many, assisting with the relief of pain.

Encouraging a woman to move instinctively seems to be the key rather than directing that one position is better than another. The midwife's role should be to support women to adopt positions they find comfortable and encourage freedom of movement. Having some basic knowledge of the differences in each position and when they might be suggested may help to promote normal birth (see Figure 5.2 and Table 5.2).

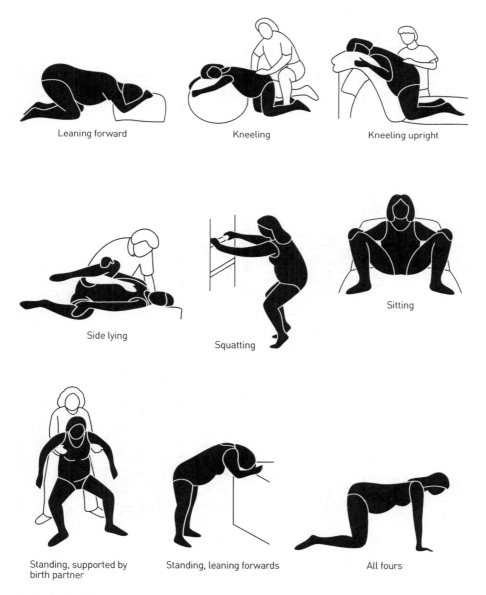

Figure 5.2: Birth positions

Position	Advantages	Disadvantages	Other information
Standing	Gravity assists decent of fetus; aligns fetus with pelvic inlet and can help flex fetal head; can relieve backache; can allow other movements such as swaying to be used at the same time	Multigravida women may birth too fast in this position	Can be supported by birth partner
Kneeling	Less pain; good for assisting rotation of baby; allows access to back for massage by partner or birth attendant	Legs may get numb after a while – providing a cushion for support can help	Kneeling over birth ball can help change position and soothe because of its gentle rolling movement.
Hands and knees	Can help rotate baby's position if needed; good for backache; can slow down a very fast birth; reduces perineal damage; optimum expansion of outlet of pelvis; allows access to back for massage by partner or birth attendant	Difficult if woman has pains in her knees	
Squatting	Aids descent of fetus; reduces likelihood of episiotomy; may enhance urge to push; may enlarge pelvic outlet	Increased blood loss	May be supported or unsupported; squatting compresses blood vessels behind knees – encourage woman to stand or sit back intermittently to reduce this

Position	Advantages	Disadvantages
Sitting at greater than 45 degrees	Increases the diameter of the pelvis at the inlet; provides some gravity	Pressure on sacrum and coccyx may reduce outlet
Side lying	Increased intact perineum rate; may increase oxygenation to fetus; can be a useful position for resting in; may promote progress; allows movement of sacrum	Lacks gravity if this is needed for descent
Dorsal position	Convenient for staff	Does not promote physiology of labour or birth; may lead to reduced placental blood flow and decelerations of fetal heart; longer labour; feelings of loss of control for woman

Table 5.2: Different birth positions: their advantages and disadvantages

Providing hydration and nutrition

Women in normal labour should eat and drink as to their appetite (Singata et al., 2010). Women in strong labour rarely wish to eat and only sip fluid. Champion (2010) suggests this is because oxytocin regulates appetite and ingested behaviours, inhibiting both food intake and gastrointestinal activity. As labour progresses and the cervix stretches and contractions increase, increased oxytocin is produced, which may lead to the lack of desire to eat in active labour. Oxytocin also has an insulin-like effect, which causes maternal blood glucose levels to decline, with a corresponding fall in fetal blood glucose levels. The maternal body responds to this by breaking down adipose tissue to release fatty acids and glycerol, leading to the production of ketones as by-products. Both the fetus and the mother use ketones as a source of energy.

Transitional phase of labour

'Transition' is the move from one phase of labour to the next. Contractions often become intense and extremely painful, with little gap in between. Many women become agitated during this stage, and their behaviour may change. There may be an accompanying rupture of membranes or large mucoid show, which may indicate rapid dilatation of the cervix. The woman may start to get an urge to bear down as the fetus rotates and descends through the birth canal. This stage usually lasts for only 15 to 20 minutes, but the woman and her partner will require intensive support from the midwife during this time. This support may involve constant presence and reassurance, eye-to-eye contact, talking in quiet soothing tones and generating an atmosphere of calm while acknowledging the extreme pain the woman is in and giving her short relevant instructions on breathing or positions as well as encouragement and praise.

Activity 5.10   *Decision-making*

Francesca is screaming loudly for pain relief, and asking you to save her as she is going to die. She has been in strong labour for six hours, and suddenly her demeanour changes. Her partner Ian pleads with you to get her an epidural.

How would you cope with this situation? What do you think is happening?

An outline answer is given at the end of the chapter.

The second stage of labour

The transition from one phase of labour to the next may not always be clinically apparent; however, midwives can look out for several physiological events.

- Uterine contractions may become expulsive; these may be heard through changes in the woman's breathing patterns, bearing down sounds or her actively stating she wishes to push.

- The forewaters may rupture, the anus may dilate and gape in response to deep engagement of the presenting part. The purple line, a pigmented line running along the anal cleft as labour progresses, may be observed to be reaching the top of the cleft.
- The Rhombus of Michaelis may present; heavy blood stained mucus ('the show') may be observed and the presenting part may become visible.
- If a vaginal examination is carried out, no cervix would be felt. Some practitioners do not trust the physiological signs, and if the fetal head is not visible may use a vaginal examination to confirm that the next phase of labour has commenced.

The second stage of labour starts after the cervix has dilated to 10 cm, and it continues until the fetus finishes moving through the vagina and is born. This stage can last from a few minutes to a few hours, having a latent phase and an active phase (NICE, 2007b). When the second stage begins, the woman may become more aware of her surroundings, alert and energetic as an urge to push intensifies and guides her to bear down and find a position that feels right. As the fetus moves through the vaginal canal, she may temporarily hold back till the body's strong urges take over and she lets go, releasing her pelvic floor and her attempts to control the process. She may grunt or moan with contractions and instinctively moves into different positions. The midwife's role when a woman is coping in this way is to monitor fetal and maternal well-being as unobtrusively as possible, providing encouragement and reassurance as needed and supporting instinctive behaviours as much as possible as long as the mother and fetus are tolerating the second stage of labour. Where progress is being made, there is no reason to intervene, and this includes time limits. During this phase of labour the fetus continues its progress through the birth canal.

Understanding the principles of the mechanism of labour can assist the midwife to facilitate normal progress and enhance the ongoing physiological processes in the second stage.

Activity 5.11 *Evidence-based practice and research*

Visit:

www.youtube.com/watch?v=Xath6kOf0NE&feature=player_detailpage

Watch the animation of the mechanism of labour.

Visit:

www.casttv.com/video/afu6jl/otpol-fteal-presentation-version-2-video

Watch and listen to the description of the mechanism of labour.

Take the opportunity to borrow a doll and pelvis, and explore how the 'baby' negotiates its way through the pelvis.

It may be helpful to revisit the anatomy of the fetal skull and maternal pelvis to do this, and the following resources will help you:

continued . . .

> **www.midirs.org/development/MIDIRSEssence.nsf/articles/90D1C687 F4ADBF63802578E2003518E9**
>
> **www.midirs.org/development/studentmidwife.nsf/article/18981B4099 E3A345802576F00040945A?OpenDocument**
>
> *As this activity is based on your own research, there is no outline answer at the end of the chapter.*

Some women start to feel like pushing or bearing down before the cervix is dilated to 10 centimetres; others feel like pushing after the cervix is completely dilated. For other women, after the cervix has dilated to 10 centimetres, it takes time for the baby to move down into the vagina, and then they feel like pushing. Until recently, women have been asked to start pushing as soon as the cervix has dilated to 10 centimetres, but as long as they do not have a temperature and the fetal heart rate is normal, there are many benefits to waiting to push until the woman feels the need to push.

Activity 5.12	Reflection

What do you think the benefits may be of waiting until the woman has the urge to bear down?

What have you observed in practice?

As this activity is concerned with your own ideas and experience, there is no outline answer at the end of the chapter.

Pushing phase

There is variation and to some extent disagreement among practitioners about how women should push. Table 5.3 summarises the differences between two different styles of pushing: open glottis pushing and closed glottis pushing (valsalva manoeuvre).

Support and care in the second stage of labour

As birth becomes imminent, the role of communication with both parents and any birth supporters becomes more crucial. Explanations should continue to be offered, and while there is usually great excitement a calm environment that continues to maintain the woman's privacy and dignity should be facilitated. While encouragement and support are key elements, the environment in the birth room should be led by the woman's needs. Some women are quiet and serene giving birth while others are noisy and vociferous. Asking the woman to change how she is reacting may be insensitive and culturally inappropriate.

	Open glottis pushing	Closed glottis pushing
Description	A health care provider and/or support person is there to encourage the woman to trust her body and to support her as she pushes, reassuring her that her sensations are normal, and reminding her to relax her perineum. The woman pushes when she feels the urge to bear down or when she feels like having a bowel movement. Most women take several breaths between pushes, probably pushing for about five seconds three to five times during each contraction. Women may grunt or make a deep noise when they are pushing. This is a sign that they are pushing well.	A health care provider and/or support person tells the woman how and when to push. The woman is asked to take a big breath and hold it before starting pushing, then to bear down as if having a bowel movement. She is encouraged to push for a count of 10, starting at the beginning of a contraction, then taking a breath and pushing again, pushing about three times with each contraction. The woman may be asked not to make any noise when she pushes.
Benefits	Blood flow to the uterus and fetus is not affected, so there is less chance of fetal heart rate abnormalities. There is less chance that woman will get so tired so she can't push any more. There is less chance of perineal trauma. Women spontaneously change position more often.	This type of pushing might shorten the time it takes to push the baby out.

Table 5.3: The differences between open glottis pushing and closed glottis pushing (valsalva manoeuvre)

(contd)

	Open glottis pushing	Closed glottis pushing
Risks	The second stage of labour may be slightly longer.	Decrease in the venous return and cardiac output leads to lowering of maternal blood pressure. Decrease in maternal blood oxygen levels and blood flow to the placenta and increase in maternal carbon dioxide levels until the woman gasps for air. Sudden increase in blood pressure can cause bursting of the tiny blood vessels in the whites of the eyes, the face and the neck (petechial haemorrhages). The blood flow to the uterus and fetus is lowered, which can raise the chance that fetal heart rate irregularities may occur, which may lead to interventions. There is a higher chance that the woman may become exhausted and not push any more. There is a higher chance of perineal trauma. There is a higher chance of difficulties in passing urine after the baby is born.

Table 5.3: Continued

Observations of maternal and fetal condition should continue as per NICE (2007b) and Trust guidelines. Maternal contractions should be assessed for length, strength and frequency by palpation; the resting phase between contractions may be longer, but strength and length may increase.

The woman should have an empty bladder, and care in the first stage of labour should have enabled this by encouraging the woman to void urine frequently as the compression of the bladder between the head and the pelvic brim may cause trauma.

Offering sips of fluid, cool cloths and wipes, and also changing wet pads or sheets can all assist with maintaining comfort. Involving birth supporters in these simple gestures can help them feel involved.

Providing all maternal observations have been normal, there is usually no need to carry these out in the second stage of labour unless there is slow progress. Recording of the maternal pulse and continual comparison to fetal heart remain vital.

To assess the well-being of the fetus once in the active phase of second stage, the recommendation is to auscultate the fetal heart after every contraction or every five minutes at least (NICE, 2007b), the same parameters being observed as discussed previously. If the membranes have ruptured, the amount and colour of the liquor should also be assessed.

As the woman continues pushing, the midwife should observe for descent of the fetal head. This can usually be seen as the **vertex** advances and is usually slower in a primigravida and more rapid in a multigravida. Descent is a good sign of progress and, provided that descent is apparent, the midwife and woman can be reassured that birth will be imminent.

Birth preparation

Key to preparation is consideration of the environment, which should be calm and warm. The midwife should ensure that any specific cultural or spiritual requests for the birth are enabled if possible. A safe clean area should be prepared to receive the baby, with sterile cord clamps and warm dry wraps for the baby available.

As the fetus descends, the midwife should put on protective equipment such as gloves and an apron. Depending on the position the woman has adopted, the midwife may subtly place a pad in place against the perineum to absorb any fluids or faecal matter.

As the head descends, the perineal muscles stretch, and the head continues to recede between contractions. During this time the midwife should observe the perineum, supporting the woman by explaining the sensations felt in the perineum and what they mean. There remains debate about whether midwives should apply pressure to the presenting part or have hands poised. There is evidence from the HOOP trial (McCandlish et al., 1998) that the hands-off technique is associated with slightly more discomfort at ten days postnatal but is associated with reduced episiotomy rates. Midwives should consider all aspects of what is happening – for example, the position of the woman, active versus spontaneous pushing, rapidity of descent – in making the decision as to whether to have hands on or hands poised.

> ### Case study
>
> *Becky is about to birth her baby. Nimisha her midwife is softly encouraging her. Nimisha has already explained to Becky what she may feel in order to prepare her and her partner. Becky had become despondent at one point as she could feel the baby's head receding following each contraction. Nimisha explained that this was a normal part of birth for a first baby and that it was enabling the perineal tissues to slowly stretch to accommodate the fetal head. Becky was reassured by this and continued to spontaneously bear down with each contraction. When the head no longer receded back and started to be born Nimisha reminded Becky about breathing gently to allow the head to be birthed slowly. Nimisha had her hands poised in order to offer support if needed. As the head was born Nimisha looked at the time and reminded Becky that the next contraction would allow the baby's head to turn a little (**restitution**) and the shoulders to be born. Nimisha was prepared to assist with this, allowing whichever shoulder presented first to be born gently over the perineum. As the remainder of baby was born, Becky was encouraged to reach down to receive her baby. Nimisha gently unwrapped a loop of cord that was around the baby's neck as both Becky and her partner were encouraged to find out what sex the baby was. Nimisha congratulated the couple as she placed a dry towel over the baby as it lay skin to skin against Becky.*

The third stage of labour

The third stage is from the birth of the baby to the birth of the placenta and membranes, and control of bleeding, and it is a continuation of the previous phases of labour.

Once the baby is born, the placenta continues to function until it separates from the uterine wall. There are currently several practices available to support separation of placenta and membranes. Current guidance (NICE, 2007b) advocates an active approach using an oxytocic drug; however, natural separation may be seen as a logical conclusion following a normal labour and birth (RCM, 2008). Fahy et al. (2010) advocate a holistic physiological approach to third-stage care as safe for women at low risk of postpartum haemorrhage, and this is supported by Dixon et al.'s (2011) systematic review of the literature related to physiological third stage (see Table 5.4).

Umbilical cord clamping

Recent recommendations support the use of delayed cord clamping in order to benefit the newborn baby (NICE, 2007b; Richmond and Wyllie, 2010). Benefits to the newborn when the cord is left to pulsate include reduced respiratory problems at birth, ongoing placental oxygenation if the transition to extra-uterine life is delayed, and increased iron content helping prevent anaemia and iron deficiency. Not only does leaving the cord to pulsate ensure that the baby receives a full complement of stem cells, it ensures that there remains optimum perfusion of all bodily organs. Leaving the cord intact promotes undisturbed time for the mother and baby, which ensures an ideal start to breastfeeding and mother–infant interaction.

Physiological birth of the placenta	Active management of the third stage of labour
Appropriate if the woman has a physiological normal labour and birth	Appropriate if the woman has had any interventions in labour or is at high risk of bleeding
Delayed cord clamping allows increased blood flow to the baby, increasing the haemoglobin and **haematocrit** without increasing the risk of neonatal jaundice	Oxytocic drug given at birth of anterior shoulder or immediately following the birth of the baby
Principle of care is watchful waiting, unhurried atmosphere, warm room, quietness	Immediate cord clamping and cutting it is not required and can be delayed for two to three minutes while oxytocic drug takes effect
No oxytocic drug is given	Placenta is delivered by controlled cord traction, traditionally guarding the uterus with one hand while gently but firmly pulling the cord of the placenta with the other. Signs of separation may be waited for prior to traction on the cord (modified Brant Andrews)
No palpation of the uterus	Placenta usually delivered within ten minutes
No cord traction	Prolonged third stage of 30 minutes (NICE, 2007b)
Skin to skin encouraged	
Breastfeeding encouraged, which increases oxytocin production	
Blood loss and signs of separation watched for – also cord lengthening, trickle of blood, woman becoming restless or having an urge to push, placenta being visible	
Upright posture may help to birth the placenta; the woman may be encouraged to give a few pushes with a contraction	
95% of women will birth placenta within one hour	
Placenta and membranes checked for completeness	Placenta and membranes checked for completeness

Table 5.4: Active management of third stage of labour vs physiological third stage

You can find out more about clamping the cord by reading the article by Buckley featured in the further reading list on page 113, or by watching a demonstration of benefits of delayed cord clamping at **www.youtube.com/watch?v=W3RywNup2CM**.

Examination of the placenta

The placenta should be carefully examined as soon as possible. Examination of the placenta may take place in front of the parents – they are often interested. Some parents may wish to keep the placenta, and the midwife's responsibility is to ensure they understand how it should be disposed of safely.

While the main reason for examining the placenta is to ensure its completeness, samples of cord blood may also be required (particularly if the mother has a rhesus negative blood group). You can find more information on this topic at **www.midwivesonline.com/parents/parents1 //121**.

Immediate post-birth care

Be guided by the parents: some wish to be left alone while others are anxious for support and guidance. Quietly ensure that both the mother and the baby are safe. Remove any wet linen towels to ensure both are warm, thereby increasing natural oxytocin levels, which play a part in facilitating breastfeeding and maternal infant interaction. Ensure the uterus is well contracted and carry out observations on both the mother and the baby at an appropriate time. The perineum needs to be examined for trauma; best practice is to ensure any suturing is completed as soon as possible, but be guided by the clinical situation and the parents' wishes.

Offering refreshments is often welcome. You will also need to complete any records (NMC, 2004b). Examination of the baby, weighing, and the administration of any drugs or labelling should be carried out in line with local guidelines but also with sensitivity to the situation. Some parents will want the baby weighed immediately; others will wish to wait. Skin-to-skin contact and breastfeeding should take priority over routine tasks (see also Chapter 7 on Neonatal care).

Prior to transferring the woman to a ward – or prior to the midwife leaving the woman's house if a home birth – temperature, pulse, blood pressure, **lochia** (discharge from the uterus following the birth) and firmness of fundus need to be assessed, and the woman must have passed urine. Parents should know how to contact the health professional/midwife at any time.

Perineal tears

Perineal injury is a serious complication of birth and can have a severe impact on the quality of life of healthy women. The prevalence of tears among women giving birth in hospital has increased over the last decade while it is lower among women who give birth at home. Many things need to be considered in order to minimise the risk to the perineum; these are not limited to the actual moment of the birth but start with the communication between the midwife and the woman (Lindgren et al., 2011). Perineal assessment following birth is needed and suturing should take place as soon as possible if required.

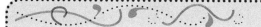

Chapter summary

The midwife's role in normal labour and birth is to provide support and guidance as well as to assess maternal and fetal well-being. The relationship between the midwife and the woman is vital in supporting and enhancing normal processes. This chapter has considered the physiology of the phases of labour and how women respond to this. It has also looked at the role and responsibilities of the midwife. The importance of maternal and fetal observations throughout the labour process has been explored from a physical and psychosocial perspective.

Activities: brief outline answers

Activity 5.1: Reflection (pages 83–4)

The advantages of a hospital birth might be: (a) feeling confident in the hospital environment if a woman has had a complicated birth dealt with well there on a previous occasion; (b) having more choice about pain relief; (c) having access to options such as birth in water. Disadvantages might be: (a) finding the hospital environment impersonal; (b) feeling that the hospital staff are the ones in control; (c) concern that she may be subject to interventions that she does not wish to have.

Advantages of a home birth might be: (a) the woman might feel more confident and comfortable in her own environment; (b) she might have had a less than enjoyable experience of a previous hospital birth; (c) previous births may have been quick, so she would feel safer at home. Disadvantages are: (a) the choice of pain relief will be less wide; (b) it will take longer to get help if there are problems with the labour. A first-time mother may find this makes her anxious.

A free-standing birth centre may be seen as a compromise – offering some of the advantages (but also potentially some of the disadvantages) of both.

A woman's choice is likely to be affected by (a) previous experiences (both her own and that of friends or family members); (b) what is available locally; (c) her own instincts about what may be best for her and her baby.

As a midwife, you need to work in partnership with women and at times be an advocate for them; part of your role in this is to give women the information they need to make the best possible choice for them. It is important to be aware, however, that the best choice for one woman will not necessarily be the best choice for another. You need to be sensitive in your listening and accept that her choice may not necessarily be the one you would make in her position. You also need to talk through with the woman what may happen if her original birth plan gets derailed by events (for example, she may be expecting a hospital birth, but her baby doesn't want to wait that long, or she may be hoping for a home birth but need to be transferred to hospital for an emergency caesarean). Changes in plan don't mean she has failed – they just mean her safety and that of her baby are being put first.

Activity 5.5: Critical thinking (page 88)

- Reassure Lucy that labour is progressing normally and that the best place for early labour is at home. Talk to her about what she has experienced so far and what strategies, if any, she has used to promote her comfort.

- Explain how she can recognise that her labour is progressing and discuss support measures to use at home such as positions, mobility, using the birth ball, getting in the bath, resting, eating and drinking normally as well as voiding urine regularly.
- Listen to her coping with contractions and gauge her response, talking through breathing techniques if needed.
- Assess fetal well-being by asking about fetal movements and their pattern over the previous hours.
- Encourage the use of simple analgesia such as paracetamol, if required.
- Ensure she has the support of family or friends at home and that she has enough privacy.
- Encourage her to call back if she requires more advice or support; offer her your name, letting her know how long you are there for so you can start to develop a relationship.

Activity 5.6: Evidence-based practice and research (page 95)

Issues that impact on the use of technology in normal pregnancies.

- Fear of litigation.
- Under-confidence in the use of intermittent auscultation, perhaps by being deskilled in its use.
- Over-confidence on the reliability of technology over traditional methods.
- Not understanding the implications of the use of technology in low-risk normal pregnancies and how this may lead to further intervention.
- Value given to being able to interpret read-out as opposed to listening and understanding intermittent auscultation.

Activity 5.7: Evidence-based practice and research (pages 95–6)

1. The transfer of oxygen and carbon dioxide between the maternal and fetal circulations depends on:
   - blood flow;
   - a high fetal haematocrit (17–19 g/dl), and the presence of fetal haemoglobin F, which help to ensure adequate oxygen content.
   Oxygen carriage to vital organs is also dependent on fetal cardiac output and adequate umbilical circulation.
2. Fetal haemoglobin has a much greater affinity for oxygen, and this facilitates oxygen transfer.
3. Fetal haemoglobin is of a higher level than adult haemoglobin – 16–19 g/dl compared to 11–13 g/dl – so it has more oxygen-carrying capacity.

Activity 5.8: Group work (pages 96–7)

- Intermittent auscultation with the Pinard or sonicaid stethoscopes is recognised as being the most beneficial method of auscultation of fetal heart rate for low-risk women in labour.
- Fetal heart rate, placental blood flow, placental soufflé and maternal pulse may be heard on auscultation.
- Practitioner can differentiate between the sounds heard by taking the maternal pulse at the same time and by recognising the normal parameters of a fetal heart rate.
- When listening with either a Pinard or sonicaid, the minimum length of listening time should be one minute with at least another 30–60 seconds to listen for variations (variability). Listening for longer can help to ensure more understanding of fetal heart rate variations.

Activity 5.10: Decision-making (page 102)

Francesca's changed demeanour may indicate transition from one phase of labour to the next. As the contractions have been very intense and painful, it is highly likely the cervix is nearing complete dilatation and the fetal head is descending through the birth canal. Understanding the physiological changes that are taking place, the midwife can offer reassurance and information to Francesca and her partner while continuing to look out for signs from Francesca such as experiencing the urge to push, stating that she wishes to open her bowels or making grunting sounds at the height of the contractions. Other signs that labour is progressing are a large blood-stained mucus 'show', the membranes rupturing, anal dilatation, contractions becoming more expulsive, and the fetal head starting to become visible.

Further reading

Buckley, S (2011) Top 10 tips for cord clamping. *Essentially MIDIRS*, 2(10): 27–31.

Chapman, V and Charles, C (2009) Water for labour and birth, in Chapman, V and Charles, C (eds) *The midwife's labour and birth handbook*, 2nd edition. Oxford: Wiley Blackwell.

An introduction to the use of water.

Fraser, D and Cooper, D (2009) *Myles' textbook for midwives*, 15th edition. Edinburgh: Churchill Livingstone.

See especially Serci, I, 'The fetus', to help you to understand the fetal circulation, and Hamilton, A, 'Comfort and support in childbirth', for an overview of pain relief methods both natural and pharmacological.

Johnson, R and Taylor, W, Chapter 9: Principles of infection control hand hygiene, and Chapter 30: Principles of intrapartum skills: first stage issues, in *Skills for midwifery practice*, 3rd edition. Edinburgh: Churchill Livingstone.

Simpkin, P and Ancheta, R (2011) Prolonged 2nd stage of labour, in *The labour progress handbook*, 3rd edition. Chichester: Wiley Blackwell.

This chapter provides a good explanation of delayed urge to push in the second stage of labour.

Walsh, D (2010) Birth environment, in Walsh, D and Downe, S, *Essential midwifery practice: intrapartum care*. Chichester: Wiley Blackwell.

Walsh, D (2012) *Evidenced based skills for normal labour and birth: a guide for midwives*, 2nd edition. Abingdon: Routledge.

See particularly the chapter on 'Rhythms in the first stage of labour', which gives an interesting discussion on the use of the partogram in labour; also the chapters covering 'Fetal heart rate monitoring in labour'.

Useful websites

www.givingbirthnaturally.com/pushing-stage.html

A website for parents, but helpful for midwives as it gives some rationales for actions that are useful to think about.

www.studentmidwife.net/educational-resources-35/midwifery-pregnancy-and-birth-videos-28/34698-vaginal-births-hands-off-hands.html

An amazing video of hands-off birth to reflect on.

www.youtube.com/watch?v=gHnFoWEVs7o&feature=related

Provides a useful review the anatomy of the placenta, membranes and cord.

http://academicobgyn.com/2011/01/30/delayed-cord-clamping-grand-rounds/

A 50-minute presentation on issues of delayed cord clamping for those that want detailed information. Another useful website is: **http://cord-clamping.com/**.

http://magazine.lamaze.org/Birth/LaborDay/tabid/71/Default.aspx

A useful detailed outline using diagrams and words of what is happening in labour and helpful to direct parents to.

www.wombecology.com/?pg=fetusejection

Gives an explanation of the physiological reflex, and suggests how you might use this information in your practice.

Chapter 6
The role of the midwife in postnatal care

Sam Chenery-Morris

NMC Standards for Pre-registration Midwifery Education

This chapter will address the following competencies:

Domain: Effective midwifery practice
Work in partnership with women and other care providers during the postnatal period to provide seamless care and interventions which:

- are appropriate to the woman's assessed needs, context and culture;
- promote her continuing health and well-being;
- are evidence based;
- are consistent with the management of risk;
- are undertaken by the midwife because she is the person best placed to do them and is competent to act;
- draw on the skills of others to optimise health outcomes and resource use.

Care will include:

- providing support and advice to women as they start to feed and care for the baby;
- providing post-operative care for women who have had caesarean and operative deliveries;
- providing pain relief to women;
- team-working in the best interests of women and their babies.

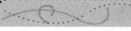

NMC Essential Skills Clusters

This chapter will address the following ESCs:

Cluster: Communication
Women can trust/expect a newly registered midwife to:

7. Provide care that is delivered in a warm, sensitive and compassionate way.
8. Be confident in their own role and within a multi-disciplinary/multi-agency team.

continued . . .

Cluster: Initiation and continuance of breastfeeding

3. Support women to breastfeed.
5. Work collaboratively with other practitioners and external agencies.
6. Support women to breastfeed in challenging circumstances.

Chapter aims

After reading this chapter you will be able to:

*   offer women ongoing postnatal care;
*   understand the needs of women and their families during this time;
*   identify women in need of additional care;
*   understand the importance of communication in your relationship with women and others during this period to maximise the experience for families.

Introduction

For the purposes of this book, postnatal care begins after the birth of the baby and placenta, and when all the documentation and assessments have been completed. Postnatal midwifery care ends when the woman is referred onwards to the care of the health visitor. Technically, however, the definition of the postnatal period is the period between the birth of the baby and placenta and the time when **haemostasis** is achieved. The period lasts approximately six to eight weeks and ends when the textbooks say the woman's body reverts back to its non-pregnant state. This is not the same as returning to its non-pregnant state as some parts of the woman's body never quite recover their elasticity following pregnancy and birth. This is not something women should be worried about – although some are – but something to be acknowledged.

The chapter continues the underlying theme of the previous chapters: that communication between you, the midwife, and the woman is paramount. The woman and her family should be at the centre of any decisions made during this period. For them to make informed choices, the midwife has to ensure the woman has the information needed to decide what is best for her and her infant and family. Care should, as always, be based on the best available evidence and tailored to meet the individual needs of the woman.

Most women have uncomplicated postnatal periods, but the midwife's role during this time is to recognise deviations from the normal and to refer women appropriately to another professional, and to support women and their families in this transition stage, whether they be single people or married couples becoming parents for the first time, or parents who are expanding their families. The main maternal postnatal complications are postpartum haemorrhage, thromboembolic disorders, infections and mental health disorders. You are strongly recommended to read the

NICE (2006) postnatal care guidance, as this gives clear guidelines about who women should be referred to and how urgently they require additional care.

Prior to discharge

Discussions about the length of a postnatal hospital stay should be made in consultation with the woman. Women are discharged into the community earlier than in previous decades. For example, a six-hour postnatal stay is now common following a vaginal birth, as is a 48-hour stay after a caesarean section. The NICE (2011) guidance states that women who have had a caesarean section who wish to be discharged, are apyrexial (that is, they have no raised temperature) and have had no complications may be discharged 24 hours after the operation.

Scenario

A primigravid woman, Charlotte, has a spontaneous vaginal birth using Entonox® for pain relief. Her baby, Noah, weighs 3.2 kg at 38 weeks gestation. He has been to the breast and latched on well. Charlotte is keen to go home even though it is only four hours since she gave birth; all her observations have been within normal limits and she is confident handling Noah. She does not want to spend her first night as a family away from her partner. Her partner is supportive and also keen for her to come home. As her midwife, you listen to her request and facilitate the discharge to home, informing Charlotte of the numbers to call should she need advice or reassurance. You tell her the signs and symptoms she needs to be aware of overnight (see below) and make arrangements for Noah to have his 48-hour examination in the community.

Before the postnatal woman and her baby are discharged from hospital, or the midwife leaves the woman's home, some important life-saving information should be shared by the midwife, should any problems occur. This information should be presented in a way that is not scary to the woman and her partner, but gives them the knowledge of what needs urgent medical attention.

These are the conditions that midwives must be alert for during the whole postnatal period. An awareness of the possibility of them arising should form the basis of the observations and discussions with women about their health and well-being during this period. All contact numbers of the midwife, GP, ward and central delivery suite should be documented in the woman's postnatal notes prior to discharge so the woman knows who to call for advice when unattended.

Prior to discharge the midwife must ensure she knows the address and contact details that the woman will be discharged to, in case this differs from her previous notes, or she is convalescing somewhere else.

Signs and symptoms	Condition
Sudden and profuse blood loss or persistent increased blood loss; faintness, dizziness or palpitations/tachycardia	Postpartum haemorrhage
Fever, shivering, abdominal pain and/or offensive vaginal loss	Infection
Headaches accompanied by one or more of the following symptoms within the first 72 hours after birth: visual disturbances; nausea, vomiting	Pre-eclampsia/eclampsia
Unilateral calf pain, redness or swelling; shortness of breath or chest pain	Thromboembolism

Table 6.1: Signs and symptoms of potentially life-threatening conditions in the postnatal period
Source: Taken from NICE, 2006, p11.

Organisation of postnatal care

Postnatal care has been described as the Cinderella service for childbearing women (Wray, 2006). This implies that women's needs during the postnatal period are not considered a priority, and that postnatal care is at risk of further reductions through budgetary constraints. As more resources for effective antenatal and intrapartum care are required to reduce risks and improve pregnancy outcomes, the focus on postnatal care is less acute. Conversations at the International Confederation of Midwives conference in Durban suggest that this UK observation may be universal (Davies, 2011a). The continuity of care model, where the same midwife cares for the woman in the antenatal and postnatal periods, may be the best use of resources, as midwives and women know each other and can work in partnership through this changing period. Facilitating this transition to parenthood is one of the pivotal roles of this period, in addition to recognising if deviations from the normal are occurring and making referrals to the appropriate health professional if necessary.

The number of postnatal visits across the UK varies; care should be tailored to the individualised woman's needs as stated in *Midwives rules and standards* (NMC, 2004a). According to the NMC, the postnatal period begins after labour, and the midwife should attend the woman and baby for a minimum of ten days; above that minimum, the midwife should attend for as long as the midwife considers necessary. There is evidence that women receive between zero and ten postnatal visits (NCT, 2010) and that only half of these visits are from midwives – the rest are from midwifery support workers. In other research (RCM, 2010), midwives acknowledged that care took place in the home, on the phone and in postnatal clinics. The majority of women were transferred to the care of the health visitor by day ten postnatally.

Historically, within the UK most postnatal care was offered in the woman's home. Recently, a radical change in the provision of postnatal care has been introduced: the postnatal clinic (Lewis, 2011). These clinics have supposedly been introduced to improve access and choice for women and utilise resources more effectively; however, they may mean that traditional relationships between women and midwives will change, and not necessarily for the better (Lewis, 2011).

There is also news that mobile phone technology may be used to support women in the postnatal period (Dabrowski, 2011). If this is used as an adjunct to, as opposed to a replacement for face-to-face midwifery visits to support the most vulnerable or hard-to-reach women, this is great. However, there is the danger that cheap technologies are used instead of expensive midwifery care in an effort to streamline services. Already there is evidence that women do not receive enough support in the postnatal period, so to reduce further this emotional, physical and informational care will leave more women feeling they have been left to their own devices (NCT, 2010). A mixed approach of some postnatal home visits and clinic appointments supported by mobile technologies is somewhat inevitable.

Midwifery postnatal care

Midwives may use almost all of their senses to evaluate whether women and their babies are thriving or not during the postnatal period.

Activity 6.1 — *Reflection*

With a fellow student, recall your five senses and consider how these may be used within a postnatal visit with a new mother and baby. As you discuss this activity together, see if your colleague has similar answers and if bouncing ideas together expands your thinking.

There are some suggested answers at the end of this chapter.

Now that you have considered how your senses are used within midwifery care, we will look at differences in the care delivered.

The philosophy of how postnatal care is implemented may alter from midwife to midwife, as each has their own set of beliefs. This can be difficult for students, as they may be working with midwives who practise in differing ways within the postnatal period. Some midwives may consider the conversation and relationship with the woman to be the most important. If the relationship is trusting and empathetic, the woman will tell the midwife everything she needs to know to evaluate whether the woman and baby are well. Other midwives may have a more structured approach to this care.

As a student midwife, it is sometimes helpful to have a routine in order to ensure that no aspect of the postnatal care is missed. This is not a checklist as such, but it aids your development as you have a rationale for each aspect of the postnatal care offered. While you are learning, therefore, a head-to-toe approach of physical and psychological postnatal care may be helpful, assessing the woman from her head to her toes and asking questions about the body systems as you work 'down' her body. Starting at the top, the head of the woman, you will ask the woman how she is feeling. Listening to her response – especially if you already have a relationship with the woman from the antenatal period – may highlight that she is well or that 'something' does not seem right with this family. Looking and listening occur as soon as you interact with this woman.

The head is, of course, where the brain is located, and in this top-to-toe assessment it is where the woman's emotional responses stem from. As a midwife, you are ascertaining how this woman is psychologically and how she is interacting with her family, including the new baby.

You may remember from the antenatal chapters a recommended NICE document, *Antenatal and postnatal mental health guidelines* (NICE 2007a). These guidelines, as the title suggests, are equally pertinent in this period. The guidelines suggest that healthcare professionals – and this includes you, the midwife – should ask women about their previous mental health to determine which women may require more support and surveillance during this time of emotional turmoil. Remember that for a woman to feel able to answer honestly when there are mental health issues to report, she needs to feel able to trust her midwife (Brealey et al., 2010). If the woman does have a history of previous mental health issues, an individualised care plan should be written in partnership with the woman and her family, and she should also be referred to services to support her care – in the first instance this is usually her GP. This topic is covered in more detail in the high-risk book in this series.

For women who have not been previously affected by mental health issues, social support should be offered by the midwife in the postnatal period. This includes asking the woman how she is feeling, coping and sleeping. It can be offered individually; equally, there are social support networks that a woman and her baby may access locally in a group format. These range from breastfeeding cafés to infant massage groups.

Activity 6.2   *Evidence-based practice and research*

Use the Internet and face-to-face contacts such as your mentor, health visitor and staff at the local children's centre to compile a list of available support groups in your local area.

Find out a little about each group, so you have the knowledge to offer women resources that they may choose to access.

A selection of possible answers is given at the end of this chapter.

Local support services may be advertised in the children's centre; see if their adverts match the details on your list, to ensure all professionals are aware of changes to groups and support sessions. There is nothing worse than recommending a group that no longer exists.

Although your role in the postnatal period is the psychological well-being of the woman, their family is part of their support network, so asking about their family might be prudent. Research reminds health professionals to explore emotions with men on their experiences of fatherhood (Chin et al., 2011). Remember that not all women have male partners and that single or lesbian women and their partners need midwifery care and support too.

Each time you ask a woman how she is, remember to listen to the way she answers, as that will give you clues, too. Often women are baby focused; they jump straight in and answer about how they are caring for their baby without considering how they are coping themselves, and not acknowledging their emotions. Your role is to listen to their responses, to allow the women to pace the postnatal communication, respond to their issues and then ask again about their well-being. Document all advice and care information given. One of the most negative points women report about postnatal care is the inconsistent advice they receive from healthcare professionals, so if we document information, there is continuity of advice even if the midwife changes, and women will feel less confused and frustrated.

Activity 6.3   *Critical thinking*

Think about the interactions you have had with women in the postnatal period, both with your mentor and perhaps when you have been alone with women in the birthing room or postnatal ward. Have you taken time to listen to these women's experiences and what care they would like? If so, was this different from your expectations or the services offered in your area? If not, try this activity next time you have the opportunity.

As this activity is based on your own experiences, there is no suggested answer at the end of this chapter.

Now that we have briefly touched on the psychological needs of women in the postnatal period, we will consider the physical needs and care you need to undertake.

There are three physiological processes happening in the postnatal period, also called the **puerperium**. These are **involution** of the uterus and genital tract, initiation and establishment of lactation and other changes to the body often under the presence of the changing endocrine system.

You will remember that hormones help sustain the pregnancy. If you need to be reminded, stop here and refer to one of the anatomy and physiology books in the further reading section in order to increase your knowledge of the endocrine effects in pregnancy so the rest of this chapter makes more sense. During the postnatal period, once the placenta has been delivered, there is a decrease in the placental hormones, most notably oestrogen and progesterone. The effects of the decrease in these hormones will be discussed as we assess each of the woman's body systems in our top-to-toe process.

The head can be assessed physically as well as psychologically. Headaches or visual disturbances may be a symptom of pre-eclampsia. Remember that although most women present with pre-eclampsia in the antenatal period, it can develop postnatally. This is a major postnatal complication, and women should be asked about the presence of headaches at each contact (NICE, 2006). If the woman reports a headache, her blood pressure must be checked – see the observations below. If this measurement is raised, she should be referred to the obstetrician for review. A woman who has had epidural analgesia may be predisposed to headaches, and extra vigilance is needed. Further assessment, usually by an anaesthetist, may be necessary.

Even if you have never met Victoria before, you can probably realise that she has a hectic life. You will probably be reassured to know that simple pain killers and some rest – if her mum is able to distract the children – would be recommended (see also the next paragraph). When her partner returns Victoria will probably also feel reassured because she will be able to share their news and their new baby.

Occasionally a woman will experience a headache with no pre-eclampsia or epidural analgesia; this, if all other observations are satisfactory, may be treated with mild pain killers such as paracetamol, which is not contraindicated even if breastfeeding. Remember that lack of sleep sometimes initiates a headache; relaxation techniques may also be advised.

Observations

The woman's upper body may be observed or touched to perform pulse, blood pressure, respiratory rate and temperature measurements. Some midwives have a belief that if all other conversations with the woman seem normal, it may not be necessary to undertake basic physical observations. Most women will tell you if they have been feeling hot or if their lochia has increased, which would indicate that observations are required. However, the latest CMACE report suggests a 'back to basics' message would save more lives (CMACE, 2011). By routinely undertaking basic observations in order to recognise and initiate treatment, fewer women may die.

The 'top ten' recommendations suggest that improving midwifery history taking, understanding normality – to know when the woman you are caring for is no longer 'normal' – and undertaking basic observations are good practice points. It is vital that common signs and symptoms in pregnancy and the postnatal period are recognised and that midwives realise that these signs may amount to a more serious diagnosis and need to be reported.

Activity 6.4   *Critical thinking*

Access the CMACE publication *Saving mothers' lives*, in particular, Chapter 13: Midwifery. It can be found here:

http://onlinelibrary.wiley.com/doi/10.1111/j.1471-0528.2010. 02847.x/abstract

Page 151 details poor midwifery care, including poor communication, inadequate documentation, failure to perform basic observations, failure to follow up the woman reporting feeling unwell and failure to visit or revisit during the postnatal period.

Reflect on what skills you need to improve to ensure you can learn from this substandard care.

As this is about your own skills, there is no suggested answer at the end of the chapter.

A minimum of one blood pressure measurement should be taken within six hours after birth (NICE, 2006). Thus, if the woman is discharged home at around six hours after birth, her blood pressure will be assessed prior to discharge and it need not be assessed again in the community the following day. However, should she exhibit any other sign or symptom of pre-eclampsia, such as a headache, it would be necessary to undertake this measurement. If the BP diastolic is 90 mmHg or greater, then a further reading is required four hours later. This may delay a woman's discharge from hospital. If it is the same or if the woman has any other signs and symptoms of pre-eclampsia, she needs to be seen urgently. In the antenatal period, you will remember that urine is tested for protein to help detect pre-eclampsia. In the postnatal period, due to the blood loss, the urine test will always show positive for protein, so it is not useful to test for proteinuria postnatally.

The back to basics campaign is particularly relevant to sepsis recognition, that is, realising a woman has an infection. A pyrexia of 38°C needs to be reported, and referral to the hospital for obstetric assessment is usual, as it is indicative of infection. Women can become seriously affected by an infection in a short period of time, so recognising and initiating treatment are of the utmost importance.

A rapid pulse rate is indicative of infection, too, as the woman's needs for oxygen circulation around the body increase. A sustained tachycardia of 100 beats per minute or more may indicate infection and needs referral as before. Once you have palpated the maternal pulse for one full minute, it is advisable to remain sitting still, holding the wrist and counting the respirations of the woman. Breathlessness or a respiratory rate of above 20 respirations per minute is also indicative of sepsis or pulmonary embolism and requires urgent attention (see Figure 6.1).

The other observations required by midwives include recognising if women are experiencing chest, epigastric or abdominal pain, diarrhoea/vomiting, uterine tenderness, renal tenderness or headache, or feeling unduly panicky or unwell; all could indicate a more serious problem.

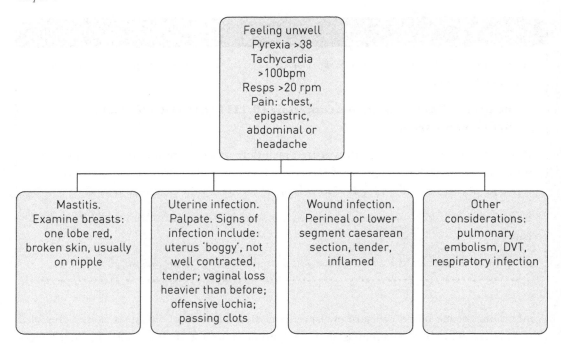

Figure 6.1: Visual representations of deviation from normal postnatal recuperation

Breasts

The breasts are next on the assessment, but although we are using the head-to-toe plan to structure this chapter, remember that if the woman is leading the postnatal consultation, she may want to talk about her breasts, their changes and feeding her baby first. Refer to the neonatal chapter for a full description of the initiation and continuance of breastfeeding. In the postnatal period, no special care of the breasts is recommended, whether the woman is breastfeeding or not. A daily bath or shower is sufficient to freshen her whole body. No creams or potions should be recommended, but a well-fitting bra is essential.

As the neonatal chapter explains, the milk will 'come in' between day two and day four, regardless of the woman's infant feeding intention. Should the woman choose not to breastfeed her baby, the symptoms of enlarged breasts, which can cause mild discomfort, will naturally decrease over the next 24–48 hours. The woman may take paracetamol to relieve her symptoms and is advised to leave the breasts alone; stimulation only increases the breast milk supply.

Women who are breastfeeding should offer the baby the breast often to relieve the same symptoms of enlarged (engorged) breasts and sometimes mild discomfort. Correct and careful positioning and attachment of the baby at the breast will reduce the likelihood of breastfeeding worries; sometimes massage of the breast is also helpful. If the woman is uncomfortable or initiates the conversation about her breast, observing the breasts and a breastfeed may be offered at each contact by the midwife. This can be both to reassure the woman and also to educate and empower her. The midwife will explain to the woman what she is looking for: intact nipples and smooth breasts indicate all is well. Red lobes or lumpy breasts could indicate a blocked milk duct, which may subside with frequent feeding or breast massage. Occasionally, a more serious infection such as mastitis or sore and cracked nipples are seen. Sore and cracked nipples usually indicate that the baby is not attached well at the breast, and extra support is offered to ensure the woman knows what correct attachment looks and feel like. The midwife should observe the feeding to reassure and support the woman.

Cabbage leaves, as well as hot and cold compresses, have been proven to be effective at relieving breast engorgement and pain during this time (Arora et al., 2008). Reminding all women that these symptoms are transitory may help them to cope with this change in their body.

Abdominal assessments

Uterus

The next landmark on the woman's body is the uterus. The uterus involutes, or decreases in size, over the first few days after birth, until it becomes a pelvic organ again (in about ten days), as opposed to an abdominal organ, and then returns to almost the same size, shape and position as it was pre-pregnancy (about six weeks after birth). Three processes take place to enable this organ to reduce in size: ischaemia, the absence of the blood supply; autolysis, the breakdown of the muscle fibres; and phagocytosis, the removal of excess elastic tissues. Refer to an anatomy and physiology textbook, as indicated in the further reading section, to enhance your knowledge of how this occurs. As for the midwifery care during this time, read on.

Whether to palpate the involuting fundus is a question that is still not resolved in midwifery circles. Some midwives feel very strongly that palpating the involuting uterus is a necessity; others feel the woman will notify the midwife of events that may indicate that involution is impaired, such as heavier or offensive lochia or pain. If these symptoms are reported, it is essential that the uterus is palpated. The differences in philosophies stem from the belief that women should reclaim their privacy during this time versus the medical model belief that birth is only a normal process after recovery has been uneventful. There is no absolute answer here – your relationship with the woman, the birth and her previous history will give you clues about her recovery and the involution of her uterus. Whether you palpate the uterus if there are no adverse symptoms is a matter of midwifery intuition as much as knowledge.

Scenario

Freya is a 22-year-old primiparous woman. She has had an uneventful pregnancy and birth with no analgesia and no sutures. She is breastfeeding her baby, William, who weighed 3.6 kg at 41 weeks. She is two days postnatal. She is happy with William's feeding and sleeping, and had two three-hour episodes of sleep last night, after which she was too excited to sleep any more. She reports that her lochia is red, but not heavy; she has taken paracetamol for general aches and pains but is comfortable now. She has passed urine several times and had her bowels open this morning. She feels well. She bathed William this morning as he had passed meconium and it was everywhere; he is now asleep on her partner's chest. What postnatal care do you feel Freya needs?

From the history Freya has given, it would seem everything is going well here. Freya seems confident and excited postnatally. There is little a midwife can add today. There is probably no need to examine Freya; her body systems seem to be working appropriately, because she has told you they are. What the midwife can offer is another visit or telephone contact tomorrow and reassurance that Freya seems well; the midwife could also ensure she knows who to call if she needs anything at any point. It might be worth reminding Freya to rest now – as the baby is asleep – or later in the day by going to bed with William to relax, even if she cannot sleep; that way, if he feeds more frequently tonight, as he may, Freya will be prepared.

The NICE (2006) guidelines remind a midwife that in the absence of abnormal vaginal loss, palpation and assessment of involution of the uterus is unnecessary. The notion of routine assessment of each woman is outdated; each woman should be assessed individually and care tailored to her needs. If the uterus is palpated because the woman either has symptoms or is worried, it should be involuting at approximately 1 centimetre per day. It is good midwifery practice to ask the woman to empty her bladder before the abdominal examination so she is more comfortable and you can more accurately assess the involution – otherwise a deviation from the midline may indicate a full bladder. Sub-involution, which is the slower-than-expected involution of the uterus, is usually associated with increased lochia – see below – although it can be due to an over-distended uterus from a twin pregnancy, polyhydramnios (increased amniotic fluid) or a large baby. Remember also that each woman's uterus will involute differently.

Abdominal pain

If the woman complains of pain when you palpate the uterus, you should consider whether there is a uterine infection. As previously said, there are many signs and symptoms of infection, and usually there are more than one present that indicate treatment is required. Pyrexia or tachycardia, heavier or offensive lochia, abdominal pain and sub-involution all indicate that the woman needs to be seen by a doctor. There are, however, differential diagnoses of abdominal pain, and the midwife has to use her clinical knowledge and judgement to decide the most likely cause of the pain.

Pain that is constant or present on abdominal palpation is unlikely to be innocuous, or not relevant. Many women experience 'afterpains' – usually women who have had a baby before. Management of afterpains should be with simple analgesics, such as paracetamol. If the woman is breastfeeding and experiencing afterpains, as soon as the baby stirs it is helpful for them to take paracetamol and go to the bathroom so they are comfortable; this will help them feed without interruption by the pain or a full bladder. In breastfeeding women, the initiation of suckling stimulates the oxytocin release that causes afterpains; generally, these diminish over the first four to seven days postnatally.

Other causes of abdominal-related pain are pelvic pain associated with a full bladder, constipation, flatus, intrauterine infection or, rarely, a pelvic vein thrombosis. Symphysis pubis pain may also exhibit.

Caesarean wound care

If the woman has had a caesarean section – at present in the UK approximately 20–25 per cent of women give birth this way – her wound should be looked at by the midwife or trained maternity support worker after 24 hours when the dressing is removed. Specifically assessing the wound for signs of infection – increased pain, redness, discharge or dehiscence (separation of the scar) – is imperative (NICE, 2011). If the woman experiences feeling hot or develops a fever, she should be referred back to the obstetrician. For their general comfort and to aid healing, women should be advised to wear loose, natural-fibred clothes.

The midwife should also be hypervigilant to many of the aspects of care in this chapter as women recovering from LSCS (lower segment caesarean section) have higher incidences of pain, urinary infections and incontinence, and venous thromboembolitic episodes, but usually have prophylactic treatment for this. They do not have higher incidences of breastfeeding issues, depression, post-traumatic stress disorder, **dysparenuia** (painful sex) or faecal incontinence, though (NICE, 2011).

Bladder care

The woman should pass urine within six hours of birth, and this should be documented by the midwife in the postnatal notes (NICE, 2006). If she does not spontaneously pass urine, the midwife must consider why this is. If the midwife has palpated the abdomen to assess the involution of the uterus, as above, she may have felt a full bladder, or alternatively have known that the bladder is not in retention, that is, retaining urine that it needs to shed.

The reason midwives need to be vigilant about bladder care is related to the anatomy and physiology of the puerperium. During the pregnancy, you may remember that there were changes in the circulating blood volume to meet the increased requirements of the woman and developing fetus. Within the first 48 hours following birth, due to the reduction in hormones, especially oestrogen, the woman's body naturally removes the excess circulating blood volume by a process of **diuresis** (increased urine production). This happens in conjunction with a decrease in progesterone, which leads any excess fluid that has been sitting in the tissues as oedema to return to the circulatory system to be excreted, too – oedema of the legs and feet may occur even if it has not been experienced in pregnancy.

During labour the bladder has been displaced into the abdomen and the urethra stretched. With this potential for bruising and the increases in urinary output, you can see the need for the midwife to be vigilant about bladder care. Early mobilisation of the woman and frequent micturition (passing of urine) prevent overdistention of the bladder and retention of urine. However, if the woman does not pass urine, a warm bath or shower may relax her to enable micturition; alternatively, bladder volume should be assessed and a catheter may be considered. This must be reported to the obstetrician, too.

Bowel care

During pregnancy the smooth muscles of the gastrointestinal tract are relaxed by the action of progesterone. Following birth this resolves, so minor disturbances experienced during pregnancy such as constipation should be resolved. Other reasons for constipation may occur with birth, and the midwife should be vigilant to these. Asking the woman explicit questions about her bowel function, including the presence of haemorrhoids, faecal incontinence and constipation, should detect if there are problems. Solutions to constipation include educating the woman about mobilisation and increasing fibre and fluid in her postpartum diet. Remember too that perineal trauma may inhibit a woman's defecation due to fear or pain. If the midwife does not directly ask about bowel function, the woman may be reluctant to mention it, or be too busy caring for her baby to notice that she may not have had her bowels open.

Perineal care

Women who have birthed their babies vaginally may have sustained perineal trauma. Perineal trauma includes labial lacerations, a tear or an episiotomy, and whether there is an observed trauma or not, women may experience perineal pain. At each contact the midwife should specifically ask the woman if she has any pain, discomfort or concerns about her perineal healing, including stinging with micturition or dysparenuia. These direct questions allow the woman without symptoms to retain her dignity and privacy as the midwife can be confident the perineum is healing well without inspection. However, if symptoms are reported, the perineum should be inspected for signs of infection, tight sutures or wound breakdown. Vaginal blood loss may be observed while observing the perineum, as may haemorrhoids or vaginal varicose veins or varicosities.

All women should be advised of adequate hygiene – hand washing before and following micturition or defecation, frequent changing of sanitary protection – and advised to be aware of signs of infection. Analgesia such as paracetamol can be suggested for pain.

Lochia

The involution of the uterus is associated with vaginal blood loss, and this loss is called lochia. The constituents of the lochia alter over the postnatal days, and this is reflected in the colour and consistency of lochia. Initially, fresh blood is lost, with decidual cells, so the lochia is bright red and called 'lochia rubra'. Over the next two or three days the lochia becomes less red, and less volume is lost; it is called 'lochia serosa', or pink loss, at this stage and is stale blood, exudate from the placental site, cervical mucous and shreds of degenerating decidua. After about ten days the loss turns clear; it is then called 'lochia alba' and consists mostly of white blood cells, mucous and other cells. The loss may last up to three weeks postnatally, but the timing will be different for each woman.

To evaluate whether this woman's loss is within normal limits, the midwife should ask questions regarding the colour and amount of lochia, whether it has increased or decreased from the previous day, and whether the woman has any concerns or noticed any offensive smell.

Legs

One of the most common causes of maternal death in the UK is thrombosis, although midwives are getting better at assessing maternal risk factors and referring women to the obstetrician for prophylactic treatment. Thromboembolitic diseases are most likely to occur in the postnatal period, especially in the first 24 hours as the diuresis alters the thickness (viscosity) of the maternal blood, so it is more likely to clot. One of the most likely places a clot will develop is in the calves of a postnatal woman; hence all women are asked if they have any pain or swelling in their legs. If the clot dislodges from the legs, it can travel to the lungs and this is a life-threatening condition, pulmonary embolism, as the clot stops the lungs from exchanging gas (oxygen).

Recognition of a deep vein thrombosis, DVT, and referral for treatment is potentially life saving. Women who are most prone to this disease are women who have had a caesarean section, are aged over 30, have had more than five babies, weigh more than 80 kg, have a personal or family history of DVT, smoke, have reduced mobility or are dehydrated or have pre-eclampsia. Many women will have prophylactic treatment in the hospital if they have two or more risk factors; some will come home on preventative treatment, which is an injection of low molecular weight heparin.

Vigilance is required by all midwives as all women can exhibit symptoms; in a CMACE report (2011), women who had fewer risk factors had more pulmonary embolisms than those with more risk factors because those at higher risk had had the preventative medicine.

Other assessments

In addition to the physical and psychological assessment of the postnatal woman, the midwife is reminded by the NICE (2006) guidance to enquire about the family's emotional attachments. This includes communicating about bonding, nurturing and caring for their infant, as well as voicing their own emotions. See the next chapter on neonatal care for more on this.

Activity 6.5	*Evidence-based practice and research*

To consolidate your learning on this chapter, look at the NCT website and their postnatal care research:

www.nct.org.uk/professional/research/pregnancy-birth-and-postnatal-care/postnatal-care

continued . . . •••

Can you reflect upon any cases you have had that resonate with the experiences of the women in this research? Think about how you can ensure women in your care are better supported.

As this is based on your own experiences, there are no suggested answers at the end of this chapter.

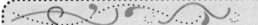

Chapter summary

This chapter has discussed the care of the woman and her family in the postnatal period. A relationship between the woman and midwife may have developed during the antenatal period, and this can be built upon in the postnatal period as the woman and her partner – if she has one – make the transition to becoming parents or extending their family. The midwife's role has been considered, as have the systems of the body that need to be evaluated to check maternal and neonatal well-being during this time. A specific pattern of postnatal care has not been suggested, as care should be individualised to each woman's needs during this time. The chapter has informed you about what you should be looking for and why during this time, although there will be differences in the provision of postnatal care across the UK.

Activities: brief outline answers

Activity 6.1: Reflection (page 119)

The five senses, you may recall, are: sight; hearing; smell; taste; and touch.

Sight is used to look at the woman and her baby, how they are interacting, what they look like and whether they seem calm. Hearing is used to listen to women and their babies, their voices as well as what they are saying or sometimes not saying. Touch is used to physically examine by palpating the involuting uterus or holding the newborn, to see whether everything feels normal. Your sense of smell may be used to indicate abnormalities such as infections in either the mother or infant. We do not use taste in contemporary midwifery; however, it has been documented that cystic fibrosis may be detected if a newborn tastes salty; nowadays the neonatal blood screening is seen as a more reliable method to detect this condition.

Activity 6.2: Evidence-based practice and research (page 120)

If a woman has a problem in the first few days or weeks of her baby's life, community midwives may offer drop-in clinics, although women should be aware that home visits are also available, should they need them.

There may be parent and toddler groups run by a local church or community centre. The National Childbirth Trust may have meetings. There may be baby breastfeeding cafés at which women can support one another with breastfeeding joys and worries.

Baby massage, signing and gymnastics offer the opportunity for parents and infants to learn a new skill together and encourage bonding; it can also be fun. There are always on-line resources for parents to find support from one another, too.

Further reading

Fraser, D and Cooper, M (2009) *Myles' textbook for midwives*, 15th edition. London: Churchill Livingstone.

Stables, D and Rankin, J (2005) *Physiology in childbearing with anatomy and related biosciences*. London: Elsevier.

These two textbooks offer further reading on the postnatal physiology and care given.

NICE (2006) *Postnatal care*. London: RCOG Press.

This is an essential document that will support your care decisions. During the course of your training it is a good idea to read it so you can provide contemporary postnatal care.

Useful website

www.nct.org.uk/professional/research/pregnancy-birth-and-postnatal-care/postnatal-care

This is the National Childbirth Trust's advice page on postnatal care.

Chapter 7
Neonatal care

Moira McLean

> **Chapter aims**
>
> After reading this chapter you will be able to:
>
> * understand normal neonatal physiology;
> * understand how a newborn baby adapts to extra-uterine life;
> * explain the knowledge and skills that midwives need for assessing the mother and baby's well-being;
> * understand the processes of initiating breastfeeding and how the midwife can promote this.

Introduction

Much of the midwife's role in the neonatal period is directed towards enabling and empowering parents to provide optimum care for their newborn baby. This chapter therefore looks at the needs of the newborn baby from initial assessment at birth. It covers the principles of adaptation to extra-uterine life, initial physical examination, facilitation of interaction between mother and baby, establishment of breastfeeding and ongoing neonatal care, including the basic principles of newborn screening.

Initial assessment

Following birth, the neonate must make complex physiological changes to enable it to survive outside the uterus. Changes to the baby's circulatory and pulmonary systems occur within the first few moments of extra-uterine life, and adaptation continues throughout the postnatal period as described in Table 7.1 and Figure 7.1.

A short time after birth, as oxygen levels increase, the ductus arteriosus starts to close; however, blood can continue to be shunted through the duct for several hours after birth, as closure is not usually completed until around 96 hours. Once the baby is born and starts to breathe, the first few breaths gradually inflate the lungs, and over the next few hours the lungs become aerated. However, inspired pressures are needed to overcome the fluid-filled airways. Before birth, when the lungs are filled with fluid, tension in the lungs is aided by the resistance of the chest wall. Lung fluid contains an important substance known as surfactant that reduces the surface tension in the lungs and stops airways collapsing on expiration. At birth, the lungs cease to breathe fluid and start to breathe gases. As the alveoli inflate, the amount of surfactant diminishes and the surface tension rises. This means that the amount of pressure required to keep the alveoli open reduces. The first breath requires pressures approximately 10 to 15 times higher than for subsequent breaths; following this first breath, the work of breathing becomes easier. The first breath helps to force the remaining fluid from the alveoli and it is absorbed by the lymphatic system. Increased pulmonary blood flow also helps alveolar expansion, and the current recommendation to delay the clamping and cutting of the cord (Richmond and Wyllie, 2010) facilitates this and ensures

In fetal life:	The lungs are collapsed and fluid filled.
	Blood flow to the lungs is minimal – only around 8% of the total cardiac output, just enough to maintains lung growth and development. Oxygenated blood from the placenta passes through the fetal heart and into the systemic circulation without entering the lungs. Four temporary anatomical structures (the umbilical vein, the ductus venosus, the foramen ovale and the ductus arteriosus) facilitate this.
	• The umbilical vein brings oxygenated blood to the fetus from the placenta. • The ductus venosus allows blood from the umbilical vein to enter the inferior vena cava. • The foramen ovale acts as a pathway for fetal blood to flow directly from the right to the left side of the heart. • The ductus arteriosus allows oxygenated blood to pass from the main pulmonary artery to the aorta.
	The increase in blood flow through the pulmonary artery to the oxygenated lungs has the effect of lowering the pressure on the right side of the heart and raising pressure on the left side of the heart, which causes the foramen ovale to close and separate the two atria. This process of closing up may take up to nine months to complete (Blackburn, 2007).
Once the baby has been born	The ductus arteriosus starts to close – a process which takes around 96 hours. During this time some blood can still be shunted through the duct.

Table 7.1: Background information: neonatal physiology

adequate blood volume that pulls the alveoli open and enhances lung compliance and gaseous exchange. Respiration is also stimulated by other sensory stimulation such as cold, light, noise and pain, as well as a rise in carbon dioxide levels. To help your understanding of this, see the further reading and useful websites lists on pages 156–7.

Respiration is irregular during the first 15 minutes of life with rates between 60 and 80 breaths per minute; however, in the first half-hour these settle to between 30 and 60 breaths per minute.

Following birth the newborn must adapt to changes in temperature and the effects of potential heat loss by conduction, convection, radiation and evaporation. The neonate has a high surface to body weight ratio, which encourages heat loss. A baby who is unable to maintain its body temperature will become exhausted by the physical effort of keeping warm, and in time this will lead to metabolic distress (WHO, 1997). Prompt and effective drying can go some way to overcome this, as can covering the infant's head.

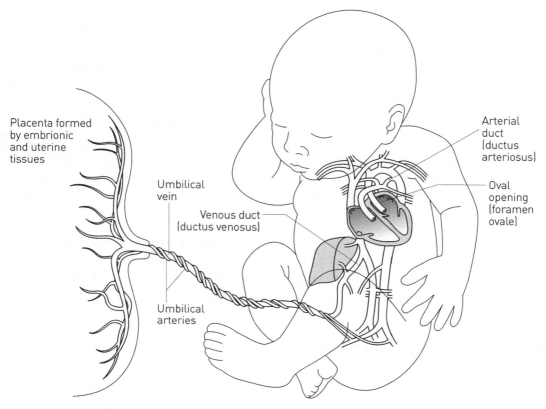

Figure 7.1: The fetal circulation

Activity 7.1   *Evidence-based practice and research*

Look up the description of neonatal physiology in:

> **http://journals.lww.com/advancesinneonatalcare/Fulltext/2010/
> 10001/Thermoregulation_and_Heat_Loss_Prevention_After.3.aspx**

> **www.neonatal-nursing.co.uk/pdf/inf_015_nor.pdf**

> **www.who.int/reproductivehealth/publications/maternal_perinatal_
> health/MSM_97_2/en/index.html**

Read in particular the section on the importance of maintaining body temperature in the first of the references above.

List the steps you as a midwife can take to ensure the optimal environment for a smooth transition to extra-uterine life.

An outline answer to this activity is given at the end of the chapter.

Blood glucose levels in the neonate are approximately 70 to 80 per cent of maternal levels. Glucose is needed for most metabolic pathways of the body, so if additional glucose is required (e.g. for keeping warm), the neonate will rapidly use its glucose stores. During the last trimester of pregnancy, the fetus stores glycogen in the liver, but this can be used up within one to three hours of birth, mainly in maintaining heat but also because the neonatal brain requires significant glucose levels. Physiologically the initial drop in blood glucose within the first hour is then accompanied by a rise in blood sugar over the subsequent three hours of age. This happens even if the infant has not been fed (Ward-Platt and Deshpande, 2005) and is accompanied by a fall in insulin, which helps preserve glucose levels. Glucose levels of between 1.2 and 2.0 mmol per litre or less in full-term infants and levels of 2.2–2.8 mmol/l in infants 24 hours old (2.2–2.8 mmol/l) have been put forward as the lowest levels acceptable before clinical intervention (Cornblath et al., 2000).

This interrelationship between the development of **hypoglycaemia** and **hypoxia** has been termed the energy triangle (Aylott, 2006). Prevention of excessive cooling after birth, maintenance of an appropriate temperature and initiation of feeding in these first few hours will reduce the infant's energy expenditure and help to ensure a smooth transition to extra-uterine life.

First steps in neonatal care

Most full-term neonates take between 30 and 90 seconds to make the first physiological adaptations. During this time parents may be anxious about the baby's well-being and why it may not be crying. The midwife's role is to be supportive, allowing transitions to take place in an unhurried environment, simultaneously observing and ensuring the baby's safety (Carter, 2003).

Case study

Julie has just given birth to her first baby, Joshua, after a straightforward labour. Pam, her midwife, explains that Julie needs to keep her baby warm and shows her how she can do this by holding baby Joshua against her body to maintain skin-to-skin contact. Julie needs to ensure that the other side of Joshua's body is covered by a towel or blanket to prevent his temperature dropping. Pam explains to Julie that keeping Joshua warm and snug will prevent him having to use up his energy (already depleted by the stress of being born) in keeping warm. It will also help them to bond. She then encourages Julie to semi-recline, with Joshua between her breasts to allow him to find her nipple. She also talks to her gently about how she might recognise when Joshua is hungry. Pam is concerned that these early moments between Julie and Joshua should be positive and helpful ones, laying the groundwork for a happy mother–baby relationship, ensuring a healthy infant and making the establishment of breastfeeding easier.

Apgar score

The Apgar scoring system is a systematic assessment using key characteristics, each giving an indication of the health of the baby (see Table 7.2). Each characteristic is scored 0 to 2, and the overall condition of the baby can be determined by calculating the score out of 10. Scoring is assessed at one minute and five minutes. A healthy baby may be born blue but will have good tone, will cry within a few seconds of delivery and will have a good heart rate within a few minutes of birth (the heart rate of a healthy newborn baby is about 120–150 per minute). A less healthy baby will be blue at birth, will have less good tone, may have a slow heart rate (less than 100 per min), and may not establish adequate breathing by 90–120 seconds. An ill baby will be born pale and floppy, not breathing and with a slow, very slow or undetectable heart rate. The heart rate of a baby is judged best by listening with a stethoscope. It can also be felt by gently palpating the umbilical cord, but a slow rate at the cord is not always indicative of a truly slow heart rate.

While the Apgar score continues to be used, it needs to be recognised that it can be subjective: factors such as the lighting in the room, skin pigmentation and the immaturity of the baby, as well as different assessments by individual practitioners, can influence the score. However, it remains a useful tool, and if the baby you have just delivered has an Apgar score of less than 5, you will need to summon help and start resuscitation whether you are attending a birth in hospital or in the community.

	Sign	Score
Appearance (colour)	Blue, pale	0
	Body pink, limited blue	1
	All pink	2
Pulse (heart rate)	Absent	0
	Less than 100	1
	Greater than 100	2
Grimace (response to stimuli)	None	0
	Grimace	1
	Cry	2
Activity (muscle tone)	Limp	0
	Some flexion of limbs	1
	Active movements, well flexed	2
Respiratory effort	None	0
	Slow, irregular	1
	Good strong cry	2

Table 7.2: Apgar scoring

Activity 7.2   *Critical thinking*

1. Is Apgar scoring used in your unit? How useful do you find it? Is there another system you might find more helpful.
2. Look again at Table 7.2. What Apgar score would you give the following babies?
   a. Baby Jakob has a pink body and blue hands and feet; he is crying and curled up against his mother. He responds briskly as you dry him.
   b. Baby Marcus is blue all over, with slow irregular breathing. His heart rate is 140 bpm, he has some flexion of his limbs and he is making a good response to tactile stimulation.

An answer to the second question of this activity is given at the end of the chapter.

Principles of resuscitation

Most babies born at term need no resuscitation and they can usually stabilise themselves during the transition from placental to pulmonary respiration very effectively. It is important, though, that the midwife pays attention to preventing heat loss and is patient about cutting the umbilical cord (Richmond and Wyllie, 2010). In the unlikely event that resuscitation is required, the Resuscitation Council Guidelines should be followed (see **www.resus.org.uk/pages/ nls.pdf**).

Umbilical cord clamping (see also Chapter 5)

Recommended practice (NICE, 2007b; Resuscitation Council, 2010) is now to delay clamping the cord after the birth of a healthy, full-term infant for at least one minute or until the cord stops pulsating, in order to improve the baby's iron status.

Breastfeeding

Many babies make a smooth transition to extra-uterine life, and the midwife can observe the baby's colour, breathing and tone, and make sure that the baby is kept warm, drying and covering the head, while the baby rests skin-to-skin with its mother. This also enables parent–infant interaction to be established (see Figure 7.2).

Skin-to-skin contact helps mothers initiate breastfeeding soon after birth as oxytocin levels are high in the first hour following birth (Nissen et al., 1996; Odent 2002). As well as encouraging the let-down reflex, the high oxytocin levels facilitate instinctive breastfeeding behaviour in both the mother and the infant (Bergman, 2008). Studies have found that infants who have had skin-to-skin contact

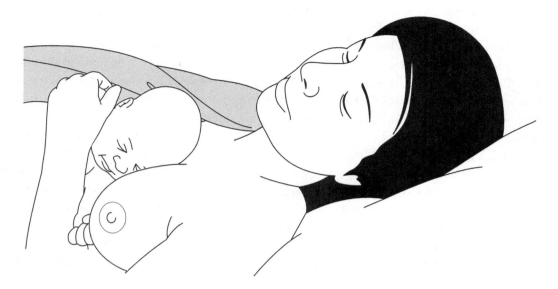

Figure 7.2: Skin-to-skin contact between mother and baby

interact more with their mothers, maintain temperature better and cry less; they are also likely to breastfeed for a longer duration (Moore et al., 2009). This suggests strongly that contact should not be interrupted to provide routine care such as weighing the infant, although Sheriden (2010) found that in hospitals mother–baby contact after birth is usually interrupted for completion of tasks.

Concept summary: biological nurturing model

Biological nurturing (BN) can be described as a 'bridging process' that minimises maternal/neonatal separation. Biological nurturing is a collective term for the natural mother–baby state and for the interactions between mother and baby that release instinctive responses to getting started with feeding. Mothers tap into what they innately know and breastfeed easily without a lot of rules about how to do it or prescriptive advice.

Biological nurturing is quick and easy. If left to their own devices, most mothers and babies automatically move into comfortable positions that work. The health care provider's role is to understand the releasing mechanisms and learn how to promote an environment that helps mothers and babies do what comes naturally.

Ideally, this period of skin-to-skin contact should last as long as the mother wishes (UNICEF, 2008). It is a good opportunity for the midwife to talk to the parents about infant feeding cues and behaviour. Feeding cues (which are reflex movements) may include sucking movements, sucking noises, lip licking, head movement from side to side, rapid eye movement and restlessness. Crying is considered to be a late sign of hunger. A baby lying against its mother's body is a baby in the right place at the right time (Colson, 2010). Continuity with the mother – familiar voice, heartbeat, odour and body spaces – optimises conditions for postnatal adaptation.

Colson (2010) goes on to cite hormonal and physiological evidence and argue that metabolic adaptation to extra-uterine life by biological nurturing reduces the risk of neonatal hypoglycaemia. Early breastfeeding patterns frequently differ in type, frequency and duration from those established later, often changing on a daily basis. For example, there is no uniformity in the first 24 hours. Colson (2010) makes a comparison between babies left in cots, who may not feed at all for eight hours or longer, and those left in contact with their mothers, who latch on and suck often, although the length of each episode may be very short. The first-day patterns are often followed, during the second postnatal day, by periods of constant sucking, suggesting that arbitrary time schedules are inappropriate (Pollard, 2012). This often coincides with the time when many mothers fear they have not got enough milk. Colson claims this fear is unsubstantiated as physiological research findings suggest that the mechanisms for mothers' breast milk production are fully developed from about four months of pregnancy, with many mothers releasing small quantities of milk/**colostrum** during pregnancy. Colson (2007) argues that the advice often given that milk 'comes in' on the third postnatal day is incorrect and suggests health professionals should instead talk about milk volume increasing to meet individual baby demands as initially babies only require small frequent colostrum feeds.

Activity 7.3 — *Evidence-based practice and research*

Take some time to read at least one of the following texts to develop your understanding of the physiology of lactation.

Inch, S (2009) Infant feeding, in Fraser, D and Cooper, M (eds) *Myles' textbook for midwives*, 15th edition. Edinburgh: Churchill Livingstone.

Pollard, M (2012) Evidence-based care for breastfeeding mothers: a resource for midwives and allied health care professionals. Abingdon: Routledge. Chapter 2: Anatomy and physiology of lactation.

Riordan, J and Wambach, K (2010) *Breast feeding and human lactation*, 4th edition. Boston MA: Jones Bartlett Publishers. Chapter 3: Anatomy and physiology of lactation.

As this activity is based on your own reading and experience, there is no outline answer at the end of the chapter.

It has been recognised that suckling is an important factor associated with milk production, promoting high concentrations of **prolactin**, which promotes the supply of milk (Noel et al., 1974; Pollard, 2012). In contrast, the release of oxytocin – which is responsible for the letdown (milk ejection) reflex – can be stimulated just by thinking about the baby, and it takes only two and a half minutes to initiate peak oxytocin levels. Prolactin is stimulated only through suckling, face- and hand-to-breast contact and active milk extraction. Prolactin peaks at 55 to 40 minutes from the start of a feed. This research indicates that initially holding the baby for long periods and breast emptying regulate the milk supply. This needs to be explained to mothers so they understand the process. Some mothers think that if their baby cries when put down, this is a sign that they do not have enough milk. In fact, however, the baby may be crying simply because it doesn't like being away from its mother. Colson (2010) suggests that during the first three postnatal days (the period of metabolic adaptation) it is not normal to put the baby down for long periods of time. She argues that parents should be told this, and reassured that a baby crying does not necessarily indicate an insufficient milk supply (see also NICE, 2008b).

There is more than one way to breastfeed. Similarly, there is no right or wrong breastfeeding position – a right position is one that works. For example, the baby does not need to be awake to latch on to the breast and feed. Often babies can self-attach to the breast, and mothers can help them to do this. Infants have reflex movements called cues (described above), indicating they are ready to feed while asleep. Knowing how to recognise these cues will increase a mother's confidence. Crying as a late hunger cue tends to make latching on difficult.

Infants do not always feed for hunger, and this 'non-nutritive sucking' is beneficial in increasing milk supply and satisfying the baby's needs. Biological nurturing can be of benefit to breastfeeding, too, particularly in the early postpartum period (Colson, 2005, 2010).

Breastfeeding positions

UNICEF (2008) recognises that the understanding of effective positioning attachment and suckling is key if health professionals are to support and empower mothers. See Figure 7.3 for some suggested breastfeeding positions.

Recommended principles include the mother adopting a position that she can sustain comfortably, allowing the baby to feed for longer to benefit from full fat milk at the end of the feed. This reduces the build-up of the feedback inhibitor of lactation (FIL), a whey protein secreted by the lactocytes, which regulates milk production (Wilde et al., 1995; Riordan and Wambach, 2010). As the alveoli distend there is a build-up of the FIL, and milk synthesis is inhibited. When breast milk is effectively removed, FIL concentrations reduce and milk synthesis resumes. This is a local mechanism that can occur in one or both breasts, exerting a negative feedback response to inhibit milk production when there is ineffective removal of breast milk (Czank et al., 2007).

It is also suggested that the head and neck should be in a straight line, enabling the infant to open its mouth wide with the tongue on the base of the mouth. This approach supports Colson's (2007) biological nurturing positions. It also avoids twisting the head and neck, and protects the airway to provide a successful suck–swallow–breathe reflex.

The baby should be placed so that it can move its head freely. Avoiding holding the back of the infant's head is critical for success in breastfeeding; the neck and shoulders should be supported so the baby can move freely and find the correct position, keeping its nose free and opening its mouth with a wide gape. Holding the back of the baby's head tends to result in the baby flexing the neck, causing an obstruction of the airway and potentially blocking the nose (Inch, 2009). If the mother tries to avoid blocking the baby's nose by pressing the breast with her fingers, she is likely to prevent milk flow and interfere with attachment. If the baby is given the freedom to extend the neck, however, it will be encouraged to approach the breast chin first, scooping the breast into its mouth and keeping its nostrils free. Pushing the head against the breast may result in breast refusal (Pollard, 2012).

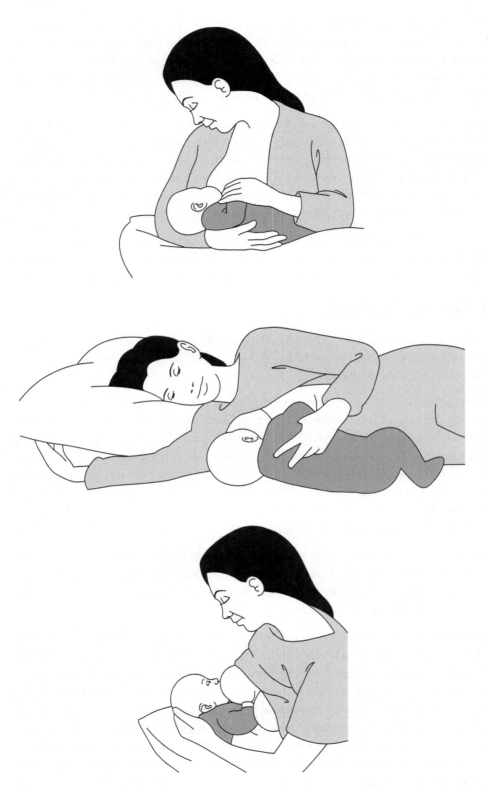

Figure 7.3: Breastfeeding positions

Bringing the infant to the breast rather than the breast to the infant is also suggested in order to avoid distorting the shape of the breast (Inch, 2009). Pointing the baby's nose to the mother's nipple to encourage the infant to tilt its head backwards may also be helpful, so encouraging the position of the tongue to remain at the base of the mouth and enabling the nipple to be at the junction of the hard and soft palate.

Activity 7.4   *Critical thinking*

Visit the following website and watch the video clip:

www.bestbeginnings.org.uk/3-birth-skin-to-skin-and-the-first-feed/e89a9720-b64a-46ec-bc5f-872045d4f864

Then think about the following.

- Was it helpful to see the positions used for skin-to-skin contact and for later feeding?
- How does the midwife teach Angela how to look for feeding cues?
- has the video given you any ideas for helping women and babies to overcome a less than perfect start?
- Do you think that encouragement from a professional (midwife, breastfeeding counsellor) helps establish the rapport between mother and baby? Do you think it helps the mother's confidence?

As this activity will be based on your own responses to the video clip, there is no outline answer at the end of the chapter.

Creating an atmosphere supportive of breastfeeding can be helpful. Encourage the mother and her partner to experiment with different ways of arranging cushions or pillows. It can be helpful to have a glass of water to hand as well. Pollard (2012) describes common positions that may be used for breastfeeding but identifies that as long as the principles discussed above are adhered to, the infant can feed in any position. The most common position is the cradle position in which the mother sits upright and the infant's neck and shoulders are supported by her forearm or bend in the elbow.

The cross-cradle position is similar except that the baby is supported by the forearm and the neck and shoulders by the mother's hand. The infant's head needs to be free to move to attain optimal attachment on the breast (Inch, 2009).

The underarm hold is suggested as particularly helpful if the mother has had a caesarean section as it avoids pressure on the wound. Again, the mother sits upright, but she holds the infant to the side, tucking the infant's trunk under her arm with its feet towards her back (Pollard, 2012).

Lying down or side lying is useful if the mother is tired or has a sore perineum. In this position, the infant faces the breast, its body in alignment and its nose to the nipple (Inch, 2009)

UNICEF (2008) states that the mother must be taught the signs of correct attachment to ensure successful breastfeeding. Go to the following website and find out what they are:

www.unicef.org.uk/BabyFriendly/Parents/Resources/Resources-for-parents/?Page=2

Write down a list of them before going to the answer at the end of the chapter.

Poor attachment at the breast can lead to sore, cracked nipples, ineffective removal and stasis of breast milk, breast engorgement, blocked ducts, mastitis and possible abscesses (UNICEF, 2008). Poor milk supply will lead some infants to feed for long periods of time, becoming unsatisfied, frustrated, reluctant to go to the breast and difficult to settle (UNICEF, 2008). Some infants will not stay at the breast long enough to receive the fatty milk that is present as the breast empties, and this will often result in the infant becoming colicky with explosive, watery, frothy stools. Ultimately, this will lead to weight loss and failure to thrive, leading the mother to give up breastfeeding. By supporting and preventing this cycle from occurring, the midwife can do much to maintain breastfeeding.

Feeding pattern

Time limits for length of feeding are difficult to estimate, as this is individual to each infant. However, understanding the basis of the physiology of how infants feed can go some way to supporting mothers in the establishment of feeding.

At the beginning of the feed, before milk ejection, the infant normally sucks rapidly with long and infrequent pauses to swallow; as the feed progresses, the bursts become slower and shorter, and the pauses longer until at the end of the feed the sucks become like flutters and the infant releases the breast. Ideally, the mother should leave the infant to release the breast automatically as the fat content of the breast milk is highest at that point. At the end of the feed, the infant will become more relaxed and let go of the breast. In the first few weeks it is normal for feeding to be as frequent as 12 times a day. Many factors affect infant feeding behaviour, including gestation, separation from the mother and any medications the mother is taking.

Sucking at the breast plays an important role in breast emptying. Geddes (2007) demonstrated that vacuum negative-pressure in the infant's mouth is essential. During sucking, the nipple/areola is drawn into the mouth by negative pressure to the anterior point of the junction of the hard and soft palate. A teat is formed and the vacuum holds it in place. The vacuum occurs as the tongue and jaw move down, drawing milk from the breast; as the tongue rises, the vacuum decreases and the milk flow reduces.

Case study

Yana is breastfeeding her first baby, Georgia. Following the birth Georgia was placed skin-to-skin and spontaneously fed on and off for about two hours. On transfer to the postnatal ward, Yana's midwife (Rachel) ensured that Georgia remained skin-to-skin against Yana's chest, thereby keeping mother and baby together. The midwife noticed Georgia spontaneously rooting and sucking throughout the next four hours while she lay 'tummy to mummy' against Yana's chest as they both rested. Rachel did not have to instruct Yana on how to breastfeed as she could see that this prolonged contact enabled Yana to develop confidence in her own and her daughter's instinctive abilities.

Expressing breast milk

UNICEF (2008) recognises the value of hand expression of milk. Women who know how to hand express can overcome many of the early challenges to breastfeeding (see Table 7.3).

Baby	Mother
Sleepy and unable to stimulate the milk supply	Needs to be reassured she is actually producing breast milk
In neonatal unit	Has full breasts, making it difficult to attach the baby effectively*
Reluctant to breastfeed and needs to be tempted	Has a blocked duct

Table 7.3: Breastfeeding challenges faced by mothers

* See: **www.unicef.org.uk/BabyFriendly/Health-Professionals/Going-Baby-Friendly/ FAQs/Breastfeeding-FAQ/Engorgement**

An understanding of how to remove milk from the breast may help mothers' understanding of attachment (UNICEF, 2008).

Activity 7.6   *Critical thinking*

Go to the website below and watch the video you find there:

www.bestbeginnings.org.uk/expressing-and-returning-to-work/ a4b9f50a-8c5d-4d04-b20f-608b17117667

continued . . .

Now consider the following questions.

- What approach could you take in teaching women to hand express?
- What differences would you note for expression on day 1 or 2 and later expression?

An outline answer to this activity is given at the end of the chapter.

Artificial feeding

UNICEF (2010) states that mothers who choose to artificial feed should be shown how to prepare a bottle of infant formula correctly. This is for reasons of hygiene (ensuring there is no cross-contamination) as well as for nutritional reasons.

Activity 7.7   *Evidence-based practice and research*

Visit the UNICEF website and read 'A guide to infant formula for parents who are bottle feeding' available at:

**www.unicef.org.uk/BabyFriendly/Resources/Resources-for-parents/
A-guide-to-infant-formula-for-parents-who-are-bottle-feeding/**

Go to the following website too:

www.nhs.uk/Planners/birthtofive/Pages/bottle-feeding.aspx

Read the bottle feeding advice there. Make notes on the key points you would include in a discussion with parents about safe formula feeding.

An outline answer to this activity is given at the end of the chapter.

Examination of the newborn

Immediately following the birth of the baby, one of the roles of the midwife is to undertake a complete top-to-toe initial examination of the newborn. The aim of this examination is to ensure normality and health. A more thorough examination, including heart, lung, eye and hip check, will be undertaken within 72 hours of birth by a midwife trained in examination of the newborn, a paediatrician or a general practitioner (NSC, 2011). This section covers the initial examination of the newborn by the midwife.

Preparation includes ensuring that the room is warm and that there is a good light source. Midwives should discuss with parents the aim of the examination and gain their consent. Involving parents in the examination provides an opportunity for health promotion and to ensure any questions or anxieties can be addressed. It also provides opportunities to observe how the mother and baby interact with each other.

The midwife can observe the baby's condition and behaviour while mother and baby are engaged in skin-to-skin contact. At the same time, the baby's neurological responses such as sucking,

Question	Answer	When to talk to your midwife
How can I tell that breastfeeding is going well?	Breast feeding is going well if: Your baby has 8 feeds or more in 24 hours Your baby is feeding for between 5 and 30 minutes at each feed Your baby is generally calm and relaxed while feeding and is content after most feeds Breastfeeding is comfortable	Your baby is sleepy and has had fewer than 6 feeds in 24 hours Your baby consistently feeds for 5 minutes or less at each feed Your baby consistently feeds for longer than 40 minutes at each feed Your baby always falls asleep on the breast and/or never finishes the feed himself Your baby comes on and off the breast frequently during the feed or refuses to breastfeed You are having pain in your breasts or nipples, which doesn't disappear after the baby's first few sucks. Your nipple comes out of the baby's mouth looking pinched or flattened on one side
Is my baby gaining the right amount of weight?	Babies lose up to 7% of birth weight normally and should have regained this by day 14, averaging a 20g weight increase a day	If more than 7% of birth weight is lost, a feeding review and well-being assessment by the midwife will be required, and if weight loss is excessive, a review by a paediatrician may be needed
How many wet and dirty nappies should my baby have?	1–2 days old: 1–2 or more per day; 1 or more dark green/black 'tar like' (called meconium) 3–4 days old: 3 or more wet nappies per day; nappies feel heavier; 2 or more dirty nappies, changing in colour and consistency – brown/green/yellow,	Fewer nappies than this, or if meconium persists after day 2

(contd)

Table 7.4: Checklist to be shared with new mothers

Source: The information in this table has been adapted from **www.unicef.org.uk/Documents/Baby_Friendly/Forms/mothers_breastfeeding_ checklist.pdf**

Question	Answer	When to talk to your midwife
	becoming looser ('changing stool') 5–6 days old: 5 or more heavy wet nappies; 2 or more yellow dirty nappies; may be quite watery 7 days to 28 days old: 6 or more heavy wet nappies; 2 or more dirty nappies, at least the size of a £2 coin; yellow and watery, 'seedy' appearance	
How do I know if my baby is swallowing correctly?	When your baby is 3–4 days old and beyond you should be able to hear your baby swallowing frequently during the feed	You cannot tell if your baby is swallowing any milk when your baby is 3–4 days old and beyond
Where should my baby sleep?	The safest place for your baby to sleep is in a cot. For the first six months, it is best for the cot to be in a room with parents, and if there is not enough space, in the next nearest room, with the doors left open (NICE, 2006)	Make sure parents have emergency numbers to call in case of SIDS or other crises
Will my baby need to be fed during the night?	A new baby will be growing and developing fast so will be using a lot of energy. This means that they will need to be fed on demand, including at night. It is also important to respond to the baby's demands for night feeding as this helps to stimulate milk flow	

Table 7.4: Continued

routing, general movement and tone can be noted. A systematic examination includes the points covered in Table 7.5.

Activity 7.8   *Evidence-based practice and research*

Read the following texts.

- Farrel, P and Sittlington, N (2009) The normal baby, in Fraser, D and Cooper, M (eds) *Myles' textbook for midwives*, 15th edition. Edinburgh: Churchill Livingstone.
- Johnson, R and Taylor, W (2012) *Skills for midwifery practice*, 3rd edition. Edinburgh: Churchill Livingstone. Chapter 37: Assessment of the baby: assessment at birth; and Chapter 38: Assessment of the baby: daily examination.

Now complete Table 7.5. Some points have already been inserted to get you started.

An answer to this activity is given at the end of the chapter.

Following examination of the newborn appropriate records should be made; these must include notification of the birth, which is a legal requirement within 36 hours of the birth.

Part of the examination includes weighing the newborn, ideally using electronic scales. Babies less than 2.5 kilograms are usually considered to be low birth weight whereas large (macrosomic) babies are those over 4.5 kilograms. Baseline length measurements may also be undertaken; the average length of a full-term baby is 40 to 55 centimetres. Head circumference is normally measured around the occipital frontal circumference, the normal range being 32 to 37 centimetres. There is debate about the best time to undertake both length and head circumference measurements, with some evidence indicating that to delay taking these measurements until the following day may provide more accurate results (NICE, 2007b).

Daily examination of the newborn

The role of the midwife includes daily examination of the newborn. It is important to talk to the parents while you are carrying out your examination, and to encourage them to be aware of what changes to expect. You can revise the topic of early development by looking at the chapters listed in the further reading section on page 156.

The checklist of questions in Table 7.4 can be given to a new mother so she can be involved in monitoring her baby's development and also so she knows when to be concerned (NICE, 2006).

All home visits should be used as an opportunity to assess relevant safety issues for all family members in the home environment and promote safety education. You can make sure you are familiar with the principles of home safety by going to **www.babycentre.co.uk/baby/ safety/** or to the RoSPA or Child Accident Prevention Trust websites, which are accessible through the Babycentre one. You should take every opportunity to promote the correct use of basic safety equipment, including, for example, infant seats and smoke alarms, as well as to educate mothers on hygiene and safe preparation of formula feeds.

Examine	Findings	Rationale
Skin colour	Most Caucasian babies are pink following birth with blue extremities (acrocyanosis). Dark-skinned babies tend to be a paler version of their parents' skin tone with lighter extremities	To ensure transition to extra-uterine life; to explain to parents to allay any anxieties
Shape of head	Midwives should observe moulding (overriding of the skull bones) and caput succedeneum (oedema of the scalp) and explain these and that they normally recede within 24 hours	To recognise normal processes and identify variations; to provide reassurance and information to parents
Eyes		
Ears	Two. Check position: in relationship to rest of head should have top of pinna above eye line	
Mouth		
Neck		
Chest		
Cord	Check for three vessels in cord	
Genitalia		
Legs	Two limbs of equal length and both moving	
Feet		
Arms		
Hands	Two hands with five digits, all separate	To ensure no webbing or accessory digits that may be an indicator of abnormality
Back		
Skin	Smooth and intact; colour appropriate for culture; acrocynosis of hands and feet	To report any irregularity, to exclude any undue trauma, and to provide explanations or reassurance to parents

Table 7.5: Initial examination of the newborn: uncompleted form

Activity 7.9   **Critical thinking**

Visit the following website:

> **http://hearing.screening.nhs.uk/public**

Familiarise yourself with the basics of newborn screening. For more detailed information and to complete the eLearning module, you will need to register at **http://cpd. screening.nhs.uk/elearning**.

Read and familiarise yourself with 'Screening tests for you and your baby', which is issued to all parents and can also be found at:

> **http://newbornphysical.screening.nhs.uk/leaflets**

Now read the following:

> **http://sarawickham.files.wordpress.com/2011/10/a1-vitamin-k-a-flaw-in-the-blueprint2.pdf**

Consider the evidence presented.

As this activity involves your own reading and research, there is no answer at the end of the chapter.

Vitamin K prophylaxis

Vitamin K is essential for the formation of prothrombin, which enables blood to clot. Haemorrhagic disease of the newborn is a rare, potentially fatal disorder associated with low vitamin K levels, and is also known as vitamin K deficiency bleeding, since it can also occur later than the first week of life. Bleeding sites include gastrointestinal, cerebral umbilical. Vitamin K deficiency bleeding affects 1 in 17,000 babies who have not had vitamin K prophylaxis, compared to between 1 in 25,000 and 1 in 70,000 babies who have had a single oral 1–2 mg dose at birth and 1 in 400,000 babies who have had a single intramuscular injection at birth (Puckett and Offringa, 2000).

Doubt exists about the optimal level of vitamin K in the newborn (Wickham, 2001). The Department of Health (1998) and NICE (2006) recommend all newborn babies be given vitamin K. In the early days and weeks following birth babies build up a supply of vitamin K from feeding. Totally breastfed babies have been found to be slightly more prone to the onset of haemorrhagic disease. In over half of these babies, however, there was an underlying cause such as mal-absorption or liver disease contributing to vitamin K deficiency (Puckett and Offringa, 2000), leading Hey (2003) to suggest that term breastfed babies are more likely to be at risk if early intake is limited or poor.

Current professional recommendations advocate the administration of vitamin K to all babies, but choice of route and whether to decline it altogether should rest with parents. As a midwife with access to relevant information, you can utilise opportunities to discuss vitamin K deficiency with the parents antenatally and postnatally to help them reach an informed and personal decision.

> ### Case study
>
> *Dianne and Gary's baby (Leo) has just been born and Usha, Dianne's midwife, has come to talk to them about vitamin K prophylaxis. Usha begins by asking them if they know anything about vitamin K. They respond that while they have heard of it they do not really understand why it may be needed. Usha continues by telling them that vitamin K is poorly transferred across the placenta, so fetal stores are low and can quickly become depleted following birth. She explains that vitamin K is needed for blood clotting and that Leo will eventually manufacture his own vitamin K in his bowel once he starts feeding. Having a low level of vitamin K, however, could lead to vitamin K deficiency bleeding. Usha tells Dianne and Gary that giving baby Leo the injection will avoid this very small risk, but she understands that injections are always upsetting for babies and their parents. She goes on to say that as their baby is in a low-risk group it would be very rare to develop bleeding, but it could have severe consequences such as brain damage should it occur. Finally, Usha asks Dianne and Gary whether they have any questions before they decide whether or not they would like Leo to have the injection.*
>
> *Do you think that Usha has used the information in the Sara Wickham article cited in Activity 7.9 effectively in her conversation with Dianne and Gary? Would you have approached the subject differently?*

Newborn blood spot screening

In addition to newborn hearing screening and physical examination, parents are offered newborn blood spot screening between five and eight days postnatally.

Currently the following conditions are screened for.

- Phenylketonuria.
- Congenital hypothyroidism.
- Sickle cell diseases.
- Cystic fibrosis.
- MCADD (Medium-chain acyl-CoA dehydrogenase deficiency).

More information can be found by visiting the following weblink: **http://newbornblood spot.screening.nhs.uk/professionals**.

Revisit this website frequently to ensure that you have the most recent evidence-based information.

Educating for parenthood

Pregnancy and infancy offer a unique opportunity to work effectively with families at risk in order to set good parenting patterns for the future and break the cycle of abuse and poor parenting.

You will need to explain to new parents that newborn babies cannot regulate their sleep/wake cycle. You also need to tell them that because infants are growing and developing fast in the early days, they will need frequent feeds to satisfy demands for growth and brain development. Find time to explain that newborn babies need comfort and reassurance that their parents are nearby.

Additionally, the safety of the newborn is critical, and the avoidance of overheating is a recognised principle in reducing sudden infant death (Blair et al., 2008).

Faure (2011) suggests that swaddling the baby can be helpful as the pressure imitates the womb environment. Swaddling also stop limbs from shooting out and limits both the startle and Moro reflexes, which are common causes of night waking in a young baby. It is important to swaddle the baby with the hands free near its face so it can suck on them to self-soothe and regulate its body temperature (Faure, 2011). Colson (2010), however, argues that swaddling is unnecessary where biological nurturing is used, and may, in fact, impede fine innate movements.

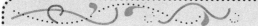

Chapter summary

This chapter has considered the adaptation to extra-uterine life made by the newborn baby and the skills and knowledge required by the midwife in order to support this. The initial assessment at birth has been explained as well as the initial steps in resuscitation, if needed. Breastfeeding has been explored with reference to relevant anatomy and physiology. The principles of hand expression of breast milk have been described, and opportunities to develop an understanding of the principles of safe artificial feeding have been offered. The principles of examination at birth and daily examination of the newborn from both a physical and psychosocial perspective have been outlined.

Activities: brief outline answers

Activity 7.1: Evidence-based practice and research (page 135)

The steps you can take to ensure the optimal environment for a smooth transition to extra-uterine life include the following.

- Close windows and doors; switch off fans to minimise drafts.
- Warm the towels, blankets and baby clothes.
- Dry the baby and cover its head.
- Enable skin-to-skin contact with the mother.

Activity 7.2: Critical thinking (page 138)

Baby Jakob's Apgar score is 9.
Baby Marcus's Apgar score is 6.

Activity 7.5: Evidence based practice and research (page 144)

Signs of a good latch include:

- wide open mouth, tongue on the base of the mouth, scooping a large mouthful of breast;
- chin indenting the breast;
- lower lip curled out and upper lip in a neutral position;
- full cheeks;
- the sound of swallowing;
- seeing milk at the sides of the mouth;
- more areola visible above the top lip than the bottom lip.

Activity 7.6: Critical thinking (pages 145–6)

You may have identified some of the following points.

In the early days, hand expressing will be far more successful than using a pump, as colostrum is much easier to express this way. Breast milk supply is linked to hormone stimulation, and the skin contact and massage involved in hand expressing is a better way to stimulate the hormones. It is also a much more effective way of removing colostrum as the colostrum is often quite thick. Hand expressing enables the mother to collect even small amounts of breast milk or colostrum, which can very easily be lost in the collecting set of a breast pump.

Wash hands with soap and water and have a clean container to collect the breast milk available. It is also helpful to place towels under the breasts. Encourage the mother to gently feel round the areola and ask her to place the thumb and first two fingers in C shape at 6 o'clock and 12 o'clock, approximately 2 to 3 centimetres above the nipple. She should then gently compress the breast and release to express the breast milk. Some mothers may need to compress the breast back to the chest wall. As the drops of milk reduce and stop, the fingers should be moved to a different position to drain all the ducts. The mother should be taught to avoid squeezing/sliding the fingers over the skin as this may cause breast tissue damage (Pollard, 2012).

As breastfeeding continues, using a pump can be helpful for collecting volumes of milk for storage for feeding the baby later. Breast massage should continue as it is essential to stimulate milk ejection; it should be performed prior to pumping (Jones and Spencer, 2008). Other ways to assist milk ejection are to express near the infant or to have a photograph or piece of the infant's clothing nearby. The same principles of hygiene are used. The mother should be encouraged to support the breast in the centre of the funnel of the breast shield, with the funnel pressing against the breast but taking care not to press too hard. Start the vacuum of the pump on minimum and gradually increase, switching the pump off before removing the shield to try to avoid breast trauma.

Activity 7.7: Evidence-based practice and research (page 146)

Principles to include when discussing safe artificial feeding with parents should include:

*   sterilisation techniques available for bottles;
*   safe making up of formula;
*   safe storage of formula;
*   safe heating of formula;
*   safely feeding the baby.

Activity 7.8: Evidence-based practice and research (page 149)

Examine	Findings	Rationale
Skin colour	Most Caucasian babies are pink following birth with blue extremities (acrocyanosis). Dark-skinned babies tend to be a paler version of their parents' skin tone with lighter extremities	To ensure transition to extra-uterine life; to explain to parents to allay any anxieties
Shape of head	Midwives should observe moulding (overriding of the skull bones) and caput succedeneum (oedema of the scalp) and explain these and that	To recognise normal processes and identify variations; to provide reassurance and information to parents

Examine	Findings	Rationale
	they normally recede within 24 hours	
Eyes	Two eyes present beneath eyelids; should be symmetrical; no discharge or swelling; should move and follow movement. Observe if epicanthic fold present	To acknowledge normal. If epicanthic fold present, consider observations on baby; may be cultural or familial, or may be indicative of abnormality
Ears	Two. Check position: in relationship to rest of head should have top of pinna above eye line	Low-set ears: be alert for other abnormalities
Mouth	Mouth opens, the lips complete and philtrum present. View palate and feel palate; observe if tongue tie present; elicit sucking reflex	To ensure intact and provide information and support to parents, referring early if any deviation
Neck	Examine creases and folds, and ensure neck moves from side to side	To ensure normality of movement
Chest	Two nipples present and symmetrical, breathing is regular with no indrawing of chest	To ensure normal physical appearance and no respiratory distress
Cord	Three vessels in cord; ensure cord not bleeding and clamp or ties secure	A small number of a babies have one umbilical artery with one or more associated congenital abnormalities
Genitalia	Female: labia majora should cover the clitoris and labia minora; white vaginal discharge normal. Male: penis present and completely covered by foreskin, urethral opening at the end of the penis and scrotum soft and covered in rugae; examine the testes to ensure descended into scrotum.	To identify sex of baby and to refer if any concerns
Anus	Ensure patent and correctly positioned	Imperforate anus is an abnormality and prompt referral is needed for early treatment

Examine	Findings	Rationale
Legs	Two limbs of equal length and both moving with good muscle tone; observe position of legs	To ensure normal
Feet	Five digits all separate	To ensure no webbing or accessory digits that may be an indicator of abnormality
Arms	Two limbs of equal length and both moving	To ensure complete
Hands	Two hands with five digits, all separate; palmar creases present	To ensure no webbing or accessory digits that may be an indicator of abnormality
Back	Palpate the length of the spine to feel all the spinous processes to ensure intact; examine cleft of the buttocks to ensure no sacral dimple	To exclude any spinal lesion
Skin	Smooth and intact; colour appropriate for culture; acrocynosis (blueness) of hands and feet; acknowledge any 'birthmarks'	To report any irregularity, to exclude any undue trauma, and to provide explanations or reassurance to parents

Table 7.5: Initial examination of the newborn: completed form

Further reading

Colson, S (2000) Womb to world: a metabolic perspective. Available at: **www.midwiferytoday.com/articles/womb.asp**.

This is a useful introduction to the metabolic changes that take place in the newborn baby.

Fraser, D and Cooper, D (2009) *Myles' textbook for midwives*, 15th edition. Edinburgh: Churchill Livingstone.

See especially Serci, I, Chapter 12, 'The fetus', to help you to understand the fetal circulation, and Farrell, P and Sittlington, N, Chapters 39 and 40 'The baby at birth' and 'The normal baby', to help you understand neonatal physiology.

Useful websites

www.cochrane.org/podcasts/most-accessed-cochrane-reviews/early-skin-skin-contact-mothers-and-their-healthy-newborn-in

This podcast reviews the evidence for skin-to-skin contact between mothers and their newborn babies.

www.indiana.edu/~anat550/cvanim/fetcirc/fetcirc.html

This website offers an animation of fetal circulation to support understanding.

www.biologicalnurturing.com/index.html

Visit this website for some lovely pictures of the biological nurturing approach to breastfeeding.

www.unicef.org.uk/BabyFriendly/Resources/AudioVideo/Baby-led-feeding

This site shows a video clip on the establishment of breastfeeding that is well worth watching.

http://vickyandjen.com/podcast_205.html

This American podcast on the art of breastfeeding includes some useful information.

www.lowmilksupply.org/

This website has some useful reviews of the physiology of lactation.

www.nspcc.org.uk/inform/publications/downloads/encouragingbetterbehaviour_wdf48121.pdf

www.nspcc.org.uk/Inform/publications/downloads/all-babies-count-parents_wdf86487.pdf

These two web links give information about support that is currently available for new parents.

Chapter 8
Medicines management in normal midwifery care

Moira McLean

This chapter will address the following ESCs:

Cluster: Medical products management

Women can trust/expect a newly registered midwife to:

3. In the course of their professional midwifery practice, supply and administer medicinal products safely and in a timely manner, including controlled drugs.
4. Keep and maintain accurate records, which includes when working within a multi-disciplinary framework and as part of the team.
5. Work within the legal and ethical framework that underpins safe and effective medicinal products management, as well as in conjunction with national guidelines and local policies.
6. Work in partnership with women to share information in assisting them to make safe and informed choices about medicinal products related to themselves, their unborn children or their babies.

Chapter aims

After reading this chapter you will be able to:

- understand legislation surrounding the administration of medicines and midwives' exempt medicines management;
- demonstrate knowledge used within normal midwifery practice and current midwives' exempt drugs (NMC, 2011).

Introduction

While midwifery practice is essentially about supporting women during normal pregnancy and birth, midwives also need to work in partnership with women to provide support in safely selecting or avoiding medications in pregnancy. This chapter will deal with the common drugs that midwives may use as part of their professional practice in providing normal midwifery care. In order to do this, midwives need to understand the professional guidance and legislation that supports their practice. Understanding the principles will help to provide safe and effective care and minimise errors.

Legislation governing the administration of drugs

The two lead Acts of Parliament that control the administration and use of medicines are the Medicines Act 1968 and the Misuse of Drugs Act 1971. The Medicines Act 1968 was introduced following a review of legislation relating to medicines prompted by the thalidomide tragedy in the 1960s. It brought together most of the previous legislation on medicines and introduced a number of other legal provisions for the control of medicines. The Act and the regulations made under the Act set out the requirements for the manufacture, sale, supply and administration of medicines. Medicinal products fall into one of three categories (see Table 8.1).

- General sale list (GSL).
- Pharmacy medicines (P).
- Prescription-only medicines (POMs).

Type of category	Availability	Examples
General sale list (GSL)	Sold through pharmacies and other (non-pharmacy) retail outlets	Paracetamol
Pharmacy medicines (P)	Supplied only through registered pharmacies by or under the supervision of the pharmacist	'Morning after' pill; Canestan
Prescription-only medicines (POMs)	Subject to additional requirements; will be supplied (e.g. penicillin) by the pharmacist on receipt of a prescription from a regular practitioner	Antibiotics

Table 8.1: The three categories of medicine in midwifery care

Midwives' exemptions

Exemptions allow certain groups of health care professionals to sell, supply and administer specific medicines directly to patients/clients. Registered midwives may supply (but not offer for sale) and administer, on their own initiative, any of the substances that are specified in medicines legislation under midwives' exemptions, provided that they do this in the course of professional midwifery practice. They may do so without the need for a medical prescription or a patient-specific written direction. If a medicine is not included in midwives' exemptions, then a prescription or a patient-specific direction is needed (NMC, 2008b). So exemptions are distinct from prescribing, which requires the involvement of the pharmacist in the sale or supply of medicine.

However, all medicines that are administered need to be recorded and documented. In a hospital environment, this is done on a prescription chart.

Activity 8.1   *Critical thinking*

When you are in your next placement, take time to notice how midwives make a record of Midwife Exempt drugs:

(a) on a prescription chart
(b) in the woman's records.

Ask your sign-off mentor to explain this to you.

No answer is given for this activity as the answer may vary depending on local policy (for example, where the information is recorded, what colour ink is used, etc.).

Midwives' exemptions fall into two main categories (MHRA, 2011).

1. All medicinal products on the general sales list and all pharmacy medicines.
2. POMs containing any of the substances (but no other prescription-only medicines) listed in Schedule 5 Article 11 (1) (A) Part one exemption from restrictions on sale or supply (see Table 8.2).

B. Prescription-only medicines containing any of the following substances	**Conditions**
Diclofenac Hydrocortisone acetate Miconazole Nystatin Phytomenadione	The sale or supply of the prescription-only medicines listed under Schedule 5 Article 11 (1) shall be only in the course of their professional practice

Table 8.2: POMS covered by Schedule 5 Article 11 (1) A Part one exemption from restrictions on sale or supply

Exemptions from restriction administration

In the course of professional practice registered midwives may also administer **parenterally** (not via the oral route) prescription-only medicines containing any of the substances listed in Part 3 Article 11 (2) – exemptions from restriction on administration. However, it is important to note that midwives may not administer any other substance specified in Column 1 of Schedule 1 of the order, even if the medicine contains a substance listed in Part 3 Article 11 (2) 2 (see Table 8.3). This means simply that it is these named drugs only. Even if a midwife knows of another drug with similar properties, he or she cannot administer it.

Prescription-only medicines for parenteral administration containing any of the following substances but no other substance specified in Column 1 of Schedule 1 of the order	Conditions
Adrenaline Anti-D immunoglobulin Carboprost Cyclizine lactate Diamorphine Ergometrine maleate Gelofusine Hartmann's solution Hepatitis B vaccine Hepatitis immunoglobulin Lidocaine Lidocaine hydrochloride Morphine Naloxone hydrochloride Oxytocins, natural and synthetic Pethidine hydrochloride Phytomenadione Prochloperazine Sodium chloride 0.9%	The administration shall be only in the course of their professional practice and in the case of lidocaine and lidocaine hydrochloride shall be only while attending on a woman in childbirth.

Table 8.3: Prescription-only medicines to which the exemption applies (Column 1 Schedule 1)

In July 2011, the legislation concerning midwives' exemptions was amended. This amendment enables student midwives to administer medicines listed on midwives' exemptions, excluding controlled drugs, under the direct supervision of a registered midwife who must be a sign-off mentor. The Medicines and Healthcare products Regulatory Authority (MHRA) made this a condition for agreeing that midwives may enable students to administer medications listed under midwives' exemptions. Although students are *not* able to administer controlled drugs in the midwives' exemptions list, they will be able to administer a controlled drug from a prescription that has been written by a medical or midwife prescriber, under the guidance and supervision of their sign-off mentor.

The MHRA has now been very specific in saying that the use of a Patient Group Direction (PGD) is not necessary for midwives to supply and/or administer any of those substances that are specified as 'midwives' exemptions'. Student midwives are *not* authorised to administer any medicine under a PGD.

Activity 8.2   *Teamwork*

Enlist the help of two or three colleagues. Individually, go to the following website:

**www.mhra.gov.uk/Howweregulate/Medicines/Availabilityprescribing
sellingandsupplyingofmedicines/ExemptionsfromMedicines
Actrestrictions/PatientGroupDirectionsintheNHS/index.htm**

Read the information on PGDs that you find there and make notes.

Meet up at a prearranged time to discuss what you have found and how you feel it relates
to the practice you have seen so far in your clinical practice placements.

As your responses to this will vary, no outline answer is given at the end of the chapter.

Patient specific directions

A patient specific direction (PSD) is a written instruction from a qualified and registered
prescriber for a medicine, including the dose route and frequency, or an appliance to be supplied
or administered to a named patient.

Student midwives and medicines administration

Standard 17 of the *Standards for pre-registration midwifery education* states that:

> *student midwives must be able, at the point of registration, to select, acquire and administer safely, a range
> of permitted drugs consistent with legislation, applying knowledge and skills to the situation which pertains
> at the time. Methods of administration include: oral, intravenous, intramuscular, topical and inhalation.*
> (NMC, 2009)

In order to achieve the standard required for registration, student midwives must be given
opportunities to participate in the administration of medicines, but this must always be under the
direct supervision of a registered midwife or nurse (NMC, 2011).

Activity 8.3   *Critical thinking*

Visit the NMC website and read the circular related to drug administration and student
midwives:

**www.nmc-uk.org/Documents/Circulars/2011Circulars/nmc
Circular07–2011-Midwives-Exemptions.pdf**

Find out whether your local Trust has specific guidance for the administration of
medications by student midwives. Does this differ for students who are already on the
nursing part of the register?

An outline answer to this activity is given at the end of the chapter.

Having reviewed the basic principles of legislation related to medicines management, we will review the principles of administering medicines safely.

Principles of administering medication

The NMC document *Standards for medicines management* (2008b) provides clear guidance on administration of medicines. Despite this, the National Patient Safety Agency (NPSA, 2009) continues to report medicine errors, 41 per cent of which are specifically related to administration. It is very important, therefore, to adhere to these guidelines in order to reduce the risk of harm to the mother or baby. Students should always be supervised in all aspects of medicines administration.

The NMC (2008b) states that the administration of medicines is an important aspect of professional practice for all individuals whose names are on the Council's register. It is not solely a mechanistic task to be performed in strict compliance with the written prescription of a medical practitioner (or independent/supplementary prescriber). It requires thought and the exercise of professional judgement.

Good practice related to drug administration involves consideration of eight main principles. These are commonly referred to as the Eight Rs.

- Right drug.
- Right route.
- Right time.
- Right patient.
- Right dose.
- Right documentation.
- Right education.
- Right effect.
  (Parboteeah, 2011)

Table 8.4 outlines the principles of safe drug administration, giving reasons why each aspect should always be applied.

Common drugs used in normal midwifery practice

While most women in normal pregnancy are fit and well, there are some drugs you may offer them as part of their care. As a student midwife you are required to know about these drugs, how they work, their dosages and side effects, as well as any contraindications to them (NMC, 2009).

The following drugs will now be introduced:

- Nitrous oxide and oxygen, also known as Entonox®
- Oxytocin and ergometrine maleate mixed, known as Syntometrine®

Drug administration principle	Rationale
Read prescription chart carefully	To check that the prescription is clear and accurate
Ensure you know what the drug is, what it is used for, the usual side effects, contraindications and any special instructions (for example, to be given with food)	To ensure there are no potential contraindications or other drug interactions
If prescription chart is unclear, do NOT administer drug. Seek guidance from prescriber	To reduce the risk of errors
Check patient details clearly written on drug chart	To ensure correct medications are given to the correct patient
Check each prescribed medication for the name of the drug route of administration, start date, signature of prescriber, any special instructions, time of administration, time due for administration (NMC, 2008b)	To ensure the correct drug is given by the correct route in the right dose at the right time
Check drug against prescription: name of the drug, the dose of the drug, any calculation, expiry date of drug (NMC, 2008b)	To ensure that the correct dose is given of an effective drug
Check patient's identity against the prescription chart and name bracelet asking patient to state the name and date of birth	To ensure the correct patient receives the correct drug (NMC, 2008b)
Obtain patient's consent and administer drug	Patient consent is required for all treatments (NMC, 2008b)
Record the drug administered (NMC, 2004b). Mentor should ensure that they countersign student signatures when supervising drug administration (NMC, 2008b, 2011)	To indicate that the dose has been given and prevent the dose being given again
If the drug is not being given for any reason, record this and inform prescriber	It may be necessary to alter the route administration or review the need for the drug (NMC, 2008b)
Note the effectiveness of the medication given, if appropriate (for example, pain relief)	To evaluate and review medication

Table 8.4 The principles of safe drug administration

- Oxytocin, also known as Syntocinon®
- Phytomenadione, also known as Konakion.

Entonox®

Midwives may assist women to self-administer Entonox® during labour, most commonly using a mouthpiece or mask to which an expiratory valve and filter is attached. This mode of administration allows the drug, which is a gas and breathed into the lungs, to be absorbed quickly into the bloodstream via the alveoli in the lungs. Although the exact pharmacokinetics of Entonox® are not known, we do know that it is not metabolised by the body but rapidly excreted through the lungs. It is also thought to enhance the release of the body's own endorphins and suppress pain signals. Entonox® works within about 30 seconds, and has very few side effects. This makes it a popular choice for relieving pain in labour.

Entonox® comes in a cylinder that will vary in colour depending on the supplier, but that is normally blue with white shoulders. Alternatively, it may be available from a piped circuit within the birthing room. It comes as a concentration of 50:50 of oxygen and nitrous oxide (BOC, 2010).

An assessment needs to be made antenatally to address whether the woman is eligible to receive Entonox®. The assessment should note any medical issues that may be affected by its use. The woman's consent, and her understanding of the drug, is also required (NMC, 2008b). Use of Entonox® needs to be signed for by the **registrant**.

Entonox® is made up of a compound of gases that will support combustion, so no naked flames, smoking or use of any grease (including hand creams) can be allowed near the apparatus. The cylinder should be stored in an identified area that is dry and well ventilated. If cylinders are transferred to the community, the midwife will ensure they have competence in its transfer. A compressed gas sign needs to be clearly displayed and the midwife needs to be aware that the cylinder gases will separate at a temperature of –6°C (Johnson and Taylor, 2010). The cylinder needs to be at room temperature for effective administration.

Activity 8.4   *Evidence-based practice and research*

Visit:

http://discover.entonox.co.uk/

Complete the learning packages relevant to childbearing. You will need to register to use this site.

There is no outline answer to this activity at the end of this chapter.

Syntometrine®

Syntometrine® is made up of ergometrine maleate 500 µg (micrograms) and oxytocin 5 international units. It is used during the third stage of labour or after the birth of the baby to reduce bleeding. The dosage is 1 ml and is administered intramuscularly, normally after the birth of the anterior shoulder of the baby. The oxytocin works within three to five minutes, causing regular uterine contractions that help to facilitate the separation and delivery of the placenta. Ergometrine works within seven minutes, causing a sustained uterine contraction that helps to reduce bleeding from the placental site. The drug is used as part of the active management of labour, and following its administration, controlled cord traction is normally applied to assist the birth of the placenta. Syntometrine® is a midwife-exempt drug and contraindications include pre-existing cardiac disease, hypertension and severe asthma (Jordan, 2010). There are several side effects, including headache, nausea, vomiting and abdominal cramps. Syntometrine® should be stored away from light, at a temperature of between 2 and 6°C. If containers of the drug are left standing at higher temperatures, they should be discarded after two months.

Activity 8.5　　　　　　　　　*Evidence-based practice and research*

On your next clinical placement, find out where Sytometrine® is stored. If this placement is in a hospital setting, then carry out the same piece of research next time you have a clinical practice placement in the community (or vice versa).

Talk to one or more colleagues who have carried out the same process of finding out, and compare notes.

As the answers to this activity will depend on your own research and experience, no outline answer is given at the end of the chapter.

Oxytocin (Syntocinon®)

Oxytocin is used to induce or augment labour and to facilitate management of the third stage of labour by reducing the amount of bleeding. It can also be used to control postpartum haemorrhage.

As a student midwife caring for women in normal labour, you are most likely to see its use in third-stage management, as current recommendations (NICE, 2007b) are to give this drug to all women in the third stage of labour in order to reduce their risk of postpartum haemorrhage. It is recommended rather than Syntometrine® because the risk of side effects is lower (NICE, 2007b).

In this context, Syntocinon® is usually administered intramuscularly in the outer thigh in the dosage of 10 international units. Its action is to enhance regular rhythmic contractions of the uterus, and this usually occurs within 3–7 minutes and lasts for 30–60 minutes. Syntocinon® should be stored at a temperature between 2 and 8°C. If stored at higher temperatures, its shelf life may be reduced to three months (Jordan, 2010).

> ## Activity 8.6   *Evidence-based practice and research*
>
> Find out what drug is used in your local Trust for third-stage management.
>
> Read the following review.
>
> Begley, C, Gyte, G, Devane, D and McGuire, W (2011) *Active versus expectant management for women in third stage of labour.* Cochrane Pregnancy and Childbirth Group. Available at: **http://onlinelibrary.wiley.com/o/cochrane/clabout/articles/PREG/frame .html**.
>
> Reflect on the evidence used to inform decision-making.
>
> *As the answer to this activity will be based on your own research and reflection, no answer is given at the end of the chapter.*

Phytomenadione

Phytomenadione is a drug offered prophylactically to prevent vitamin K deficiency bleeding (VKDB), which is a rare but potentially fatal bleeding disorder (Jordan, 2010). The Department of Health (DH, 1998) and NICE (2006) advocate that all newborns should receive a dose of konakion as a matter of routine, but, as with all medications, informed consent is required. Parents should be given a choice about whether the drug should be administered to their newborn and, if so, what route would be most effective.

> ## Activity 8.7   *Communication*
>
> Go to the following website to read the guidance from the Department of Health:
>
> **www.dh.gov.uk/en/Publicationsandstatistics/Lettersandcirculars/ Professionalletters/Chiefmedicalofficerletters/DH_4004993**
>
> Then read the article by Harvey (2008) which you will find listed in the further reading section on page 172.
>
> Now turn back to the section on vitamin K prophylaxis on pages 151–2 of Chapter 7. Re-read this section, particularly the case study featuring Dianne, Gary and baby Leo. Think about what information you would give to parents to enable them to make an informed choice about whether to consent to their baby having an injection of konakion.
>
> *An outline answer to this activity is given at the end of the chapter.*

Phytomenadione: what is recommended

While all Trusts may have their own guidance, it is usual to recommend that healthy neonates of 36 weeks gestation and older receive either:

- 1 mg administered by intramuscular injection at birth or soon after birth;

or

- 2 mg orally at birth or soon after birth. The oral dose should be followed by a second dose of 2 mg at between four and seven days.

The ampoule contents should be clear at the time of use, and it should be stored below 25°C and protected from light.

The majority of healthy newborns will receive the standard dose of 1 mg, and as the volume of this is so small, it is recommended that 1 ml with a 0.01 graded syringe is used to ensure accuracy of dosage (**www.medicines.org.uk/emc/medicine/17299/PIL/konakion%20mm%20paediatric**).

Further doses

Babies who are given vitamin K by mouth and who are breast-fed (not given formula milk) may need more doses of vitamin K by mouth.

Bottle-fed babies given the two doses of vitamin K by mouth do not need any more doses of vitamin K. This is because it is included in formula milk.

As konakion is usually administered to newborns, it requires two qualified practitioners to witness its dosage and administration.

Case study: vitamin K prophylaxis

Ruby was born at home at 38 weeks gestation. Her parents, Damian and Flora, have discussed prophylactic vitamin K antenatally with their community midwife. After reading around the topic, they have decided to accept this for their daughter.

Carla the midwife removes the ampoule from its packet, checks the drug name and expiry date with Greta the student she is mentoring, and Francine the second midwife. She supports Greta to calculate the correct dosage from the 2 mg in 0.2 ml ampoule. Greta correctly draws up the liquid using a 1 ml graduated syringe ensuring she has 0.1 ml of clear, pale yellow solution. This is checked by Carla (who is Greta's sign-off mentor) and witnessed by Francine. The needle is changed for an orange needle suitable for injecting neonates. Greta gains verbal consent from the parents, tells them what she is going to do and explains that baby Ruby may cry a little. Then, while being carefully observed by Carla, Greta injects the dose of phytomenadione gently into the vastus lateralis muscle of baby Ruby's thigh. Greta disposes of the sharps carefully and correctly, then records on the neonatal prescription chart in the mother's notes, and on the paediatric child record, that the injection was given. This is countersigned by Carla, her sign-off mentor.

Ruby is cuddled by her parents.

Lidocaine hydrochloride

Lidocaine hydrochloride (commonly referred to as lidocaine), a midwife-exempt drug, is a rapid-acting local anaesthetic that midwives use most commonly prior to performing an episiotomy and prior to perineal repair. Lidocaine can also be used to provide rapid local anaesthesia prior to cannulation and prior to the insertion of urinary catheters.

Lidocaine for perineal infiltration is supplied as a clear solution in sterile ampoules. The plain lidocaine (0.5 per cent 10 ml or 1 per cent 5 ml solution) should be drawn up from the ampoule into a sterile syringe using an 18G (green) needle and aseptic technique. Infiltration of the perineum with lidocaine is associated with initial stinging followed by loss of sensation to pain in the injected area. The anaesthetic effect may last for 30–60 minutes. There may be a continued awareness of touch/pressure in an effectively anaesthetised area. There may be transient local swelling and erythema at the injection site.

It is rare for there to be any more lasting or pronounced side effects with this amount and route of administration; however, inadvertent intravascular injection may cause dizziness or pins and needles. If this occurs, stop injecting and calmly call for assistance. Lidocaine is rapidly metabolised and any symptoms should resolve in 15–20 minutes.

Allergy to plain lidocaine is very rare. Symptoms include excessive pain, itching or swelling at the injection site. Breathlessness and collapse with tachycardia and hypotension suggest anaphylaxis (Jordan, 2010).

Midwives and complementary therapies

Pregnant women are increasingly choosing to use complementary therapies, so you are certain to encounter them at some stage during your practice if you haven't already done so. As a midwife, you need to be aware of your role in supporting the woman and her choices during pregnancy. Midwives who wish to include complementary therapies as part of their practice should undertake training in a specific therapy. If you are providing midwifery care for a client who wishes to use complementary therapy, you will need to ensure you have sufficient knowledge to talk to her about her choices.

The NMC guidance related to complementary therapies identifies that the registrant should successfully have completed a training course in complementary or alternative therapies before applying the specialist knowledge and skill to their practice (NMC, 2008b). Midwives have a responsibility to ensure that no complementary therapy causes harm to mothers or babies; they should aim to ensure that women make an informed choice at all times. This will take into consideration any other medication or any other conditions the woman may have. If a midwife wishes to use complementary therapies within their practice, they should discuss them with their employer and ensure they are familiar with any local guidance (Tiran, 2010). The midwife has a legal duty to obtain the consent of the mother to any procedures, and to ensure her wishes and choices are respected as much as possible. In addition, all midwives should keep clear records of any discussions or agreements with the mother involving the use of complementary therapies.

Activity 8.8   *Evidence-based practice and research*

Start to maintain a Midwifery Drug Formulary to enable you to develop your knowledge and understanding about the drugs used in pregnancy and childbirth. This specimen table gives you some headings and other information to get you started.

As this activity is based on your own experience, there is no outline answer at the end of the chapter.

Drug name	Dosage	Type of drug (e.g. midwife exempt/ POM/GSL)	Uses	How it works	Contra-indications	Side effects	Midwife's responsibilities
para-cetamol	?	GSL	Pain relief		Liver problems		

Table 8.5: My midwifery drug formulary

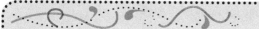

Chapter summary

This chapter has considered the principles of safe drug administration and reviewed the medicines that are currently available as midwife-exempt drugs. Some of the most common drugs in midwifery practice and how you may see them used in practice have been explained. Your role as a student midwife has been discussed in the context of the safe and appropriate administration of drugs.

Activities: brief outline answers

Activity 8.3: Critical thinking (page 163)

As a student you cannot administer a drug that is not prescribed (even though paracetamol is a drug that is available over the counter).

If you are a student in this position, an appropriate response would be to explain to your mentor that you are not able to give the paracetamol, at the same time as acknowledging Fiona's need for analgesia. Explain to Fiona that you are in the process of ensuring she receives analgesia as soon as possible.

As a qualified midwife, it is your responsibility to record the paracetamol on the drug administration chart, checking when Fiona last received paracetamol and ensuring she had no allergies. Once all the appropriate checks have been undertaken to administer the paracetamol, the time the drug has been given must be recorded on the drug administration chart. As a mentor you should not have given the student this responsibility as all aspects of drug administration need to be overseen, checked and countersigned. All student midwives are supernumerary in status and require drug administration in midwifery settings to be supervised.

Activity 8.7: Communication (page 168)

To insure that an informed choice has been made, the following points should be discussed with the parents and made available to them in a format that they can understand; they should also be given time in which to make their decision.

* What vitamin K is.
* What vitamin K deficiency bleeding is and how it may affect the baby.
* The percentage chance of their baby getting this without prophylaxis compared with the percentage chance with prophylaxis by the route they choose.
* The ways in which vitamin K can be given.
* The side effects of the drug and the route used.
* What to look out for in their baby if they decide not to have the injection.

Further reading

Harvey, B (2008) Newborn vitamin K prophylaxis: developments and dilemmas. *British Journal of Midwifery*, 16(8): 516–519.

This is a good summary of the issues surrounding vitamin K prophylaxis.

Lapham, R and Agar, H (2003) *Drug calculations for nurses: a step by step approach*, 2nd edition. London: Hodder Arnold.

Lawson, E and Hennefer, D (2010) *Medicines management in adult nursing*. Exeter: Learning Matters.

This book gives the principles of medicines management and safe administration. Even though it is targeted at nurses rather than midwives, the principles are broadly the same.

Waugh, S (2010) Drug calculations, in Starkings, S and Krause, L, *Passing calculations tests for nursing students*. Exeter: Learning Matters.

These two books will help you practise your drug calculations and will be particularly useful if you struggle with arithmetic.

Useful website

http://skills.library.leeds.ac.uk/web_based_resources/mathssolutions/index.html

This useful resource demonstrates both visually and verbally how maths examples are worked out.

Glossary

acceleration   a transient increase of the fetal heart rate by 15 beats or more, lasting 15 seconds or more.

active phase of labour   the phase of labour in which contractions are occurring regularly, with around three to four contractions every ten minutes. The cervix is progressively dilating and the woman is usually moving around to find positions of comfort.

advocacy   helping the woman articulate her wishes to others.

amenorrhoea   absence of menstrual period in a woman of reproductive age, possibly indicative of pregnancy or lactation.

anaemia   reduction in the number of red blood cells or haemoglobin (Hb) concentration of the blood. A woman with an Hb level below 10.5 dl/g is considered anaemic.

asymptomatic bacteriuria   bacterial infection in the urine that exhibits without symptoms (usual symptoms include pain, frequency of micturition (passing urine) or raised temperature).

asynclitic   with the parietal bone/side of the head leading.

auscultation   listening to the internal sounds of the body; in midwifery the fetal heart rate is listened for.

autonomy   the capacity of rational individuals to make decisions. This applies equally to the women midwives care for and to midwives' own practice and their ability to make informed decisions.

baseline rate   the mean rate when the fetal heart rate is stable, excluding accelerations and decelerations. It is determined over a time period of 5 or 10 minutes and expressed in beats per minute (bpm). Normal baseline fetal heart rate is 110–160 bpm.

baseline variability   the normal fluctuation in the baseline of the fetal heart rate (FHR) occurring in a one-minute period by assessing the highest and lowest reading. Normal baseline variability ranges between 5 and 25 bpm between contractions.

beneficence   the promotion of well-being for others.

beta-human chorionic gonadotrophin   a hormone produced during the early stages of pregnancy.

birth centre alongside consultant unit   a midwifery-led unit that is housed within a consultant unit. This may be in the same building or on the same floor. The unit ideally is staffed by midwives who have a philosophy of promoting normal birth and who work together as a team within that defined area.

brim of the pelvis   the circle of the pelvic bone made up of the sacral promontory, sacral ala or wing, sacroiliac joint, ileopectineal line, ileopectineal eminence, superior ramus of pelvic bone, upper inner body of pubic bone, upper border of symphysis pubis.

cannula (cannulated)   a small plastic tube inserted with a needle into a vein to take a blood sample and through which to administer medication.

caput succedaneum   soft oedematous swelling on the top of the fetal skull where it has been pressing on the cervix; usually disappears after 24 hours.

cardiotocograph (CTG)   a machine that electronically records the fetal heart rate and frequency of uterine contractions; often called a CTG machine; the recording is also called a CTG (*cardiotocography*).

chromosomal make-up   the number and structure of genes in the human; some excess numbers are associated with trisomies such as Down's syndrome, and structural chromosomal abnormalities such as missing lengths occurring, for instance in Cri du chat.

colostrum   the fluid in the breasts during pregnancy and in the first three days following birth that contains immunoglobulins and high levels of protein and vitamin A and K.

contraction   the shortening of muscle fibres.

deceleration   a transient episode of the slowing of the fetal heart rate below the baseline level by more than 15 bpm, lasting 15 seconds or more.

diagnostic test   a medical test that states or detects whether a person has a disease or not.

dilatation   increasing widening of the external opening of the cervix increasingly dilates as a result of the contraction and retraction of the uterine muscles.

diuresis   increased urine production, usual following birth.

dysparenuia   painful sexual intercourse usually due to medical or psychological disorders and usually only found in women.

effacement   shortening of the cervix, resulting in the loss of the cervical canal, as the internal opening of the cervix dilates and forms part of the lower uterine segment.

electronic fetal monitoring (EFM)   a method for examining the condition of a fetus in the uterus by recording the pattern of the fetal heart rate.

embryo   the term used to define a developing baby from conception to ten weeks gestation (remember that this is eight weeks post-conception).

emergency caesarean section (ECV)   a caesarean section that was not planned before the onset of labour.

external cephalic version   the process by which a fetus lying in the breech position around 36 weeks gestation is turned to a cephalic presentation by a doctor using their hands on the maternal abdomen.

fallopian tubes   thin tubes connecting the ovaries and uterus in the female reproductive system.

fertilisation   also known as conception, where the gametes, the egg and sperm, come together to create a new life; usually occurs in the fallopian tubes.

fetal alcohol syndrome   permanent central nervous system damage in the developing fetus in response to prolonged exposure to maternal alcohol consumption.

fetus   the term used to describe the developing baby from eleven weeks gestation (nine weeks after conception) until birth.

free-standing birth centre   a birth centre that is independent from hospital, often staffed and run by midwives supporting women with low-risk pregnancy for labour and birth.

fundus   the top of the uterus.

gestation period   the time it takes for a baby to develop. This differs between species: in humans from conception to birth is approximately 266 days, or 38 weeks, remembering that the last menstrual period occurs two weeks before conception.

haematocrit   a measure of the percentage of red blood cells to the total blood volume.

haemoglobin   the iron-containing oxygen transporting protein of the red blood cell. In healthy pregnant women an Hb level of above 10.5 dl/g is desired.

haemoglobinopathies   the collective term for inherited single-cell gene disorders; see *sickle cell anaemia* and *thalassaemia*.

haemostasis   the process that causes bleeding to stop.

hand-held notes   also called maternal records; the record of a woman's pregnancy, visits, observations, communications and tests, held by the woman and taken to each appointment.

hypoglycaemia   a low level of glucose in blood in the neonate.

hypoxia   a decreased level of oxygen in body tissues.

iatrogenic   hospital-induced harm, usually an infection following the use of technologies such as the insertion of a cannula or the artificial rupture of the membranes. Usually no harm is intended, but the nature of the intervention has implicit risks that must be discussed with women so that they can make informed choices for care.

implantation   the stage where the embryo attaches to the uterine wall approximately nine days after conception.

involution   the shrinking of an organ; following pregnancy, the uterus and related structures shrink back to their previous shape and size.

justice   the obligation to treat others fairly.

latent phase of labour   sometimes called the pre-labour phase. Deciding the start of labour can be difficult, and many women experience a long latent phase prior to labour becoming established. There is general agreement that this phase of labour requires support and encouragement, but that it is best for the woman to be in her own home where she can relax.

lochia   discharge from the uterus following the birth.

membrane sweeping   vaginal examination and stimulation of the cervix and membranes in order to initiate prostaglandin hormone release and start labour in post-term women.

MEOWS (modified early obstetric warning score)   a chart on which maternal observations of blood pressure, pulse, temperature, respiratory rate and urinary output can be recorded. Its aim is to identify promptly women who become unwell in order to enable prompt referral, and treatment. This chart encompasses actions to be taken should any of the observations fall outside normal parameters.

micturition   the ejection or passing of urine from the bladder to the outside world.

midwifery-led care   care led exclusively by a midwife – for women whose pregnancies are considered to be of low obstetric risk.

moulding   overlapping of the fetal skull bones as they pass through the birth canal.

multigravida   the medical term referring to a woman who has been pregnant at least once before; some midwives prefer the term parous, meaning giving birth, as opposed to gravid, which is about the pregnant uterus; hence multiparous (has given birth before as opposed to multigravida, has been pregnant before).

non-maleficence   the principle of not doing harm to others.

nuchal translucency measurement   an ultrasound measurement of the thickness of the soft tissue at the back of the developing fetus's neck; a higher measurement is indicative of an abnormality within the fetus.

nulliparous   refers to a woman who has never given birth before.

obstetrician (or consultant)   the senior specialist doctor who is the lead professional in high-risk pregnancies. They are responsible for planning care that is not normal, such as raised blood pressure or decreased fetal growth. There are other consultants involved in midwifery care, such as paediatricians (baby doctors) and anaesthetists (doctors who administer analgesia for operations or procedures) as well as medical consultants who may be specialists in diabetes or other medical diseases.

occipito anterior position   the position when the occipital region of the fetal skull presents towards the front of the maternal pelvis, usually indicating that the head is well flexed with a smaller diameter presenting.

ovulation   the release of the ova (egg) from the ovary, prior to conception.

parenterally   given into the skin/muscle, usually by injection.

partogram   the visual display of part of the woman's progress on labour in the form of a structured graphical representation which may have alert and action lines.

pathological   relating to the study of a disease process, the opposite of *physiological*, which is a natural process.

pelvic cavity   extends from the brim of the pelvis to the pelvic outlet and is formed by the hollow of the sacrum; the posterior wall is concave and approximately 10 cm in length .The anterior wall is formed by the symphis pubis and is approximately 4 cm long.

physiological   relating to the science of the function of living things; in human biology, the study of normal bodily processes, such as pregnancy.

Pinard stethoscope   traditional instrument used to auscultate the fetal heart; may be made of wood, metal or plastic.

placenta   the organ that develops during pregnancy connecting the fetus to the uterine wall. This organ is responsible for gaseous exchange, nutrient uptake and waste product elimination during pregnancy.

pre-eclampsia   a medical condition occurring during pregnancy, usually from 20 weeks gestation or later, causing maternal blood pressure elevation and excretion of protein in the urine. There is no known cure except birth; pre-eclampsia may occur postnatally too.

primigravida   a woman experiencing her first pregnancy.

prolactin   hormone released from anterior pituitary gland in response to suckling or nipple stimulation. It is essential to the establishment and maintenance of breast milk production.

prophylactic anti-D   preventative anti-D treatment offered to women who are rhesus negative at 28 weeks of pregnancy to reduce the chance of the effects of potential blood mixing between the fetus and mother, where the fetus has rhesus positive blood.

proteinuria   protein in the urine.

puerperium   the postnatal period, usually lasting six weeks after birth when the body returns to a non-pregnant state.

purple line   the presence of a purple line during labour, seen to rise from the anal margin and extend between the buttocks as labour progresses has been reported. Recent research (Shepherd et al., 2010) shows medium positive correlation between its length and both cervical dilatation and station of the fetal head. Where the line is present, it may provide a useful guide of labour progress alongside other measures.

quadruple screening test   the most accurate screening test for assessing a woman's risk of a pregnancy complicated by fetal anomaly.

registrant   practitioner on the nursing and midwifery register.

restitution   untwisting of the fetal head to enable realignment of the head and shoulders in preparation for delivery of the shoulders and body.

rhesus negative   the diagnosis that the maternal blood does not have the rhesus factor or D antigen. Pregnant women with this blood status are offered prophylactic anti-D to prevent any future pregnancies resulting in a baby with haemolytic disorder of the newborn.

rhesus positive   the diagnosis that the maternal blood has the rhesus factor, also called the D antigen.

Rhombus of Michaelis   a diamond-shaped protrusion on the woman's lower back that becomes visible as the bones adjust to allow the baby's further descent into the pelvis. It is most visible when the mother leans forward and reaches her arms out. It can also be felt on the woman's back as a curved area of tissue just below her waist. A woman may suddenly grasp both sides of the back of her pelvis as the ilea are pushed out and she is suddenly aware of those muscles that have never been stretched before.

risk   the chance of a negative event happening; in midwifery each pregnancy is categorised as low or high risk, based on the maternal medical, social and obstetric history and current pregnancy events. Almost every human activity has some risk attached; pregnancy is considered more risky for some women than for others, but remember that the absolute risk of some negative event happening in the UK is small.

salutogenesis   the study of well-being in times of stress; can be applied to midwifery to promote well-being during the 'uncertain' period of pregnancy, with all the decisions and choices experienced by women and their partners.

screening   a strategy used to detect diseases in populations; all pregnant women are offered screening tests, from blood pressure measurements to ultrasound scans. If on screening a test result is not as expected, diagnostic tests can be offered.

screening test   a specific programme that screens for a certain disease, such as chlamydia in the under 25s or the newborn blood spot for all neonates, which screens for five conditions.

sickle cell anaemia   an inherited condition where the red blood cells are characteristically hard and sickle shaped, thus affecting their ability to transport oxygen in times of stress.

sonicaid or Doppler device   electronic instrument using ultrasound waves to auscultate the heart.

statutory   regulated by law, in this case the professional regulatory body for midwifery, the Nursing and Midwifery Council (NMC).

symphysis-fundal height (SFH)   the measurement from the top of the uterus (fundus) to the pubic bone (symphysis pubis). Used as a screening tool to detect small or large fetal growth in utero from 24 weeks gestation.

thalassaemia   an inherited condition where there is a reduced rate of making haemoglobin, causing anaemia in varying degrees.

transitional phase of labour   a phase that occurs towards the end of the first phase of labour; contractions become expulsive and the woman's behaviour changes – she may feel she cannot go on and often asks for pain relief. This phase usually lasts 15 to 20 minutes just before the woman wishes to bear down.

triple screening test   a second trimester screening test offered to women after 13 weeks gestation; the test compares three results to give a risk that a woman is pregnant with a fetus with Down's syndrome.

ultrasound   a medical imaging technique able to 'visualise' internal organs, including the developing fetus.

vertex   the highest point of the fetal skull. It lies on the sagittal suture midway between the parietal eminence. The tempo vertex is also used to describe an area bounded by the anterior and posterior fontanelles and the parietal eminences.

vitamin K prophylaxis   administration of a dose of vitamin K to newborn babies to prevent them from having haemorrhagic disorders of the newborn, a rare bleeding disorder. It is offered throughout the UK and many parts of the globe routinely, but considered to be controversial and unnecessary by some.

References

AIMS (2012) Top ten tips for what women want from their midwives. *Essentially MIDIRS*, 3(3): 27–31.

Alfirevic, Z and Gould, D (2006) Immersion in water during labour and birth. Royal College of Obstetricians and Gynaecologists/Royal College of Midwives – Joint statement No. 1. Available from: www.rcog.org.uk/index.asp?PageID=546.

Alfirevic, Z, Devane, D and Gyte, GM (2006) Continuous cardiotocography (CTG) as a form of electronic fetal monitoring (EFM) for fetal assessment during labour. *Cochrane Database of Systematic Reviews*, Issue 3.Art.No.:CD006066.DOI: 10.1002/14651858.CD006066.

Anderson, T (2010) Feeling safe enough to let go: the relationship between a woman and her midwife in the second stage of labour, in Kirkham, M (ed.) *The midwife-woman relationship*, 2nd edition. Basingstoke: Palgrave Macmillan.

Antonovsky, A (1996) The salutogenic model as a theory to guide health promotion. *Health Promotion International*, 11(1): 11–18.

Arora, S, Vatsa, M and Dadhwal, V (2008) A comparison of cabbage leaves *vs* hot and cold compresses in the treatment of breast engorgement. *Indian Journal of Community Medicine*, 33: 160–162.

Aylott, M (2006) The neonatal energy triangle. Part 1: Metabolic adaptation. *Paediatric Nursing*, 18(6): 38–42.

Bates, C (1997) *Debating midwifery: normality in midwifery*. London: Royal College Midwives.

Beake, S, Rose, V, Bick, B, Weavers, A and Wray, J (2010) A qualitative study of the experiences and expectations of women receiving in-patient postnatal care in one English maternity unit. *BMC Pregnancy and Childbirth*, 10(70): 1471.

Beauchamp, T and Childress, J (2008) *Principles of biomedical ethics*, 6th edition. Oxford: Oxford University Press.

Bergman, N (2008) Breastfeeding in perinatal neuroscience, in Genna, CW (ed.) *Supporting suckling skills in breastfeeding infants*. London: Jones and Bartlett.

Blackburn, ST (2007) Maternal, fetal and neonatal physiology: a clinical perspective, 3rd edition. St Louis MO: Saunders.

Blair, P, Mitchell, E, Heckstall-Smith, M and Fleming, PJ (2008) Head covering – a major modifiable risk factor for sudden infant death syndrome: a systematic review. *Archives of Disease in Childhood*, 93(9): 778–783.

Blix, E, Reinar, LM, Klovning, A and Øian, P (2005) Prognostic value of the labour admission test and its effectiveness compared with auscultation only: a systematic review. *BJOG: An International Journal of Obstetrics and Gynaecology*, 112: 1595–1604.

BOC (British Oxygen Company) (2010) Emergency services. Available at: www.boconline.co.uk/products/products_by_industry/emergency_services.asp (accessed 21 November 2011).

Brealey, S, Hewitt, C, Green, J, Morrell, J, and Gilbody, S (2010) Screening for postnatal depression: is it acceptable to women and healthcare professionals? A systematic review and meta-analysis. *Journal of Reproductive and Infant Psychology*, 28(4): 328–344.

Bruggemann, O, Parpinelli, M, Osis, M, Cecatti, J and Neto, ASC (2007) Support to woman by a companion of her choice during childbirth: a randomized controlled trial. *Reproductive Health*, 4: 5.

Bryar, R and Sinclair, M (2011) *Theory for midwifery practice*, 2nd edition. Basingstoke: Palgrave Macmillan.

Carper, B. (1978) Fundamental patterns of knowing in nursing. *ANS: Advances in Nursing Science*, 1(1): 13–23.

Carter, C S (2003) Developmental consequences of oxytocin. *Physiology Behavior*, 79(3): 383–397.

Cash, R, Manogaran, M, Sroka, H and Okun, N (2010) An assessment of women's knowledge of and views on the reporting of ultrasound soft markers during the routine anatomy ultrasound examination. *Journal of Obstetrics and Gynaecology Canada*, 32(2): 120–125.

Champion, P (2010) Nourishment for birth. *Essentially MIDIRS*, 1(1): 39–42.

Chin, R, Daiches, A and Hall, P (2011) A qualitative exploration of first-time fathers experiences if becoming a father. *Community Practitioner*, 84(7): 19–23.

Cluett, ER, Nikodem, VC, McCandlish, R and Burns, E (2004) Immersion in water in pregnancy, labour and birth (Cochrane Review). *The Cochrane Library*, Issue 2. Available at: www.cochrane.org/cochrane/revabstr/AB000111.htm.

CMACE (2011) Saving mothers' lives: reviewing maternal deaths to make motherhood safer: 2006–08. The Eighth Report on Confidential Enquiries into Maternal Deaths in the United Kingdom. *British Journal of Obstetrics and Gynaecology*, 118 (Supplement 1): 1–203.

CMACE and RCOG (2010) *Management of women with obesity in pregnancy*. London: Centre for Maternal and Child Enquiries (CMACE) and Royal College of Obstetricians and Gynaecologists (RCOG).

Coad, J (2005) *Anatomy and physiology for midwives*. 2nd edition. Edinburgh: Mosby.

Colson, S (2000) Womb to world: a metabolic perspective. Available at: www.midwiferytoday.com/articles/womb.asp.

Colson, S (2005) Bringing nature to the fore. *The Practising Midwife*, 8(11): 2–6.

Colson, S (2007) Biological nurturing. (2) The physiology of lactation revisited. *The Practising Midwife*, 10(10): 14–19.

Colson, S (2010) *An introduction to biological nurturing: new angles on breastfeeding*. Amarillo TX: Hale Publishing.

Cornblath, M, Hawdon, JM, Williams, AF, Aynsley-Green, A, Ward-Platt, MP, Schwartz R and Kalhan, SC (2000) Controversies regarding definition of neonatal hypoglycemia: suggested operational thresholds. *Pediatrics*, 105(5): 1141–1145.

Crowther, C, Enkin, M, Keirse, M and Brown, I (2000) Monitoring progress in labour, in Enkin, M, Keirse, M, Neilson J, Crowther, C, Duley, L, Hodnett, E and Hofmeyr, J (eds) *A guide to effective care in pregnancy and childbirth*, 3rd edition. Oxford: Oxford University Press.

Crowther, S (2010) Blood tests for investigating maternal wellbeing. 2. Testing for anaemia in pregnancy. *The Practising Midwife*, 13(10): 48–52.

Czank, C, Henderson, J and Kent, J (2007) Hormonal control of the lactation cycle, in Hale, T and Hartmann, P (eds) *Textbook of human lactation*. Amarillo TX: Hale Publishing.

Dabrowski, R (2011) The future of postnatal care. *Midwives*. Online RCM magazine. Available at: www.rcm.org.uk/midwives/news/the-future-of-postnatal-care/.

Davies, L (2011a) Care in the postnatal period. Part 1. *Essentially MIDIRS*, 2(10): 38–42.

Davies, L. (2011b) Is vaginal examination in normal labour essential? *MIDIRS* 2(4): 38–42.

Deery, R (2005) An action-research study exploring midwives' support needs and the affect of group clinical supervision. *Midwifery*, 21(2): 161–165.

Devane, D, Lalor, JG, Daly, S, McGuire, W and Smith, V (2012) Comparing electronic monitoring of the baby's heartbeat on a woman's admission in labour using cardiotocography (CTG) with intermittent monitoring. *Cochrane Database of Systematic Reviews 2012*, Issue 2. Art. No.: CD005122. DOI: 10.1002/14651858.CD005122.pub4.

DH (Department of Health) (1998) *Vitamin K for newborn babies*. Ref No PL/CMO/98/3 PL/CNO/98/4. London: Department of Health

DH (2004) *National service framework for children, young people and maternity services*. London: Department of Health.

DH (2006) *NHS maternity statistics, England: 2004–05*. London: The Information Centre, Community Health Statistics. Available at: www.ic.nhs.uk/pubs/maternityeng2005.

DH (2007a) *Maternity matters: choice access and continuity of care in a safe service*. London: Department of Health.

DH (2007b) *Women's experiences of maternity care in the NHS in England*. London: Department of Health.

DH (2009) *The pregnancy book*. London: Department of Health.

DH (2010) *Survey of women's experiences of maternity services 2010*. London: Quality Care Commission.

Dixon, L, Fullerton, JT, Begley, C, Kennedy, H and Guilliland, K (2011) Systematic review: the clinical effectiveness of physiological (expectant) management of the third stage of labour following a physiological labor and birth. *International Journal of Childbirth* 1(3): 179–195.

Dodwell, M and Newburn, M (2010) *Normal birth as a measure of the quality of care: evidence on safety, effectiveness and women's experiences*. London: NCT.

Downe, S (2008) *Normal childbirth, evidence and debate*, 2nd edition. London: Churchill Livingstone Elsevier.

Downe, S and McCourt, C (2008) From being to becoming: reconstructing childbirth knowledge, in Downe, S (ed.) *Normal childbirth: evidence and debate*, 2nd edition. Edinburgh: Churchill Livingston.

Draycott, T, Lewis, G and Stephens, I (2011) Executive summary; Centre for Maternal and Child Enquiries (CMACE). *BJOG* 118(Suppl.1): e12–e21.

Edwards, N (2000) Women planning all births: the war news on the relationships with the midwives, in Kirkham, M (ed.) *The midwife-mother relationship*. London: Macmillan.

England, P and Horowitz, R (2007) *Birthing from within: an extra ordinary guide to childbirth preparation*. London: Souvenir Press.

Enkin, M, Keirse, MJNC, Renfrew, M and Neilson, J (2000) *A guide to effective care in pregnancy and childbirth*, 3rd edition. Oxford: Oxford University Press.

Everett-Murphy, K, Paijmans, J, Steyn, K, Matthews, C, Emmelin, M and Peterson, Z (2011) Scolders, carers or friends: South African midwives' contrasting styles of communication when discussing smoking cessation with pregnant women. *Midwifery*, 27(4): 517–524.

Fahy, K, Hastie, C, Bisits, A, Marsh, C, Smith, L and Saxton, A (2010) Holistic physiological care compared with active management of the third stage of labour for women at low risk of postpartum haemorrhage: a cohort study. *Women and Birth*, 23: 146–152.

Faure, M (2011) *The baby sense secret*. London: Penguin Books.

Feinstein, NF, Sprague, A and Trepanier, MJ (2000) Fetal heart rate auscultation: comparing auscultation to electronic monitoring. *AWHONN Lifelines*, 4(3): 35–44.

Fraser, D. and Cooper, M (eds) (2009) *Myles' textbook for midwives*, 15th edition. London: Churchill Livingstone.

Geddes, D (2007) Gross anatomy of the lactating breast, in Hale, T and Hartmann, P (eds) *Textbook of human lactation*. Amarillo TX: Hale Publishing.

Gibbon, K (2010) It's more than just talking. *Midwives*, 2: 36–37.

Gould, D (2011) Negative attitudes and behaviours are eroding our professional status. *British Journal of Midwifery* 19(10): 618.

Green, J, Coupland, V and Kitzinger, J (1998) *Great expectations: a prospective study of women's expectations and experiences of childbirth*. Hale: Books for Midwives Press.

Green, J, Spiby, H, Hucknall, C and Richardson Foster, H (2011) Converting the policy into care: women's satisfaction with the early labour telephone component of the All Wales Clinical Pathway for Normal Labour. *Journal of Advanced Nursing* doi: 10.1111/j.1365–2648.2011.05906.x.

Gunn, J (2010) Blood tests for investigating maternal wellbeing (3). Blood group and red blood cell antibody screening. *The Practising Midwife*, 13(11): 46–49.

Hackshaw, A, Rodeck, C and Boniface, S (2011) Maternal smoking in pregnancy and birth defects; a systematic review based on 173,687 malformed cases and 11.7 million controls. *Human Reproductive Update*, 17(5): 589–604.

Hall, J (2010) Midwifery basics: Blood tests for investigating maternal wellbeing. *The Practising Midwife*, 13(9): 40–42.

Hargreaves, K, Cameron, M, Edwards, H, Gray, R and Deane, K (2011) Is the use of symphysis-fundal height measurement and ultrasound examination effective in detecting small or large fetuses? *Journal of Obstetrics and Gynaecology*, 31(5): 380–383.

Hatem, M, Sandall, J, Devane, D, Soltani, H and Gates, S (2008) Midwife-led versus other models of care for childbearing women. *Cochrane Database of Systematic Reviews*, 4. Art. No.: CD004667. DOI:10.1002/14651858.CD004667.pub2.

Hey, E (2003) Vitamin K: can we improve on nature? *MIDIRS Midwifery Digest* 13(1): 7–12.

Hodnett, ED, Gates, S, Hofmeyr, GJ, Sakala, C and Weston, J (2011) Continuous support for women during childbirth. *Cochrane Database of Systematic Reviews* (2),art.no.CD003766,pub.3. http://onlinelibrary.wiley.com/o/cochrane/clsysrev/articles/CD003766/frame.html.

Hollowell J, Puddicombe D, Rowe, R, Linsell, L, Hardy, P, Stewart, M et al. (2011) *The birthplace national prospective cohort study: perinatal and maternal outcomes by planned place of birth*. Birthplace in England research programme. Final report part 4. NIHR Service Delivery and Organisation programme; 2011.

Hunter, B (2004) The importance of emotional intelligence. *British Journal of Midwifery*, 12(10): 604–606.

ICM (International Confederation of Midwives) (2011) ICM *International definition of the midwife*. The Hague, Netherlands: ICM.

Inch, S (2009) Infant feeding, in Fraser, D and Cooper, M (eds) *Myles' textbook for midwives*, 15th edition. Edinburgh: Churchill Livingstone.

Johnson, R and Taylor, W (2010) *Skills for midwifery practice*, 3rd edition. Edinburgh: Churchill Livingstone.

Jones, E and Spencer, S (2008) Optimising the provision of human milk in preterm infants. *MIDIRS Midwifery Digest*, 18(1): 118–121.

Jordan, S (2010) *Pharmacology for midwives: the evidence base for safe practice*, 2nd edition. Basingstoke: Palgrave Macmillan.

Keeling, J and Mason, T (2011) Postnatal disclosure of domestic violence; comparison with disclosure in the first trimester of pregnancy. *Journal of Clinical Nursing*, 20(1–2): 103–110.

Kemp, J and Sandall, J (2010) Normal birth, magical birth: the role of the 36-week birth talk in caseload midwifery practice. *Midwifery*, 26(2): 211–221.

Lamaze International (2012) The Lamaze approach to birth. Available at: www.lamaze.org

Leap, N (2012) The power of words revisited. *Essentially MIDIRS*, 3(1): 17–20.

Leap, N, Dodwell, M and Newburn, M (2010a) Working with pain in labour: an overview of evidence. *New Digest*, 49: 22–26.

Leap, N, Sandall, J, Buckland, S and Huber, U (2010b) Journey to confidence: women's experiences of pain in labour and relational continuity of care. *Journal of Midwifery and Women's Health*, 55(3): 234–242.

Leslie, K and Arulkumaran, S (2011) Intrapartum fetal surveillance. *Obstetrics, Gynaecology and Reproductive Medicine*, 21(3): 59–67.

Lewis, L (2011) Postnatal clinics: the way forward? *Essentially MIDIRS*, 2(6): 32–36.

Lindgren, HE, Brink, A and Klinberg-Allvin, M (2011) Fear causes tears; perineal injuries and home birth settings. A Swedish interview study. *BMC pregnancy and childbirth*, 11(6).

Mainstone, A (2004) The use of Doppler in fetal heart rate monitoring. *British Journal of Midwifery*, 12(2): 78–83.

Mandruzzato, G, Alfirevic, Z Chervernak, F, Gruenebaum, A, Heimstad, R, Heinonen, S, Levene, M, Salvesen, K, Saugstad, O, Skupski, D and Thilaganathan, B (2010) Guidelines for the management of postterm pregnancy. *Journal of Perinatal Medicine* 38(2): 111–120.

Marmott, M. (2001) *Fair society, healthy lives: the Marmott Review*. London Health Observatory.

McCandlish, R, Bowler, U and van Asten, H (1998) A randomised controlled trial of care of the perineum during second stage of normal labour. *British Journal of Obstetrics and Gynaecology*, 105(12): 1262–1272.

Medforth, J, Battersby, S, Evans, M, Marsh, B and Walker, A (2006) *Oxford handbook of midwifery*. Oxford: Oxford University Press.

Mehrabian, A (1971) *Silent messages*. Belmont CA: Wadsworth.

MHRA (Medicines and Healthcare Products Regulatory Agency) (2011) Midwives: exemptions. Available at: www.mhra.gov.uk/Howweregulate/Medicines/Availabilityprescribingsellingandsupplyingofmedicines/ExemptionsfromMedicinesActrestrictions/Midwives/index.htm.

Midwifery 2020 (2010) *Core role of the midwife workstream. Final report*. London: Midwifery 2020.

Moore, E, Anderson, G and Bergman, N (2009) Early skin to skin contact for mothers and their healthy newborn infants. *Cochrane Database Systematic Reviews* Issue 3. Art. No.: CD003519. DOI: 10.1002/14651858.CD003519.pub2.

NCT (National Childbirth Trust) (2006) Creating a better birth environment tool kit. Available at: www.nct.org.uk/professional/birth-environment.

NCT (2010) Left to your own devices: the postnatal care experiences of 1260 first-time mothers. London: NCT.

NICE (National Institute for Health and Clinical Excellence) (2006) *Routine postnatal care of mothers and their babies*. London: NICE.

NICE (2007a) *Antenatal and postnatal mental health guidance*. London: NICE.

NICE (2007b) *Clinical Guideline 55 Intrapartum care*. London: NICE.

NICE (2008a) *Antenatal care: routine care for the healthy pregnant woman*. London: RCOG Press.

NICE (2008b) *Improving the nutrition of pregnant and breastfeeding mothers and children in low-income households*. London: NICE.

NICE (2008c) *Induction of labour*. London: NICE.

NICE (2008d) Preg*nancy (rhesus negative women): routine anti-D*. London: NICE.

NICE (2010a) *Dietary interventions and physical activity interventions for weight management before, during and after pregnancy*. London: NICE.

NICE (2010b) *Quitting smoking in pregnancy and following childbirth*. London: NICE.

NICE (2010c) *Weight management before, during and after pregnancy*. London: NICE.

NICE (2011) *Caesarean section*. London: NICE.

Nissen, E, Uvana-Moberg, K and Svensson, K (1996) Different patterns of oxytocin, prolactin but not cortisol release during breastfeeding in women delivered by caesarean section or by the vaginal route. *Early Human Development*, 45: 103–118.

NMC (Nursing and Midwifery Council) (2004a) *Midwives rules and standards*. London, NMC.

NMC (2004b) *Guidelines for records and record keeping*. London: NMC.

NMC (2007) *Standards for the supervised practice of midwives*. London, NMC.

NMC (2008a) *The code: standards of conduct, performance and ethics for nurses and midwives*. London, NMC.

NMC (2008b) *Standards for medicines management*. Full content/summary booklet and DVD. London: Nursing and Midwifery Council.

NMC (2009) *Standards for pre-registration midwifery education*. London: NMC.

NMC (2011) Changes to midwives exemptions. Circular 07/2011 Nursing and Midwifery Council. Available at: www.nmc-uk.org/Documents/Circulars/2011Circulars/nmcCircular07-2011-Midwives-Exemptions.pdf.

Noel, GL, Suh, HK and Frantz, AG (1974) Prolactin release during nursing and breast stimulation in postpartum and nonpostpartum subjects. *Journal of Clinical Endocrinology and Metabolism*. March, 38(3): 413–423.

Nolan, M and Smith, J (2010) Women's experiences of following advice to stay at home in early labour. *British Journal of Midwifery*, 18(5): 286–291.

NPSA (National Patient Safety Agency (2009) *Safety in doses – medication safety – incidents in the NHS*, 4th report from Patient Safety Observatory. London: NPSA

NSC (Newborn Screening Centre) (2011) Website. Available at: http://newbornbloodspot.screening.nhs.uk/aboutus (accessed 29 December 2011).

Odent, M (2002) The first hour following birth. *Midwifery Today*, 61. Available at: www.midwiferytoday.com/articles/firsthour.asp.

Parboteeah, S (2011) Administration of medicines, in Hodgson, R and Marjoram, B (eds) *Foundations of nursing practice: themes, concepts and frameworks*. Basingstoke: Palgrave Macmillan.

Pollard, M (2012) Evidence-based care for breastfeeding mothers: a resource for midwives and allied healthcare professionals. London: Routledge.

Pollock, K (2011) How midwives' discursive practices contribute to the maintenance of the status quo in English maternity care. *Midwifery*, 27(5): 612–619.

Puckett, RM and Offringa, M (2000) Prophylactic vitamin K for vitamin K deficiency bleeding in neonates. *Cochrane Database of Systematic Reviews* 2000, Issue 4. Art. No.: CD002776. DOI: 10.1002/14651858. CD002776, accessed 1 January 2012.

Rattray, J, Flowers, K, Miles, S and Clarke, J (2011) Foetal monitoring: a woman-centred decision-making pathway. *Women and Birth*, 24: 65–71.

RCM (Royal College of Midwives) (2008) Evidence-based guidelines for midwifery-led care in labour. London: RCM. Available online through the RCM website: www.rcm.org.uk

RCM (2010) *The Royal College of Midwives' audit of midwifery practice*. London: RCM.

Redshaw, M, Rowe, R, Schroeder, L, Puddicombe, D, Macfarlane, A and Newburn, M (2011) Mapping maternity care. The configuration of maternity care in England. Birthplace in England research programme. Final report part 3. NIHR service delivery and Organisation programme 2011. Available at: www.sdo.nihr.ac.uk/projdetails.php?ref08-1604-140.

Resuscitation Council (2010) Newborn life support. Resuscitation Council UK. Available at: www.resus.org.uk.

Richmond, S and Wyllie, J (2010) Newborn life support in resuscitation guidelines. Resuscitation Council UK. Available at: www.resus.org.uk/pages/guide.htm#updates (accessed 12 December 2011).

Rimmer, A (2009) Prolonged pregnancy and disorders of uterine action, in Fraser, D and Cooper, M (eds) *Myles' text book for midwives*. Edinburgh: Churchill Livingstone.

Riordan, J and Wambach, K (2010) *Breast feeding and human lactation*, 4th edition. Boston MA: Jones Bartlett Publishers.

Robinson, M, Pennell, C, McLean, N, Oddy, W and Newham, J (2011) The over-estimation of risk in pregnancy. *Journal of Psychosomatic Obstetrics and Gynecology*, 32(2): 53–58.

Rogers, C (1986) Reflection of feelings. *Person-Centred Review*, 1(4): 375–377.

Sandall, J, Devane, D, Soltani, H, Hatem, M and Gates, S (2010) Improving quality and safety in maternity care: the contribution of midwife-led care. *Journal of Midwifery and Women's Health*, 55(3): 255–261.

Scammell, M. (2011) The swan effect in midwifery talk and practice: a tension between normality and the language of risk. *Sociology of Health and Illness*, 33(7): 987–1001.

Selo-Ojeme, D, Rogers, C, Mohanty, A, Zaidi, N, Villar, R and Shangaris, P (2011) Is induced labour in the nullipara associated with more maternal and perinatal morbidity? *Archives of Gynecology and Obstetrics*, 284(2): 337–341.

Shepherd, A, Cheyne, H, Kennedy, S, McIntosh, C, Styles, M and Niven, C (2010) The purple line as a measure of labour progress: a longitudinal study. *BMC Pregnancy and Childbirth*, 54: 1

Sheriden, V (2010) Organisational culture and routine midwifery practice on labour ward: implications for mother baby contact. *Evidence-based midwifery*, 8(3): 76–84.

Simkin, P and Ancheta, R (2011) *The labor progress handbook*, 3rd edition. Chichester: Wiley Blackwell.

Singata, M, Tranmer, J and Gyte, G (2010) Restricting oral fluid and food intake during labour. *Cochrane database of systematic reviews*, issue 1.

Skirton, H and Barr, O (2010) Antenatal screening and informed consent; a cross-sectional survey of parents and professionals. *Midwifery*, 26(6): 596–602.

Sparks, T, Cheung, Y, McLaughlin, B, Esakoff, TF and Caughey, AB (2011) Fundal height: a useful tool for fetal growth? *Journal of Maternal-Fetal and Neonatal Medicine*, 24(5): 708–712.

Stables, D and Rankin, J (2005) *Physiology in childbearing with anatomy and related biosciences*. London: Elsevier.

Theodosius, C (2008) *Emotional labour in health care: the unmanaged heart of nursing*. London: Routledge.

Tiran, D (2010) Avoiding the Chinese Whispers effect in maternity complimentary therapies: educational issues for midwives. *MIDIRS Midwifery Digest*, 20(1): 15–19.

UNICEF (2008) Guidance notes for implementing baby friendly initiative education standards: higher education institutions. London: UNICEF UK Baby Friendly Initiative. Available at: www.baby friendly.org.uk.

UNICEF (2010) The health professional's guide to: A guide to infant formula for parents who are bottle feeding. Available at: www.unicef.org.uk/BabyFriendly/Resources/Resources-for-parents/A-guide-to-infant-formula-for-parents-who-are-bottle-feeding/ (accessed 3 January 2012).

Walsh, D (2007) *Evidence-based care for normal labour and birth: a guide for midwives*. Oxford: Routledge.

Walsh, D (2012) *Evidence and skills for normal labour and birth: a guide for midwives*, 2nd edition. London: Routledge.

Ward-Platt, M and Deshpande, S (2005) Metabolic adaptations at birth. *Seminars in Fetal and Neonatal Medicine*. 10: 341–350.

WHO (World Health Organization) (1996) Care in normal birth: a practical guide. Available online at: http://whqlibdoc.who.int/hq/1996/WHO_FRH_MSM_96.24.pdf.

WHO (1997) Thermal protection of the newborn: a practical guide. Available at: www.who.int/reproductivehealth/publications/maternal_perinatal_health/MSM_97_2/en/index.html.

Wickham, S (2001) Vitamin K: a flaw in the blueprint. *Midwifery Today*, 56: 39–41.

Wilde, C, Addey, C, Boddy, L and Peaker, M (1995) Autocrine regulation of milk secretion by a protein in milk. *Biochemistry Journal*, 1(305): 51–58.

Wray, J. (2006) Postnatal care: Is it based on ritual or a purpose? A reflective account. *British Journal of Midwifery*, 14(9): 520–526.

Index

Engineering Fundamentals

Engineering Fundamentals

Roger Timings

Newnes

OXFORD AMSTERDAM BOSTON LONDON NEW YORK PARIS
SAN DIEGO SAN FRANCISCO SINGAPORE SYDNEY TOKYO

Newnes
An imprint of Elsevier Science
Linacre House, Jordan Hill, Oxford OX2 8DP
225 Wildwood Avenue, Woburn, MA 01801-2041

First published 2002

British Library Cataloguing in Publication Data
A catalogue record for this book is available from the British Library

ISBN 0 7506 5609 3

For information on all Newnes publications
visit our website at www.newnespress.com

Typeset by Laserwords Private Limited, Chennai, India.
Printed and bound in Great Britain by MPG Books Ltd, Bodmin, Cornwall

Contents

Preface

This book is designed to provide an accessible course in the basic engineering principles and applications required in a wide range of vocational courses. No prior knowledge of engineering is assumed.

I trust that *Engineering Fundamentals* will be found to be a worthy successor to my previous introductory books on general and mechanical engineering. As well as offering up-to-date best practice and technical information, this new title has been fully matched to the latest courses, in particular Level 2 NVQs within the Performing Engineering Operations scheme from EMTA and City & Guilds (scheme 2251). Guidance on the depth of treatment has been taken from the EMTA *Industry Standards of Competence* documents. EMTA are the NTO for the development of NVQs (the UK's National Vocational Qualifications) in all aspects of engineering.

All the chapters end with a selection of exercises. These will help with assessing the trainees' performance criteria for the underpinning knowledge and understanding that is an essential part of their training.

Finally, the author and publishers are grateful to Training Publications Ltd and Pearson Educational Ltd for allowing the reproduction and adaptation of their illustrations and material in this text.

Roger Timings

Acknowledgements

The author and publishers wish to thank the following organisations for permission to reproduce their copyright material:

British Standards Institution (BSI): Figures 1.6, 1.7, 1.8, 1.9, 1.32, 5.7, 5.8, 5.9, 5.10, 5.11, 5.12, 5.17, 5.33, 9.2, 9.8, 9.9, 9.10, 9.11, 9.12.

Cincinnati Milacron Ltd: Figure 11.2(c and d).

Myford Ltd: Figure 5.21.

Pearson Education Ltd: Figures 1.5, 1.12, 1.13, 1.14, 1.15, 1.17, 1.22, 1.25(b), 1.27, 1.29, 1.30, 1.31, 2.1, 2.2, 2.3, 3.1, 3.2, 3.3, 3.4, 3.5, 3.6, 3.7, 3.8, 4.1, 4.2, 4.3, 4.4, 4.5, 4.6, 4.7, 4.8, 4.11, 4.12, 4.13, 4.15, 4.17, 4.18, 4.19, 4.20, 4.21, 4.22, 4.23, 4.24, 4.25, 4.26, 5.1, 5.2, 5.3, 5.4, 5.5, 5.6, 5.13, 5.14, 5.15, 5.16, 5.18, 5.19, 5.20, 5.22, 5.23, 5.24, 5.27, 5.28, 5.29, 5.30, 5.31, 5.32, 5.24, 5.25, 5.26, 6.1, 6.4, 6.5, 6.8, 6.9, 6.10, 6.11, 6.12, 6.13, 6.14, 6.15, 6.16, 6.17, 6.19, 6.20, 6.21, 6.22, 6.23, 6.25, 6.26, 6.27, 6.28, 6.29, 6.30, 6.31, 6.32, 7.1, 7.5(a & b), 7.7, 7.8, 7.9, 7.11, 7.14, 7.15, 7.16, 7.17, 7.18, 7.19, 7.20, 7.22, 7.23, 7.24, 7.25, 7.26, 7.27, 7.28, 7.29, 7.30, 7.31, 7.32, 7.33, 8.1, 8.2, 8.3, 8.4, 8.5, 8.6, 8.7, 8.8, 8.9, 8.12, 8.13, 8.16, 8.17, 8.18, 8.19, 8.20, 8.21, 8.24, 8.26, 8.27, 8.28, 8.32, 8.33, 8.34, 8.35, 8.36, 8.37, 8.38, 8.39, 8.40, 8.41, 8.42, 87.43, 9.1, 9.3, 9.4, 9.5, 9.6, 9.7, 9.13, 9.14, 9.15, 9.16, 9.17, 9.18, 9.19, 9.29, 9.21, 9.22, 10.3, 10.4, 10.5, 10.6, 10.7, 10.8(a), 10.9(a), 10.10(a), 10.11, 10.13, 10.14, 10.16, 10.17, 10.18, 10.19, 10.20, 10.21, 10.22, 10.23, 10.24, 10.25, 10.26, 10.27, 10.28, 10.29, 10.30, 10.31, 10.32, 10.33, 10.34, 10.35, 10.36(b), 10.37, 10.38, 10.39, 10.40, 10.41, 10.42, 10.43, 10.44, 10.45, 10.46, 10.47, 10.48, 10.49, 10.50, 10.51, 10.52, 10.53, 10.54, 10.55, 10.56, 10.57, 10.58, 10.59, 11.4, 11.5, 11.6, 11.7, 11.8, 11.9, 11.10, 11.11, 11.12, 11.13, 11.14, 11.15, 11.23, 11.24, 11.25, 11.26, 11.27, 11.29, 11.30, 11.31, 11.32, 11.33, 11.34, 11.35, 11.36, 11.37, 12.1, 12.2, 12.3, 12.4, 12.6, 12.7, 12.8, 12.9, 12.10, 12.12, 12.13, 12.14, 12.15.

Richard Lloyd (Galtona) Ltd: Figure 11.3 (a and b).

Silvaflame Co. Ltd: Figures 10.1, 11.1(b).

Spear and Jackson plc (Moore and Wright, James Neil, Neil Magnetics): Figures 6.2, 6.3, 6.7, 6.18, 7.4, 7.6, 7.10, 12.16, 12.17, 12.18.

Training Publications Ltd: Figures 1.1, 1.2, 1.3, 1.4, 1.10, 1.11, 1.18, 1.19, 1.20, 1.21, 1.23, 1.24, 1.25(a), 1.26, 1.28, 1.33, 4.9, 4.16, 5.25, 5.26, 6.24, 7.2, 7.3, 7.5(c), 7.12, 7.13, 7.21, 8.10, 8.11, 8.14, 8.15, 8.22, 8.23, 8.25, 8.29, 8.30, 8.31, 10.12, 10.27, 11.16, 11.17, 11.18, 11.19, 11.20, 11.21(b), 11.22(b), 11.28, 12.11, 12.19, 12.20, 12.21.

WDS (Production Equipment) Ltd: Figures 10.15, 10.36(a), 11.21(a), 11.22(a), 12.5.

600 Group (Colchester Lathes): Figures 10.2, 10.25, 10.26.

1 General health and safety (engineering)

When you have read this chapter you should understand:

- The statutory requirements for general health and safety at work.
- Accident and first aid procedures.
- Fire precautions and procedures.
- Protective clothing and equipment.
- Correct manual lifting and carrying techniques.
- How to use lifting equipment.
- Safe working practices.

1.1 Health, safety and the law

1.1.1 Health and Safety at Work, etc. Act

It is essential to observe safe working practices not only to safeguard yourself, but also to safeguard the people with whom you work. The Health and Safety at Work, etc. Act provides a comprehensive and integrated system of law for dealing with the health, safety and welfare of workpeople and the general public as affected by industrial, commercial and associated activities.

The Act places the responsibility for safe working equally upon:

- the employer;
- the employee (that means you);
- the manufacturers and suppliers of materials, goods, equipment and machinery.

1.1.2 Health and Safety Commission

The Act provides for a full-time, independent chairman and between six and nine part-time commissioners. The commissioners are made up of three trade union members appointed by the TUC, three management members appointed by the CBI, two local authority members, and one independent member. The commission has taken over the responsibility previously held by various government departments for the control of most occupational health and safety matters. The commission is also responsible for the organization and functioning of the Health and Safety Executive.

1.1.3 Health and Safety Executive

The inspectors of the Health and Safety Executive (HSE) have very wide powers. Should an inspector find a contravention of one of the provisions of earlier Acts or Regulations still in force, or a contravention of the Health and Safety at Work, etc. Act, the inspector has three possible lines of action available.

Prohibition Notice

If there is a risk of serious personal injury, the inspector can issue a *Prohibition Notice*. This immediately stops the activity that is giving rise to the risk until the remedial action specified in the notice has been taken to the inspector's satisfaction. The prohibition notice can be served upon the person undertaking the dangerous activity, or it can be served upon the person in control of the activity at the time the notice is served.

Improvement Notice

If there is a legal contravention of any of the relevant statutory provisions, the inspector can issue an *Improvement Notice*. This notice requires the infringement to be remedied within a specified time. It can be served on any person on whom the responsibilities are placed. The latter person can be an employer, employee or a supplier of equipment or materials.

Prosecution

In addition to serving a Prohibition Notice or an Improvement Notice, the inspector can prosecute any person (including an employee – you) contravening a relevant statutory provision. Finally the inspector can seize, render harmless or destroy any substance or article which the inspector considers to be the cause of imminent danger or personal injury.

Thus every employee must be a fit and trained person capable of carrying out his or her assigned task properly and safely. Trainees must work under the supervision of a suitably trained, experienced worker or instructor. By law, every employee must:

- Obey all the safety rules and regulations of his or her place of employment.

- Understand and use, as instructed, the safety practices incorporated in particular activities or tasks.

- Not proceed with his or her task if any safety requirement is not thoroughly understood; guidance must be sought.

- Keep his or her working area tidy and maintain his or her tools in good condition.

- Draw the attention of his or her immediate supervisor or the safety officer to any potential hazard.

- Report all accidents or incidents (even if injury does not result from the incident) to the responsible person.

- Understand emergency procedures in the event of an accident or an alarm.

- Understand how to give the alarm in the event of an accident or an incident such as fire.

- Co-operate promptly with the senior person in charge in the event of an accident or an incident such as fire.

Therefore, safety, health and welfare are very personal matters for a young worker, such as yourself, who is just entering the engineering industry. This chapter sets out to identify the main hazards and suggests how they may be avoided. Factory life, and particularly engineering, is potentially dangerous and you must take a positive approach towards safety, health and welfare.

1.1.4 Further legislation and regulations concerning safety

In addition to the Health and Safety at Work, etc. Act, the following are examples of legislation and regulations that also control the conditions under which you work and the way in which you work (behaviour).

- Factories Act 1961

- Safety Representatives and Safety Committees Regulations 1977

- Notification of Accidents and General Occurrences Regulations 1980

- Management of Health and Safety at Work Regulations 1992

- Protection of Eyes Regulations 1974

- Electricity at Work Regulations 1989

- Low Voltage Electrical Equipment (Safety) Regulations 1989. This includes voltage ranges of 50 volts to 1000 volts (AC) and 75 volts to 1500 volts (DC)

- Abrasive Wheels Regulations 1970

- Noise at Work Regulations 1989

You are not expected to have a detailed knowledge of all this legislation, but you are expected to know of its existence, the main topic areas that it covers, and how it affects your working conditions, your responsibilities, and the way in which you work. There are many other laws and regulations that you will come across depending upon the branch of the engineering industry in which you work.

1.2 Employers' responsibilities

All employers must, by law, maintain a safe place to work. To fulfil all the legal obligations imposed upon them, employers must ensure that:

- The workplace must be provided with a safe means of access and exit so that in the case of an emergency (such as fire) no one will be trapped. This is particularly important when the workplace is not at ground level. Pedestrian access and exits should be segregated from lorries delivering materials or collecting finished work. The premises must be kept in good repair. Worn floor coverings and stair treads are a major source of serious falls.

- All plant and equipment must be safe so that it complies with the *Machinery Directive*. It must be correctly installed and properly maintained. The plant and any associated cutters and tools must also be properly guarded.

- Working practices and systems are safe and that, where necessary, protective clothing is provided.

- A safe, healthy and comfortable working environment is provided, and that the temperature and humidity is maintained at the correct levels for the work being undertaken.

- There is an adequate supply of fresh air, and that fumes and dust are either eliminated altogether or are reduced to an acceptable and safe level.

- There is adequate and suitable natural and artificial lighting, particularly over stairways.

- There is adequate and convenient provision for washing and sanitation.

- There are adequate first aid facilities under the supervision of a qualified person. This can range from a first aid box under the supervision of a person trained in basic first aid procedures for a small firm, to a full scale ambulance room staffed by professionally qualified medical personnel in a large firm.

- Provision is made for the safe handling, storing, siting, and transportation of raw materials, work in progress and finished goods awaiting delivery.

- Provision for the safe handling, storing, siting, transportation and use of dangerous substances such as compressed gases (e.g. oxygen and acetylene), and toxic and flammable solvents.

- There is a correct and legal system for the reporting of accidents and the logging of such accidents in the *accident register*.

- There is a company policy for adequate instruction, training and supervision of employees. This must not only be concerned with safety procedures but also with good working practices. Such instruction and training to be updated at regular intervals.

- There is a safety policy in force. This safety policy must be subject to regular review. One of the more important innovations of the Health and Safety at Work, etc. Act is contained in section 2(4) which provides for the appointment of safety representatives from amongst the employees, who will represent them in consultation with the employers, and have other prescribed functions.

- Where an employer receives a written request from at least two safety representatives to form a *safety committee* the employer shall, after consulting with the applicants and representatives of other recognized unions (if applicable) whose members work in the workplace concerned, establish a safety committee within the period of three months after the request. The employer must post a notice of the composition of the committee and the workplaces covered. The notice must be positioned where it may be easily read by the employees concerned.

- Membership of the safety committee should be settled by consultation. The number of management representatives should not exceed the number of safety representatives. Where a company doctor, industrial hygienist or safety officer/adviser is employed they should be ex-officio members of the committee.

- Management representation should be aimed at ensuring the necessary knowledge and expertise to provide accurate information on company policy, production needs and technical matters in relation to premises, processes, plant, machinery and equipment.

1.3 Employees' responsibilities

All employees (including you) are as equally responsible for safety as are their employers. Under the Health and Safety at Work, etc. Act, employees are expected to take reasonable care for their own health and safety together with the health and safety of other people with whom they work, and members of the public who are affected by the work being performed.

Further, the misuse of, or interference with, equipment provided by an employer for health and safety purposes is a criminal offence. It is up to all workers to develop a sense of *safety awareness* by following the example set by their instructors. Regrettably not all older workers observe the safety regulations as closely as they should. Take care who you choose for your 'role model'. The basic requirements for safe working are to:

- Learn the safe way of doing each task. This is usually the correct way.
- Use the safe way of carrying out the task in practice.
- Ask for instruction if you do not understand a task or have not received previous instruction.
- Be constantly on your guard against careless actions by yourself or by others.
- Practise good housekeeping at all times.
- Co-operate promptly in the event of an accident or a fire.
- Report all accidents to your instructor or supervisor.
- Draw your instructor's or your supervisor's attention to any potential hazard you have noticed.

1.4 Electrical hazards

The most common causes of electrical shock are shown in Fig. 1.1. The installation and maintenance of electrical equipment must be carried out only by a fully trained and registered electrician. The installation and equipment must conform to international standards and regulations as laid down in safety legislation and the codes of practice and regulations published by the Institution of Electrical Engineers (IEE).

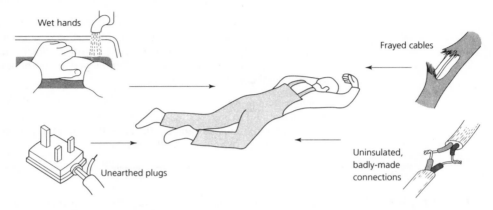

Figure 1.1 *Causes of electric shock*

An electric shock from a 240 volt single-phase supply (lighting and office equipment) or a 415 volt three-phase supply (most factory machines) can easily kill you. Even if the shock is not sufficiently severe to cause death, it can still cause serious injury. The sudden convulsion caused by the shock can throw you from a ladder or against moving machinery. To reduce the risk of shock, all electrical equipment should be earthed or double insulated. Further, portable power tools should be fed from a low-voltage transformer at 110 volts. The power tool must be suitable for operating at such a voltage. The transformer itself should be protected by a circuit breaker containing a residual current detector.

The fuses and circuit breakers designed to protect the supply circuitry to the transformer react too slowly to protect the user from electric shock. The electrical supply to a portable power tool should, therefore, be protected by a residual current detector (RCD). Such a device compares the magnitudes of the current flowing in the live and neutral conductors supplying the tool. Any leakage to earth through the body of the user or by any other route will upset the balance between these two currents. This results in the supply being immediately disconnected. The sensitivity of residual current detectors is such that a difference of only a few milliamperes is sufficient to cut off the supply and the time delay is only a few microseconds. Such a small current applied for such a short time is not dangerous.

In the event of rendering first aid to the victim of electrical shock, great care must be taken when pulling the victim clear of the fault which caused the shock. The victim can act as a conductor and thus, in turn, electrocute the rescuer. If the supply cannot be quickly and completely disconnected, always pull the victim clear by his or her clothing which, if dry, will act as an insulator. If in doubt, hold the victim with a plastic bag or cloth known to be dry. Never touch the victim's bare flesh until the victim is clear of the electrical fault. Artificial respiration must be started immediately the victim has been pulled clear of the fault or the live conductor.

1.5 Fire fighting

Fire fighting is a highly skilled operation and most medium and large firms have properly trained teams who can contain the fire locally until the professional brigade arrives. The best way you can help is to learn the correct fire drill, both how to give the alarm and how to leave the building. It requires only one person to panic and run in the wrong direction to cause a disaster.

In an emergency never lose your head and panic.

Smoke is the main cause of panic. It spreads quickly through a building, reducing visibility and increasing the risk of falls down stairways. It causes choking and even death by asphyxiation. Smoke is less dense near the floor: as a last resort crawl. To reduce the spread of smoke and fire, keep fire doors closed at all times but never locked. The plastic materials used in the finishes and furnishings of modern buildings give off highly toxic fumes. Therefore it is best to leave the building as quickly as possible and leave the fire fighting to the professionals who have breathing apparatus. *Saving human life is more important than saving property.*

If you do have to fight a fire there are some basic rules to remember. A fire is the rapid oxidation (burning) of flammable materials at relatively high temperatures. Figure 1.2 shows that removing the air (oxygen), or the flammable materials (fuel), or lowering the temperature will result in the fire ceasing to burn. It will go out. It can also be seen from Fig. 1.2 that different fires require to be dealt with in different ways.

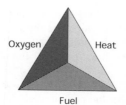

Oxygen — Heat

Fuel

The 3 essentials to start a fire

Note: Once the fire has started it produces sufficient heat to maintain its own combustion reactions and sufficient surplus heat to spread the fire

Remove heat

When solids are on fire remove heat by applying water

Remove oxygen

Liquids, such as petrol etc. on fire can be extinguished by removing oxygen with a foam or dry powder extinguisher

Remove fuel

Electrical or gas fires can usually be extinguished by turning off the supply of energy

Figure 1.2 *How to remove each of the three items necessary to start a fire. (Note: Once the fire has started it produces sufficient heat to maintain its own combustion reaction and sufficient surplus heat to spread the fire)*

1.5.1 Fire extinguishers

The normally available fire extinguishers and the types of fire they can be used for are as follows.

Water

Used in large quantities water reduces the temperature and puts out the fire. The steam generated also helps to smother the flames as it displaces the air and therefore the oxygen essential to the burning process. However, for various technical reasons, water should be used only on burning solids such as wood, paper and some plastics. A typical hose point and a typical pressurized water extinguisher is shown in Fig. 1.3.

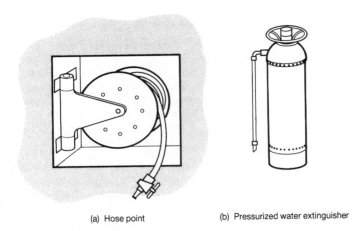

(a) Hose point   (b) Pressurized water extinguisher

Figure 1.3 *Hose point (a) and pressurized water extinguisher (b)*

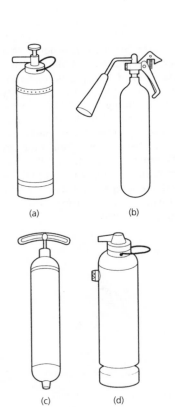

(a)   (b)

(c)   (d)

Figure 1.4 *Fire extinguishers: (a) foam; (b) CO₂; (c) vaporizing liquid; (d) dry powder*

Foam extinguishers

These are used for fighting oil and chemical fires. The foam smothers the flames and prevents the oxygen in the air from reaching the burning materials at the seat of the fire. Water alone cannot be used because oil floats on the water and this spreads the area of the fire. A typical foam extinguisher is shown in Fig. 1.4(a).

Note: Since both water and foam are electrically conductive, do not use them on fires associated with electrical equipment or the person wielding the hose or the extinguisher will be electrocuted.

Carbon dioxide (CO_2) extinguishers

These are used on burning gases and vapours. They can also be used for oil and chemical fires in confined places. The carbon dioxide gas replaces the air and smothers the fire. It can be used only in confined places, where it cannot be displaced by draughts.

Note: If the fire cannot breathe neither can you, so care must be taken to evacuate all living creatures from the vicinity before operating the extinguisher. Back away from the bubble of CO_2 gas as you operate the extinguisher, do not advance towards it. Figure 1.4(b) shows a typical CO_2 extinguisher.

Vaporizing liquid extinguishers

These include CTC, CBM and BCF extinguishers. The heat from the fire causes rapid vaporization of the liquid sprayed from the extinguisher and this vapour displaces the air and smothers the fire. Since a small amount of liquid produces a very large amount of vapour, this is a very efficient way of producing the blanketing vapour. Any vapour that will smother the fire will also smother all living creatures which must be evacuated before using such extinguishers. As with CO_2 extinguishers always back away from the bubble of vapour, never advance into it. Vaporizing liquid extinguishers are suitable for oil, gas, vapour and chemical fires. Like CO_2 extinguishers, vaporizing liquid extinguishers are safe to use on fires associated with electrical equipment. A typical example of a vaporizing liquid extinguisher is shown in Fig. 1.4(c).

Dry powder extinguishers

These are suitable for small fires involving flammable liquids and small quantities of solids such as paper. They are also useful for fires in electrical equipment, offices and kitchens since the powder is not only non-toxic, it can be easily removed by vacuum cleaning and there is no residual mess. The active ingredient is powdered sodium bicarbonate (baking powder) which gives off carbon dioxide when heated. A typical example of a dry powder extinguisher is shown in Fig. 1.4(d).

1.5.2 General rules governing the use of portable extinguishers

- Since fire spreads quickly, a speedy attack is essential if the fire is to be contained.
- Sound the alarm immediately the fire is discovered.
- Send for assistance before attempting to fight the fire.
- Remember
  (a) Extinguishers are provided to fight only small fires.
  (b) Take up a position between the fire and the exit, so that your escape cannot be cut off.
  (c) *Do not* continue to fight the fire if
     (i) it is dangerous to do so
     (ii) there is any possibility of your escape route being cut off by fire, smoke, or collapse of the building

      (iii)   the fire spreads despite your efforts

      (iv)   toxic fumes are being generated by the burning of plastic furnishings and finishes

      (v)   there are gas cylinders or explosive substances in the vicinity of the fire.

If you have to withdraw, close windows and doors behind you wherever possible, but not if such actions endanger your escape. Finally, ensure that all extinguishers are recharged immediately after use.

1.6 Fire precautions and prevention

1.6.1 Fire precautions

It is the responsibility of employers and their senior management (duty of care) to ensure the safety of their employees in the event of fire. The following precautions should be taken.

- Ensure ease of exit from the premises at all times – emergency exits must not be locked or obstructed.

- Easy access for fire appliances from the local brigade.

- Regular inspection of the plant, premises and processes by the local authority fire brigade's fire prevention officer. No new plant or processes involving flammable substances should be used without prior notification and inspection by the fire prevention officer.

- The above point also applies to the company's insurance inspector.

- Regular and frequent fire drills must be carried out and a log kept of such drills including the time taken to evacuate the premises. A roll call of all persons present should be taken immediately the evacuation is complete. A meeting of the safety committee should be called as soon as possible after a fire drill to discuss any problems, improve procedures and to learn lessons from the exercise.

1.6.2 Fire prevention

Prevention is always better than cure, and fire prevention is always better than fire fighting. Tidiness is of paramount importance in reducing the possibility of outbreaks of fire. Fires have small beginnings and it is usually amongst accumulated rubbish that many fires originate. So you should make a practice of constantly removing rubbish, shavings, off-cuts, cans, bottles, waste paper, oily rags, and other unwanted materials to a safe place at regular intervals. Discarded foam plastic packing is not only highly flammable, but gives off highly dangerous toxic fumes when burnt.

    Highly flammable materials should be stored in specially designed and equipped compounds away from the main working areas. Only minimum quantities of such materials should be allowed into the workshop at a time,

and then only into *non-smoking zones*. The advice of the local authority
fire brigade's fire prevention officer should also be sought.

It is good practice to provide metal containers with air-tight hinged lids
with proper markings as to the type of rubbish they should contain since
some types of rubbish will ignite spontaneously when mixed. The lids
of the bins should be kept closed so that, if a fire starts, it will quickly
use up the air in the bin and go out of its own accord without doing any
damage.

1.7 Accidents

Accidents do not happen, they are caused. There is not a single accident
that could not have been prevented by care and forethought on somebody's part. Accidents can and must be prevented. They cost millions of
lost man-hours of production every year, but this is of little importance
compared with the immeasurably cost in human suffering.

In every eight-hour shift nearly one hundred workers are the victims
of industrial accidents. Many of these will be blinded, maimed for life,
or confined to a hospital bed for months. At least two of them will die.
Figure 1.5 shows the main causes of accidents.

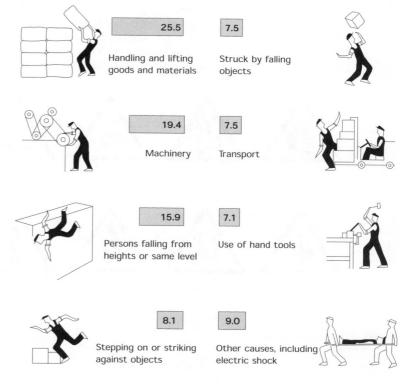

Figure 1.5 *Average national causes of industrial accidents (by per cent of all accidents)*

1.7.1 Accident procedure

You must learn and obey the accident procedures for your company.

- Report all accidents, no matter how small and trivial they seem, to your supervisor, instructor or tutor. Record your report and details of the incident on an accident form.
- Receive first-aid treatment from a *qualified* person, or your company's medical centre, depending upon the size of your company and its policy.

It is important that you follow the procedures laid down by your company since the accident register has to be produced on request by any HSE inspector visiting your company. Failure to log all accidents is an offence under the Health and Safety at Work, etc. Act and can lead to prosecution in the courts. Also if at some future date you had to seek compensation as a result of the accident, your report is important evidence.

1.7.2 Warning signs and labels

You must be aware of the warning signs and their meanings. You must also obey such signs. To disregard them is an offence under the Health and Safety at Work, etc. Act. Warning signs are triangular in shape and all the sides are the same length. The background colour is *yellow* and there is a *black* border. In addition to warning signs there are also *warning labels*. Figure 1.6 shows some typical warning signs and warning labels. It also gives their meanings.

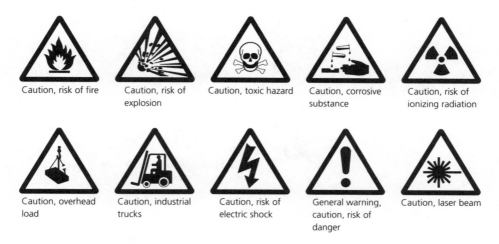

Figure 1.6 *Warning signs*

Prohibition signs

You can recognize these signs as they have a red circular band and a red crossbar on a white background. Figure 1.7 shows five typical prohibition

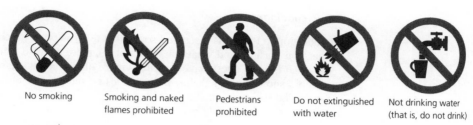

Figure 1.7 *Prohibition signs*

signs. These signs indicate activities that are *prohibited* at all times. They *must be obeyed*, you have no option in the matter. To disregard them is an offence in law, as you would be putting yourself and others at considerable risk.

Mandatory signs

You can recognize these signs as they have a blue background colour. The symbol must be white. Figure 1.8 shows five typical mandatory signs. These signs indicate things that *you must do* and precautions that *you must take*. These signs *must be obeyed*, you have no option in the matter. To disregard them is an offence in law as, again, you would be putting yourself at considerable risk.

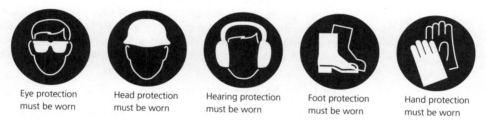

Figure 1.8 *Mandatory signs*

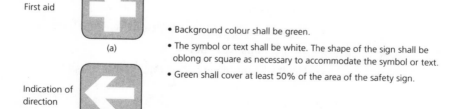

First aid

(a)

Indication of direction

(b)

- Background colour shall be green.
- The symbol or text shall be white. The shape of the sign shall be oblong or square as necessary to accommodate the symbol or text.
- Green shall cover at least 50% of the area of the safety sign.

Figure 1.9 *Safe condition signs*

Safe condition signs

In addition to the signs discussed so far that tell you what to look out for, what you must do and what you must not do, there are also signs that tell you what is safe. These have a white symbol on a green background. The example shown in Fig. 1.9(a) indicates a first aid post or an ambulance room. The example shown in Fig. 1.9(b) indicates a safe direction in which to travel.

1.8 First aid

Accidents can happen anywhere at any time. They can happen in the home and in the streets as well as in the workshops of industry. The injuries caused by such accidents can range from minor cuts and bruises to broken bones and life threatening injuries. It is a very good idea to know what to do in an emergency.

- You must be aware of the accident procedure.
- You must know where to find your nearest first aid post.
- You must know the quickest and easiest route to the first aid post.
- You must know who is the *qualified* first aid person on duty (if he/she is a part-time person, then where he/she can be found).

First aid should be administered only by a qualified person. Unfortunately in this day and age, more and more people are being encouraged to seek compensation through the courts of law. Complications resulting from amateurish but well-intentioned and well-meaning attempts at first aid on your part could result in you being sued for swingeing damages.

1.8.1 In the event of an emergency

If you are first on the scene of a serious incident, but you are not a trained first aider:

- Remain calm.
- Get help quickly by sending for the appropriate skilled personnel.
- Act and speak in a calm and confident manner to give the casualty confidence.
- Do not attempt to move the casualty.
- Do not administer fluids.
- Hand over to the experts as quickly as possible.

Minor wounds

Prompt first aid can help nature heal small wounds and deal with germs. If you have to treat yourself then wash the wound clean and apply a plaster. However, you must seek medical advice if:

- there is a foreign body embedded in the wound;
- there is a special risk of infection (such as a dog bite or the wound has been caused by a dirty object);
- a non-recent wound shows signs of becoming infected.

Sometimes there can be *foreign bodies* in minor wounds. Small pieces of glass or grit lying on a wound can be picked off with tweezers or rinsed off with cold water before treatment. However, you MUST NOT try to remove objects that are embedded in the wound; you may cause further tissue damage and bleeding.

1. Control any bleeding by applying firm pressure on either side of the object, and raising the wounded part.
2. Drape a piece of gauze lightly over the wound to minimize the risk of germs entering it, then build up padding around the object until you can bandage without pressing down upon it.
3. Take or send the casualty to hospital.

Bruises

These are caused by internal bleeding that seeps through the tissues to produce the discoloration under the skin. Bruising may develop very slowly and appear hours, even days, after injury. Bruising that develops rapidly and seems to be the main problem will benefit from first aid. Caution, bruises may indicate deeper injury. Seek professional advice.

Minor burns and scalds

These are treated to stop the burning, to relieve pain and swelling and to minimize the risk of infection. If you are in any doubt as to the severity of the injury seek the advice of a doctor.

Do not

- Break blisters or interfere with the injured area; you are likely to introduce an infection.
- Use adhesive dressings or strapping.
- Apply lotions, ointments, creams or fats to the injury.

Note: Chemical burns to the skin and particularly the eyes require immediate and specialist treatment. Expert attention must be obtained *immediately.*

Foreign bodies in the eye

Foreign bodies in the eye can lead to blurred vision with pain or discomfort. They can also lead to redness and watering of the eye. A speck of dust or grit, or a loose eyelash floating on the white of the eye, can generally be removed easily. However, a foreign body that adheres to the eye, penetrates the eyeball, or rests on the coloured part of the eye should NOT be removed by a first aider. DO NOT touch anything sticking to, or embedded in, the eyeball or the coloured part of the eye. Cover the affected eye with an eye pad, bandage both eyes, then take or send the casualty to hospital.

1.9 Personal protection

1.9.1 Appearance

Clothing

For general workshop purposes a boiler suit is the most practical and safest form of clothing. However, to be completely effective certain precautions must be taken as shown in Fig. 1.10.

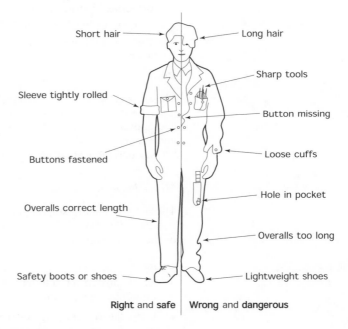

Figure 1.10 *Correct and incorrect dress*

Long hair

- Long hair is liable to be caught in moving machinery such as drilling machines and lathes. This can result in the hair and scalp being torn away which is extremely dangerous and painful. Permanent disfigurement will result and brain damage can also occur.

- Long hair is also a health hazard, as it is almost impossible to keep clean and free from infection in a workshop environment. Either adopt a short and more manageable head style or some sort of head covering that will keep your hair out of harm's way. Suitable head protection is discussed in Section 1.10.

Sharp tools

Sharp tools protruding from the breast pocket can cause severe wounds to the wrist. Such wounds can result in paralysis of the hand and fingers.

Buttons missing and loose cuffs

Since the overalls cannot be fastened properly, it becomes as dangerous as any other loose clothing and is liable to be caught in moving machinery. Loose cuffs are also liable to be caught up like any other loose clothing. They may also prevent you from snatching your hand away from a dangerous situation.

Hole in pocket

Tools placed in a torn pocket can fall through onto the feet of the wearer. Although this may not seem potentially dangerous, it could cause an accident by distracting your attention at a crucial moment.

Overalls too long

These can cause you to trip and fall, particularly when negotiating stairways.

Lightweight shoes

The possible injuries associated with lightweight and unsuitable shoes are:

* puncture wounds caused by treading on sharp objects;

* crushed toes caused by falling objects;

* damage to your Achilles tendon due to insufficient protection around the heel and ankle. Suitable footwear for workshop use is discussed in Section 1.13.

1.9.2 Head and eye protection

As has already been stated, long hair is a serious hazard in a workshop. If it becomes entangled in a machine, as shown in Fig. 1.11, the operator can be scalped. If you wish to retain a long hairstyle in the interests of fashion, then your hair must be contained in a close fitting cap. This also helps to keep your hair and scalp clean and healthy.

When working on site, or in a heavy engineering erection shop involving the use of overhead cranes, all persons should wear a safety helmet complying with BS 2826. Even small objects such as nuts and bolts can cause serious head injuries when dropped from a height. Figure 1.12(a) shows such a helmet. Safety helmets are made from high impact resistant

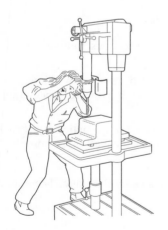

Figure 1.11   *The hazard of long hair*

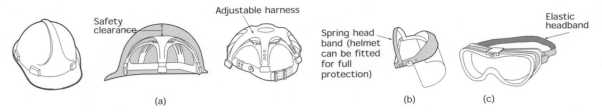

Figure 1.12 *Head and eye protection: (a) a typical fibre-glass safety helmet made to BS 2826; (b) plastic face safety visor for complete protection against chemical and salt-bath splashes; (c) transparent plastic goggles suitable for machining operations*

plastics or from fibre-glass reinforced polyester mouldings. Such helmets can be colour coded for personnel identification and are light and comfortable to wear. Despite their lightweight construction, they have a high resistance to impact and penetration. To eliminate the possibility of electric shock, safety helmets have no metal parts. The harness inside a safety helmet should be adjusted so as to provide ventilation and a fixed safety clearance between the outer shell of the helmet and the wearer's skull. This clearance must be maintained at 32 millimetres. The entire harness is removable for regular cleaning and sterilizing. It is fully adjustable for size, fit and angle to suit the individual wearer's head.

Whilst it is possible to walk about on an artificial leg, nobody has ever seen out of a glass eye. Therefore eye protection is possibly the most important precaution you can take in a workshop. Eye protection is provided by wearing suitable visors as shown in Fig. 1.12(b) or goggles as shown in Fig. 1.12(c).

Eye injuries fall into three main categories:

- Pain and inflammation due to abrasive grit and dust getting between the lid and the eye.

- Damage due to exposure to ultraviolet radiation (arc-welding) and high intensity visible light. Particular care is required when using laser equipment.

- Loss of sight due to the eyeball being pierced or the optic nerve being cut by flying splinters of metal (swarf), or by the blast of a compressed air jet.

Where eye safety is concerned, prevention is better than cure. There may be no cure!

1.9.3 Hand protection

Your hands are in constant use and, because of this, they are constantly at risk handling dirty, oily, greasy, rough, sharp, hot and possibly corrosive and toxic materials. Gloves and 'palms' of a variety of styles and types of materials are available to protect your hands whatever the nature of the work. Some examples are shown in Fig. 1.13. In general terms, plastic gloves are impervious to liquids and should be worn when handling

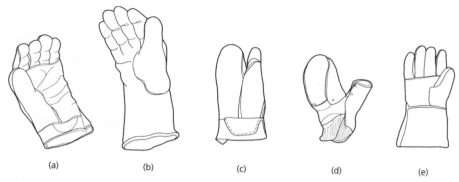

Figure 1.13 *Gloves suitable for industrial purposes: (a) leather glove with reinforced palm – ideal for handling steel sheet and sections; (b) gauntlet – available in rubber, neoprene or PVC for handling chemical, corrosive or oily materials; (c) heat resistant leather glove – can be used for handling objects heated up to 360°C; (d) chrome leather hand-pad or 'palm' – very useful for handling sheet steel, sheet glass, etc.; (e) industrial gauntlets – usually made of leather because of its heat resistance; gauntlets not only protect the hands but also the wrists and forearms from splashes from molten salts and hot quenching media*

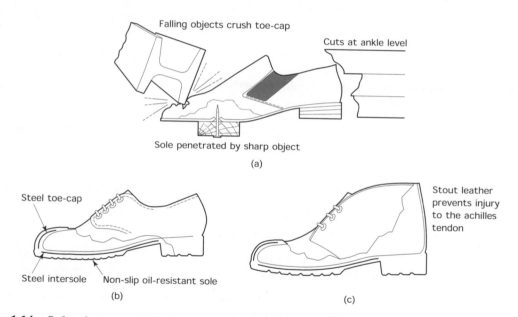

Figure 1.14 *Safety footwear: (a) lightweight shoes offer no protection; (b) industrial safety shoe; (c) industrial safety boot*

oils, greases and chemicals. However, they are unsuitable and even dangerous for handling hot materials. Leather gloves should be used when handling sharp, rough and hot materials. NEVER handle hot workpieces and materials with plastic gloves. These could melt onto and into your flesh causing serious burns that would be difficult to treat.

Where gloves are inappropriate, as when working precision machines, but your hands still need to be protected from oil and dirt rather than from cuts and abrasions, then you should use a barrier cream. This is a mildly antiseptic cream that you can rub well into your hands before work. It fills the pores of your skin and prevents the entry of oils and dirt that could cause infection. The cream is water-soluble and can be removed by washing your hands with ordinary soap and water at the end of the shift. Removal of the cream carries away the dirt and sources of infection.

DO NOT use solvents to clean your hands except under medical supervision. As well as removing oils, greases, paints and adhesives, solvents also remove the natural protective oils from your skin. This leaves the skin open to infection and can lead to cracking and sores. It can also result in sensitization of the skin and the onset of industrial dermatitis.

1.9.4 Foot protection

The dangers associated with wearing unsuitable shoes in a workshop have already been discussed. The injuries that you can suffer when wearing lightweight, casual shoes are shown in Fig. 1.14. This figure also shows some examples of safety footwear as specified in BS 1870. Such safety footwear is available in a variety of styles and prices. It looks as smart as normal footwear and is almost as comfortable.

1.10 Hazards in the workplace

1.10.1 Health hazards

Noise

Excessive noise can be a dangerous pollutant of the working environment. The effects of noise can result in:

- Fatigue leading to careless accidents.
- Mistaken communications between workers leading to accidents.
- Ear damage leading to deafness.
- Permanent nervous disorders.

Noise is energy and it represents waste since it does not do useful work. Ideally it should be suppressed at source to avoid waste of energy and to improve the working environment. If this is not possible then you should be insulated from the noise by sound absorbent screens and/or ear protectors (earmuffs).

Narcotic (anaesthetic) effects

Exposure to small concentrations of narcotic substances causes headaches, giddiness and drowsiness. Under such conditions you are obviously prone to accidents since your judgement and reactions are adversely affected. A worker who has become disorientated by the inhalation of narcotics is a hazard to himself or herself and a hazard to other workers.

Examples of narcotic substances are to be found amongst the many types of solvent used in industry. Solvents are used in paints, adhesives, polishes and degreasing agents. Careful storage and use is essential and should be carefully supervised by qualified persons. Fume extraction and adequate ventilation of the workplace must be provided when working with these substances. Suitable respirators should be available for use in emergencies.

Irritant effects

Many substances cause irritation to the skin both externally and internally. External irritants can cause industrial dermatitis by coming into contact with your skin. The main irritants met within a workshop are oils (particularly cutting oils and coolants), adhesive, degreasing solvents, and electroplating chemicals. Internal irritants are the more dangerous as they may have long-term and deep-seated effects on the major organs of the body. They may cause inflammation, ulceration, internal bleeding, poisoning and the growth of cancerous tumours. Internal irritants are usually air pollutants in the form of dusts (asbestos fibres), fumes and vapours. As well as being inhaled, they may also be carried into your body on food handled without washing. Even the cutting oils used on machine tools can be dangerous if you allow your overalls to become impregnated with the spray. Change your overalls regularly.

Systemic effects

Toxic substances, also known as *systemics*, affect the fundamental organs and bodily functions. They affect your brain, heart, lungs, kidneys, liver, central nervous system and bone marrow. Their effects cannot be reversed and thus lead to chronic ill-health and, ultimately, early death. These toxic substances may enter the body in various ways.

- Dust and vapour can be breathed in through your nose. Observe the safety codes when working with such substances and wear the respirator provided no matter how inconvenient or uncomfortable.

- Liquids and powders contaminating your hands can be transferred to the digestive system by handling food or cigarettes with dirty hands. Always wash before eating or smoking. Never smoke in a prohibited area. Not only may there be a fire risk, but some vapours change chemically and become highly toxic (poisonous) when inhaled through a cigarette.

- Liquids, powders, dusts and vapours may all enter the body through the skin:

  (a) directly through the pores;

  (b) by destroying the outer tough layers of the skin and attacking the sensitive layers underneath;

  (c) by entering through undressed wounds.

Regular washing, use of a barrier cream, use of suitable protective (plastic or rubber) gloves, and the immediate dressing of cuts (no matter how small) are essential to proper hand care.

1.10.2 Personal hygiene

Personal hygiene is most important. It ensures good health and freedom from industrial diseases. It is also more pleasant for those who work with you if they do not have to put up with unpleasant and unnecessary body odours. There is nothing to be embarrassed about in rubbing a barrier cream into your hands before work, about washing thoroughly with soap and water after work, or about changing your overalls regularly so that they can be cleaned. Personal hygiene can go a long way towards preventing skin diseases, both irritant and infectious. Your employer's safety policy should make recommendations on dress and hygiene and they should provide suitable protective measures. As previously mentioned, dirty and oil soaked overalls are a major source of skin infection. Correct dress not only makes you look smart and feel smart, it helps you to avoid accidents and industrial diseases. This is why overalls should be regularly changed and cleaned. Finally, you must always wash your hands thoroughly before handling and eating any food, and when going to the toilet. If your hands are dirty and oily it is essential to wash them *before* as well as after.

1.10.3 Behaviour in workshops

In an industrial environment reckless, foolish and boisterous behaviour such as pushing, shouting, throwing things, and practical joking by a person or a group of persons cannot be tolerated. Such actions can distract a worker's attention and break his or her concentration. This can lead to scrapped work, serious accidents and even fatalities.

Horseplay observes no safety rules. It has no regard for safety equipment. It can defeat safe working procedures and undo the painstaking work of the safety officer by the sheer foolishness and thoughtlessness of the participants. Accidents resulting from horseplay are caused when:

- A person's concentration is disturbed so that they incorrectly operate their machine or inadvertently come into contact with moving machinery or cutters.
- Someone is pushed against moving machinery or factory transport.
- Someone is pushed against ladders and trestles upon which people are working at heights.
- Someone is pushed against and dislodges heavy, stacked components.
- Electricity, compressed air or dangerous chemicals are involved.

1.10.4 Hazards associated with hand tools

Newcomers to industry often overlook the fact that, as well as machine tools, badly maintained and incorrectly used hand tools can also represent a serious safety hazard.

The time and effort taken to fetch the correct tool from the stores or to service a worn tool is considerably less than the time taken to recover from injury. Figure 1.15 shows some badly maintained and incorrectly used hand tools. Chipping screens, as shown in Fig. 8.10 (see p. 225), should be used when removing metal with a cold chisel to prevent injury from the pieces of metal flying from the cutting edge of the chisel. For this reason, goggles should also be worn and you should never chip towards another worker.

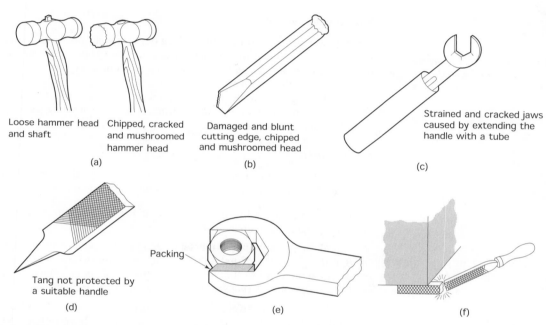

Figure 1.15 *Hand tools in a dangerous condition and misused: (a) hammer faults; (b) chisel faults; (c) spanner faults; (d) file faults; (e) do not use oversize spanner and packing – use the correct size of spanner for the nut or bolt head; (f) do not use file as a lever*

1.10.5 Hazards associated with machine tools

Metal cutting machines are potentially dangerous.

- Before operating any machinery be sure that you have been fully instructed in how to use it, the dangers associated with it, and that you have been given permission to use it.

- Do not operate a machine unless all the guards and safety devices are in position and are operating correctly.

- Make sure you understand any special rules and regulations applicable to the particular machine you are about to use, even if you have been trained on machines in general.

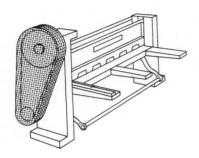

Figure 1.16 *Typical transmission guard for a belt driven machine*

- Never clean or adjust a machine whilst it is in motion. Stop the machine and isolate it from the supply.

- Report any dangerous aspect of the machine you are using, or are about to use, immediately and do not use it until it has been made safe by a suitably qualified and authorized person.

- A machine may have to be stopped in an emergency. Learn how to make an emergency stop without having to pause and think about it and without having to search for the emergency stop switch.

Transmission guards

By law, no machine can be sold or hired out unless all gears, belts, shafts and couplings making up the power transmission system are guarded so that they cannot be touched whilst they are in motion. Figure 1.16 shows a typical transmission guard.

Sometimes guards have to be removed in order to replace, adjust or service the components they are covering. This must be done only by a qualified maintenance mechanic.

Cutter guards

The machine manufacturer does not normally provide cutter guards because of the wide range of work a machine may have to do.

- It is the responsibility of the owner or the hirer of the machine to supply their own cutter guards.

- It is the responsibility of the setter and/or the operator to make sure that the guards are fitted and working correctly before operating the machine, and to use the guards as instructed. It is an offence in law for the operator to remove or tamper with the guards provided.

- If ever you are doubtful about the adequacy of a guard or the safety of a process, consult your instructor or your safety officer without delay.

The simple drilling machine guard shown in Fig. 1.17(a) covers only the chuck and is suitable only for jobbing work when small diameter drills are being used. The drill chuck shown in Fig. 1.17(b) is used for larger

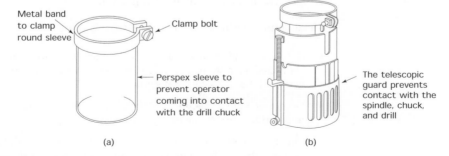

Metal band to clamp round sleeve — Clamp bolt

Perspex sleeve to prevent operator coming into contact with the drill chuck

The telescopic guard prevents contact with the spindle, chuck, and drill

(a)   (b)

Figure 1.17 *Drill chuck guards: (a) simple; (b) telescopic*

drills and for drills which are mounted directly into the drilling machine spindle. It covers the whole length of the drill and telescopes up as the drill penetrates into the workpiece.

Guards for use with milling machines, centre lathes, and grinding machines will be dealt with in the later chapters specifically relating to the use of such machines and their special hazards.

1.11 Manual lifting

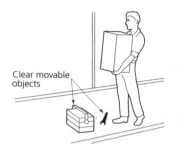

Figure 1.18 *Obstructions to safe movement must be removed*

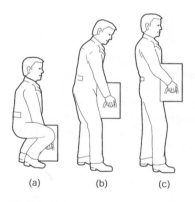

Figure 1.19 *Correct manual lifting: (a) keep back straight and near vertical; (b) keep your spine straight; (c) straighten your legs to raise load*

1.11.1 Individual lifting

In the engineering industry it is often necessary to lift fairly heavy loads. As a general rule, loads lifted manually should not exceed 20 kg. Mechanical lifting equipment should be used for loads in excess of 20 kg. However, even lifting loads less than 20 kg can cause strain and lifting loads incorrectly is one of the major causes of back trouble. If the load is obviously too heavy or bulky for one person to handle, you should ask for assistance. Even a light load can be dangerous if it obscures your vision as shown in Fig. 1.18. All movable objects that form hazardous obstructions should be moved to a safe place before movement of the load commences.

As has already been stated, it is important to use the correct lifting technique. This is because the human spine is not an efficient lifting device. If it is subjected to heavy strain, or incorrect methods of lifting, the lumbar discs may be damaged causing considerable pain. This is often referred to as a 'slipped disc' and the damage (and pain) can be permanent.

The correct way to lift a load manually is shown in Fig. 1.19. You should start the lift in a balanced squatting position with your legs at hip width apart and one foot slightly ahead of the other. The load to be lifted should be held close to your body. Make sure that you have a safe and secure grip on the load. Before taking the weight of the load, your back should be straightened and as near to the vertical as possible. Keep your head up and your chin drawn in, this helps to keep your spine straight and rigid as shown in Fig. 1.19(a). To raise the load, first straighten your legs. This ensures that the load is being raised by your powerful thigh muscles and bones, as shown in Fig. 1.19(b), and not by your back. To complete the lift, raise the upper part of your body to a vertical position as shown in Fig. 1.19(c).

To carry the load, keep your body upright and hold the load close to your body. If the load has jagged edges wear protective gloves and if hazardous liquids are being handled wear the appropriate protective clothing as shown in Fig. 1.20.

1.11.2 Manual lifting (team)

When a lifting party is formed in order to move a particularly large or heavy load the team leader is solely responsible for the safe completion of the task. The team leader should not take part in the actual lifting but should ensure that:

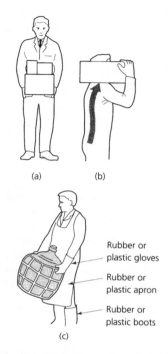

(a)   (b)

(c)

Rubber or
plastic gloves

Rubber or
plastic apron

Rubber or
plastic boots

Figure 1.20 *Correct carrying: (a) keep body upright and load close to body; (b) let your bone structure support the load; (c) wear appropriate clothing*

- Everyone understands what the job involves and the method chosen for its completion.

- The area is clear of obstructions and that the floor is safe and will provide a good foothold.

- The members of the lifting party are of similar height and physique, and that they are wearing any necessary protective clothing. Each person should be positioned so that the weight is evenly distributed.

- The team leader takes up a position which gives the best all round view of the area and will permit the development of any hazardous situation to be seen so that the appropriate action can be taken in time to prevent an accident.

- Any equipment moved in order to carry out the operation is put back in its original position when the task has been completed. This sequence of events is shown in Fig. 1.21.

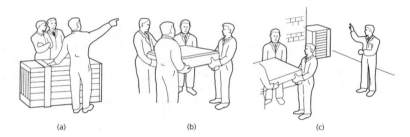

(a)   (b)   (c)

Figure 1.21 *Team lifting*

Loads that are too heavy to be lifted or carried can still be moved manually by using a crowbar and rollers as shown in Fig. 1.22. The rollers should be made from thick walled tubes so that there is no danger of trapping your fingers if the load should move whilst positioning the rollers. Turning a corner is achieved by placing the leading roller at an angle. As the load clears the rearmost roller, this roller is moved to the front, so that the load is always resting on two rollers, whilst the third roller is being positioned.

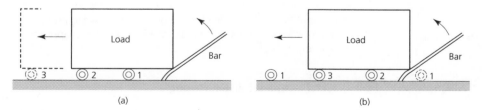

(a)   (b)

Figure 1.22 *Use of rollers: (a) load is rolled forward on rollers 1 and 2 until it is on rollers 2 and 3, roller 1 is moved to the front ready for next move*

1.12 Mechanical lifting equipment

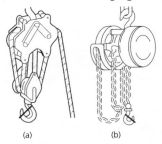

Figure 1.23 *Manual lifting equipment: (a) rope pulley blocks (snatch blocks); (b) chain blocks (geared)*

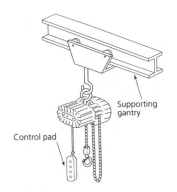

Figure 1.24 *Powered lifting equipment*

1.13 Use of lifting equipment

Mechanical lifting equipment can be classified according to the motive power used to operate it.

1.12.1 Manual (muscle power)

Examples of this type of equipment are shown in Fig. 1.23. Rope pulley blocks (snatch blocks) are light and easily mounted. However, the tail rope has to be tied off to prevent the load falling when the effort is removed. Some rope blocks have an automatic brake which is released by giving the tail rope a sharp tug before lowering the load. They are suitable for loads up to 250 kg. Chain pulley blocks are portable and are used for heavier loads from 250 kg to 1 tonne. They also have the advantage that they do not run back (overhaul) when the effort raising the load is removed.

1.12.2 Powered

An example of an electrically powered hoist is shown in Fig. 1.24. Powered lifting equipment is faster and can raise greater loads than manually operated chain blocks.

1.12.3 Safety

Only fully competent persons (i.e. trained and authorized) are permitted to operate mechanical lifting equipment. Trainees can use such equipment only under the close supervision of a qualified and authorized instructor.

1.13.1 Lifting a load

Before lifting a load using a mechanical lifting device you should:

- Warn everyone near the load and anyone approaching the load to keep clear.
- Check that all slings and ropes are safely and securely attached both to the load and to the hook.
- Take up the slack in the chain, sling or rope gently.
- Raise the load slowly and steadily so that it is just off the ground.
- Check that the load is stable and that the sling has not become accidentally caught on a part of the load incapable of sustaining the lifting force.
- Stand well back from the load and lift steadily.

1.13.2 Lowering a load

Before lowering a load:

- Check that the ground is clear of obstacles and is capable of supporting the load.

- Place timbers under the load as shown in Fig. 1.25(a) so that the sling will not be trapped and damaged. This will also facilitate the removal of the sling.

- Lower the load until it is close to the ground and then gently ease it onto the timbers until the strain is gradually taken off the lifting equipment. It may be necessary to manually guide the load into place as shown in Fig. 1.25(b), in which case safety shoes and protective gloves should be worn.

- Never work under a suspended load. Always lower the load onto suitable supports as shown in Fig. 1.25(c).

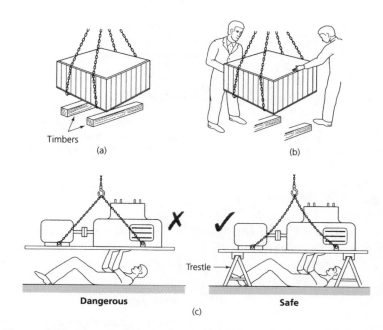

Figure 1.25 *Care when lowering a load: (a) lower onto timbers; (b) guide by hand; (c) never work under a suspended load*

1.14 Accessories for lifting equipment

Hooks

These are made from forged steel and are carefully proportioned so that the load will not slip from them whilst being lifted. The hooks of lifting gear are frequently painted bright yellow to attract attention and to prevent people walking into them.

Slings

These are used to attach the load to the hook of the lifting equipment. There are four types in common use. They must all be marked with tags stating their safe working load (SWL).

- Chain slings (Fig. 1.26(a)) – as well as general lifting, only this type of sling is suitable for lifting loads having sharp edges or for lifting hot materials.

- Wire rope slings (Fig. 1.26(b)) – these are widely used for general lifting. They should not be used for loads with sharp edges or for hot loads; nor should they be allowed to become rusty. Further, they should not be bent round a diameter of less than 20 times the diameter of the wire rope itself.

- Fibre rope slings (Fig. 1.26(c)) – fibre rope slings may have eyes spliced into them or, more usually, they are endless as shown. They are used for general lifting, and are particularly useful where machined surfaces and paintwork have to be protected from damage.

- Belt or strap slings – because of their breadth they do not tend to bite into the work and cause damage to the surface finish of the work. Rope and belt slings themselves must be protected from being cut or frayed by sharp edges as shown in Fig. 1.26(d). This packing also prevents the fibres of the slings from being damaged by being bent too sharply around the corners of the object being lifted.

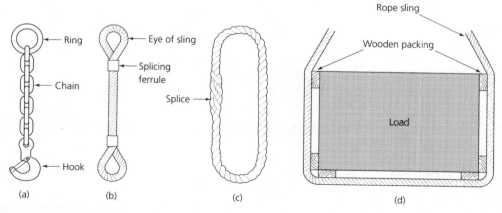

Figure 1.26 *Types and care of slings*

Care of slings

Wire rope and fibre rope slings must not be shortened by knotting since this damages the fibres causing them to fracture. Chain slings must not be shortened by bolting the links together.

Condition of slings

All slings must be checked before use for cuts, wear, abrasion, fraying and corrosion. Damaged slings must never be used and the fault must be reported.

Length of slings

Rope or chain slings must be long enough to carry the load safely and with each leg as nearly vertical as possible as shown in Fig. 1.27(a). The load on a sling increases rapidly as the angle between the legs of the sling becomes greater. This is shown in Fig. 1.27(b).

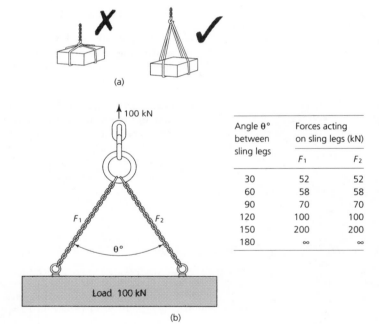

Angle $\theta°$ between sling legs	Forces acting on sling legs (kN)	
	F_1	F_2
30	52	52
60	58	58
90	70	70
120	100	100
150	200	200
180	∞	∞

Figure 1.27 *Length of slings: (a) correct length; (b) incorrect length*

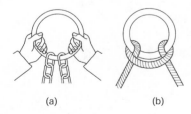

Figure 1.28 *Use of rings: (a) with 2 leg chain sling; (b) with a rope sling*

Rings

These are used for ease of attachment of the sling to the crane hook. They also prevent the sling being sharply bent over the hook. Figure 1.28(a) shows a chain sling fitted with a suitable ring at one end. Figure 1.28(b) shows how a ring is used in conduction with a rope sling.

Eyebolts and shackles

Forged steel eyebolts to BS 4278 are frequently provided for lifting equipment and assemblies such as electric motors, gearboxes, and small machine tools. An example of the correct use of an eyebolt is shown in Fig. 1.29(a), whilst Fig. 1.29(b) shows how eyebolts must never be used. Forged steel shackles are used to connect lifting accessories together. In the example shown in Fig. 1.29(c), the eye of a wire rope sling is connected to an eyebolt using a shackle.

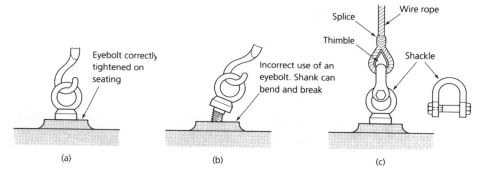

Figure 1.29 *Use of eyebolts: (a) correct use; (b) incorrect use; (c) a shackle connects the eye of the sling to an eye bolt*

1.15 Useful knots for fibre ropes

It is useful to know about the knots that can be tied in fibre ropes when moving and securing loads. Knots must never be tied in wire ropes as they are not sufficiently flexible and permanent damage will be caused. Some widely used knots are as follows.

Reef knot

This is used for joining ropes of equal thickness (Fig. 1.30(a)).

Clove hitch

This is used for attaching a rope to a pole or bar (Fig. 1.30(b)).

Single loop

This is used to prevent fibre ropes from slipping off crane hooks (Fig. 1.30(c)).

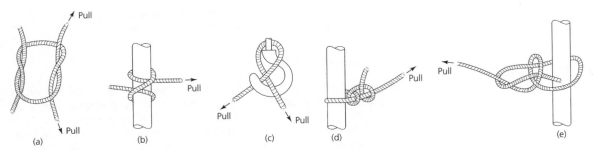

Figure 1.30 *Useful knots for fibre ropes: (a) reef knot; (b) clove hitch; (c) single loop; (d) two half hitches; (e) bowline*

Half hitches

Two half hitches can be used to secure a rope to a solid pole or for securing a rope to a sling (Fig. 1.30(d)).

Bowline

This is used to form a loop which will not tighten under load (Fig. 1.30(e)).

1.16 Transporting loads (trucks)

Various types of truck are used for transporting loads around workshops and factory sites. Only manually propelled trucks will be considered. Power-driven trucks are beyond the scope of this book. The simplest sort of truck is the hand truck (sack truck) shown in Fig. 1.31(a). It uses the principle of levers to raise the load ready for wheeling away. Quite heavy loads can be moved quite easily with this type of truck.

Platform or flat trucks are used with various wheel arrangements so that they can be steered. The type shown in Fig. 1.31(b) requires the load to be placed over the wheels so that the truck is balanced for ease of movement. The type shown in Fig. 1.31(c) has a wheel at each end and the load does not have to be so carefully balanced. Only one end wheel is in contact with the ground at any one time. Also the end wheels can slide. This facilitates steering. A heavier duty 'turntable' type truck is shown in Fig. 1.31(d). This has four wheels in the conventional position and the front wheels can be turned so that the truck can be steered.

Whichever type of truck you use there are two safety points you should observe.

- Stack the load on the trolley so that you can see where you are going in order to avoid a collision, particularly if people are working on ladders or steps along the route you are taking.

- Balance the load so that it will not topple off the truck or overturn the truck when you are turning a corner.

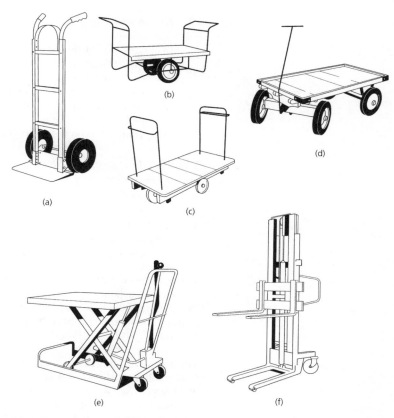

Figure 1.31 *Types of trucks: (a) sack truck; (b) two-wheeled platform truck (balanced); (c) sliding wheel platform truck; (d) heavy duty, turntable platform type truck; (e) elevating table truck; (f) stacking truck*

1.17 Inspection (lifting equipment)

It is a legal requirement under the Health and Safety at Work, etc. Act that all lifting equipment is regularly inspected by qualified engineers specializing in such work and that the results of such inspections are recorded in the register provided. If an inspector condemns any item of equipment it must be taken out of service immediately and either rectified or destroyed. If rectified, it must be reinspected and approved by a qualified inspector before being taken back into service. The inspector will, on each visit, also confirm the safe working load (SWL) markings for each piece of equipment. No new item of lifting equipment must be taken into service until it has been inspected and certificated.

Exercises   **1.1**   *Health and Safety at Work, etc. Act and other important industrial legislation*
   (a)   (i)   What do the initials HSE stand for?
          (ii)   What is a Prohibition Notice?
          (iii) What is an Improvement Notice?
          (iv)   Who issues the notices in (ii) and (iii) above?
   (b)   As an employee you also have duties under the Act. Copy out and complete Table 1.1 by writing brief comments regarding your duties in the following circumstances.

TABLE 1.1   *Exercise 1.1(b)*

Circumstances	*Duties*
You are uncertain how to operate a machine needed to complete your task	
You need to carry some sheet metal with very sharp edges	
You are working on site and you have mislaid your safety helmet	
You find that the belt guard has been removed from a machine you have been told to use	
You have spilt hydraulic oil on the floor whilst servicing a machine	
The earth wire has come disconnected from a portable power tool you are using	
Your supervisor has told you to clear up the rubbish left by another worker	
You find someone smoking in a prohibited area	

TABLE 1.2   *Exercise 1.1(c)*

Situation	*Appropriate industrial regulations*
Use of grinding machines and abrasive wheels	
Eye protection	
Electrical control equipment, use and maintenance	
Use of substances that can be harmful to health (solvents, etc.)	
Safe use of power presses	
Protection against high noise levels	
Safe use of milling machines	
Use of protective clothing	

(c)   Copy out and complete Table 1.2 by adding the name of the most appropriate industrial regulation(s) for each of the situations given.

(d)   Copy out and complete Fig. 1.32 by stating:
  (i)   the category of sign (e.g. warning sign, mandatory sign, etc.);
  (ii)   the meaning of sign;
  (iii)   where it would be used.

Sign	Meaning	Category	Where used
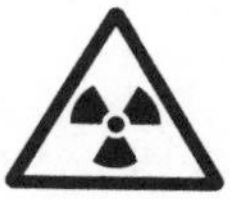			
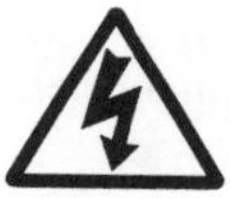			
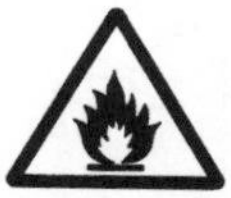			
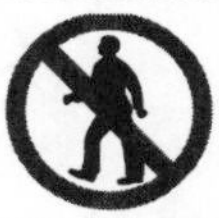			
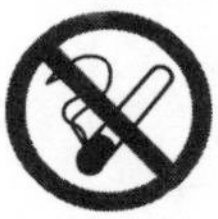			
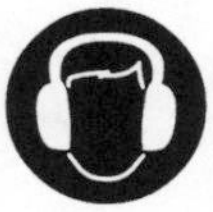			
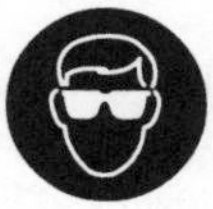			

Figure 1.32   *Exercise 1.1(d)*

1.2   *Electrical hazards*
  (a)   Explain why portable electrical equipment should be:
    (i)   earthed unless it is 'double insulated';
    (ii)   operated from a low-voltage supply;

        (iii)   protected by an earth leakage isolator incorporating a residual current detector.

(b)   When you are issued with portable electrical equipment from the stores you should make a number of visual checks before accepting and using the equipment. Describe these checks.

(c)   If the checks you made in (b) above showed the equipment to be faulty, what action should you take?

(d)   In the event of a workmate receiving a severe electric shock that renders him/her unconscious, what emergency action should you take.

1.3   *Fire hazards*

(a)   List THREE main causes of fire on industrial premises.

(b)   If you detect a fire in a storeroom at work, what action should you take?

(c)   Figure 1.33 shows some various types of fire extinguisher.

        (i)   State the types of fire upon which each extinguisher should be used and any precautions that should be taken.

        (ii)   State the colour coding that identifies each type of fire extinguisher.

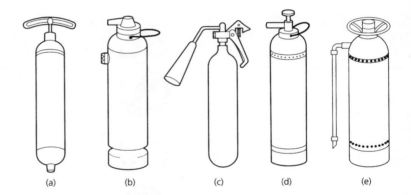

    (a)   (b)   (c)   (d)   (e)

Figure 1.33   *Exercise 1.3(c)*

1.4   *Accidents*

(a)   Why should all cuts, bruises and burns be treated by a qualified first aider, and what risks does a well-meaning but unqualified person run in attempting first aid?

(b)   Apart from rendering first aid what other action must be taken in the event of an accident?

(c)   State how you would identify a first aid post.

(d)   What action should you take if you come across someone who has received a serious accident (broken bones, severe bleeding, partial or complete loss of consciousness, etc.)?

(e)   Briefly describe the accident reporting procedures for your place of work or training workshop.

1.5 *Working environment*

    (a)   Copy out and complete Table 1.3 by stating the type of working environment in which you would need to use the following items of safety clothing and equipment listed in the table.

TABLE 1.3 *Exercise 1.5(a)*

Clothing/equipment	Situation/environment
Ear protectors	
Overalls	
PVC apron	
Leather apron	
Leather gloves	
PVC/rubber gloves	
Safety helmet	
Clear goggles	
Visor	
Barrier cream	
Safety boots	
Goggles with filter lenses	

    (b)   With the aid of a sketch explain what is meant by:
       (i)   a transmission guard;
      (ii)   a cutter guard.

    (c)   For each of the examples listed below, sketch an appropriate item of safety equipment and state how it works.
       (i)   A travelling chip guard on a lathe.
      (ii)   A milling-cutter guard where the machine is being operated by a skilled operator.
     (iii)   A drill chuck guard.
     (iv)   A chipping screen.
      (v)   An interlocked transmission guard.

1.6 *Lifting and carrying*

    (a)   State the maximum recommended weight that may be lifted without the aid of mechanical lifting equipment.

    (b)   With the aid of sketches show the correct and incorrect way to lift a load.

    (c)   What precautions should be taken when carrying loads?

    (d)   What precautions should be taken when moving a heavy load with a lifting team?

    (e)   Lifting equipment should be marked with its SWL.
       (i)   State what these initials stand for.
      (ii)   State how often lifting equipment needs to be tested and examined.
     (iii)   State what records need to be kept.

2   Establishing effective working relationships

When you have read this chapter you should understand how to:

- Create and maintain effective working relationships with supervisory staff.
- Create and maintain working relationships with other people, members of the same working groups and other employees in the same organization.

2.1   Basic relationships

Even the smallest businesses have to communicate with, and relate to, a surprising number of people either through necessity or because it is the law. This is shown in Fig. 2.1.

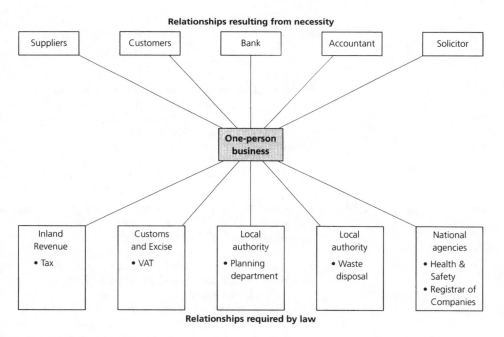

Figure 2.1   *Structure of relationships*

In the first group (*necessity*) are your suppliers of raw materials and tools and equipment used in production. Also you have to deal with the customers who buy your products and the transport organizations who deliver your products to your customers. You also need a bank and since, from time to time, you may need an overdraft, it's as well to maintain good relationships with your bank manager. There is no law that says you have to have suppliers, customers and bankers but you would not get far in business without them.

There is no law that says you need a solicitor or an accountant. However, you will require a solicitor to draw up all the documents required when setting up the business and when problems arise with customers, suppliers and the local authority (e.g. noise complaints from the neighbours). You will require an accountant to audit your accounts, advise on financial matters, sort out your tax returns, make sure that you avoid overpayment of tax, and to deal with the Customs and Excise officials over your VAT payments and returns. Therefore it is a *necessity* that you make every effort to maintain *good working relationships* with them.

In the second group (*law*) you have to communicate with such persons as local authority inspectors (planning officers, etc.), tax inspectors, VAT inspectors, and health and safety inspectors. These people have the power of the legal system behind them so it pays to maintain *good working relationships* with them.

In our working lives we have constantly to relate to and communicate with other people. For example, we have to exchange technical data, implement management decisions and safety policy, and relate to other people within the company and also to people such as customers and buyers who work outside the company. In this section we are concerned mainly with the people with whom you will work on a daily basis; not only your workmates but also your immediate supervisors and managers.

Having made the point that no one can work in isolation even if they are the sole proprietor of a one person firm, let's consider the situation if you are an employer or an employee in a small, medium or large company. Like it or not, you are going to be one of a team. Like it or not, you are going to have to communicate, participate and co-operate. You are going to have to maintain *good working relationships*. When dealing with other people, you can adopt one of two possible attitudes. You can either *confront* them or you can *co-operate* with them.

2.1.1 Confrontation

Confrontation is how the aggressive, bullying person works. A confrontational person demands and threatens to get his or her own way. It may work in the short term as long as the aggressor has the whip hand. However, such aggressive bullies never win the respect of the people with whom they work. They can never rely upon the loyalty of the people they have continually confronted when a favour is required. It would be no good expecting 'goodwill' co-operation when an extra effort is required to complete an urgent order on time.

2.1.2 Co-operation

This is how sensible, civilized people work. They collaborate and help each other. In this way they gain respect for each other. This results in the development of efficient working relationships and efficient working practices. In an emergency everyone can be relied upon to make a maximum effort and to help each other.

2.1.3 'Reading' people

As you become more experienced in dealing with people, you will realize that the most important skill is learning to 'read' their moods. You must be able to realize with whom you can have a joke and with whom you can't. You need to know who only wants a 'yes or no' answer and who prefers to discuss a problem. You need to know when to be friendly and when to be aloof, when to offer a word of sympathy or advice, and when to leave somebody alone to get over a bad mood.

2.2 Relationships with managers, supervisors and instructors

You are *employed* by the firm for whom you work, but you are *responsible* to your immediate superior. Depending on the structure of the company your immediate superior may be an instructor, a charge-hand, a foreman or forewoman, a supervisor, a manager or, in a very small firm, the 'Boss' himself.

Figure 2.2 shows the structure of a training department for a large company. The structure will vary from firm to firm but, whatever the size of the company and the structure of its training facilities, it is always

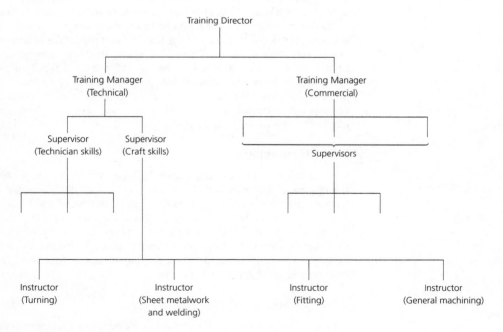

Figure 2.2 *Training personnel structure*

a good idea to find out what the structure is. You need to know who influences your training package, who trains you and who is responsible for your welfare, discipline and assessment. The change from the school environment to the adult working environment often poses unforeseen problems. It is essential to know who you should turn to when you need advice.

First and foremost, it is most important that you get on well with your instructor, your supervisor and your training manager. Each of them will require a different approach. This is not only because they are different people, but also because they have a different status and a different level of importance in the company. Let's now see how you can make a 'good impression' on these people and establish good working relationships with them. For example:

- Develop a habit of good time-keeping and regular attendance, even under difficult conditions.

- Be neat and tidy in your appearance.

- Keep your work area neat and tidy and your tools and instruments in good condition.

- Keep your paperwork up to date, fill it in neatly and keep it clean in a plastic folder.

- File your paperwork systematically so that you can produce it for your instructor or your training manager on demand. 'Attention to detail' always makes a good impression.

- Be reliable so that people quickly find that they can depend upon you.

- Be conscientious: always try your hardest and do your best.

- Reasonable requests for information should be dealt with promptly, accurately and in a co-operative manner providing they do not unduly interfere with or interrupt your work.

- If responding to any request is going to take time and interrupt your work, or if it requires you to leave your working area, always seek permission from your supervisor or instructor before carrying out the request. Always turn your machine off before leaving it.

- If you are in the middle of an intricate piece of work that requires your full concentration, don't just down tools, but ask politely if you may complete your task before responding to the request.

- No matter how tired you are or how inconvenient, trivial and un-necessary the request may seem to you, always try to be cheerful, help-ful and efficient. NEVER answer in a surly, unco-operative, couldn't care less, any old time will do, manner.

Your relationships with other people, particularly your instructor, must be a dialogue of instruction and advice. If you are in doubt you must always discuss your problem with your instructor until you are certain that you fully understand what you have to do. Your instructor is also there to help you with any personal problems you may have or problems with other people with whom you have to work. He or she wants to get to know you as a person so that they can get the best from you and help you to make a success of your training.

Should your instructor be talking to another trainee or his supervisor or manager, don't just barge in, either get on with another job and come back later or wait to one side, respectfully, until it is your turn. Be patient, on no account should you try and start work on a job or on a machine without instruction just because your instructor is busy and you are tired of waiting for him or her.

2.3 Attitude and behaviour

2.3.1 Attitude

When you enter the world of industry you are a very new, very unimportant and very expendable member of the workforce. You know little or nothing about the skills of engineering so, if you are going to complete your training successfully and become a useful member of the company and of society as a whole, you've got a great deal to learn.

Your training is a major investment for your employer. Therefore employers need to train and employ reliable people who they can rely upon and who will give them a reasonable return for their investment in time and money. Those who demonstrate good attitudes are the most likely to succeed. It is no good being the most skilful apprentice or trainee if you are also the most temperamental. Whilst high levels of skill are important, so is consistency, reliability, loyalty and the ability to work in a team.

The greatest incentive to learning a trade is the earning power it gives you. To learn a trade you need the skilled help and advice of a lot of people. You must respect their skill and experience if you are to get their help and advice in return.

Apart from the advice already given, here are some further suggestions.

- Dress in the way recommended by your company. Many firms provide smart overalls bearing the company logo. Do not turn up to work looking scruffy. For example, a long hairstyle not only gives a bad impression it can also be very dangerous (see 1.9).

- For hygiene reasons change into clean overalls daily if possible. Dirty, oily overalls can cause serious hygiene and health problems. A tidy person has a tidy and receptive mind.

- Listen carefully to the instructions your instructor gives to you, particularly safety instructions. Never operate a machine or carry out a process if you are in doubt; always check again with your instructor.

- Keep a log of the operations you are taught and the work you do because your practical skill training has to be assessed in order for you to obtain your certification. Since you may have to present your logbook at a future job interview it is worthwhile spending some time on it. Keep it neat and clean in a plastic folder.

- Show consistency, commitment and dedication in carrying out the tasks set you. Work to as high a standard as you can and always be trying to improve your standards. Have pride in your work, you never know who is going to look at it. This applies not only to the production of components and assemblies but equally to organizational tasks.

2.3.2 Behaviour

In an industrial environment horseplay and fooling around infers reckless and boisterous behaviour such as pushing, shouting, throwing things and practical joking by a person or a group of persons. Engineering equipment is potentially very dangerous and this sort of behaviour cannot be tolerated in an industrial environment.

As well as the negative attitude to behaviour just described, there are positive attitudes to be taken as well. For example, keep your workstation clean and tidy, also clean up any spillages immediately and keep the area where you are working swept clear of swarf and other rubbish. Use the waste bins provided.

2.4 Implementing company policy

Company policy may be dictated by the 'Boss' in a small company or it may be set by the board of directors in a large company. These people are not free agents and they have to abide by national and international laws and guidelines in setting out a strategy for the company. They have to consider the demands of the shareholders, and they are also responsible for the success, profitability and growth of the company upon which the job security and rewards of all who work for the company depend. For these reasons company policy should be understood and obeyed. In successful companies this is not an entirely autocratic process and there are various committee structures through which ideas from the shop floor can be fed back up the command chain to the senior management. This is particularly true for safety issues.

2.4.1 Health, safety and personal hygiene

Health, safety and personal hygiene were dealt with in detail in Chapter 1. These issues were given a whole chapter to themselves because they are so important. All engineering and manufacturing companies are legally bound by the provisions of the Health and Safety at Work, etc. Act of 1974, and other related legislation. The safety policy of your company must take on board all the requirements of such legislation.

Instructors and training managers have a vital part to play in fulfilling their obligations under such safety legislation and in anticipating and averting dangerous situations. Equally, by their manner in handling equipment and tools they must set a good example to their trainees and encourage attitudes of care and confidence.

Personal hygiene is most important. There is nothing to be embarrassed about in rubbing a barrier cream into your hands before work. There is nothing to be embarrassed about in washing thoroughly with soap and hot water after work, or about changing your overalls regularly so that they can be cleaned, or about wearing protective plastic or rubber gloves to protect your hands from chemicals and solvents. Personal hygiene can go a long way towards preventing skin diseases, both irritant and infectious.

2.4.2 Communications

No company can exist without lines of communications both internal and external. Without internal lines of communication the company policy could not be communicated to the workforce, nor would the senior management know if their policies were being carried out. Figure 2.3 shows a typical management structure for a company.

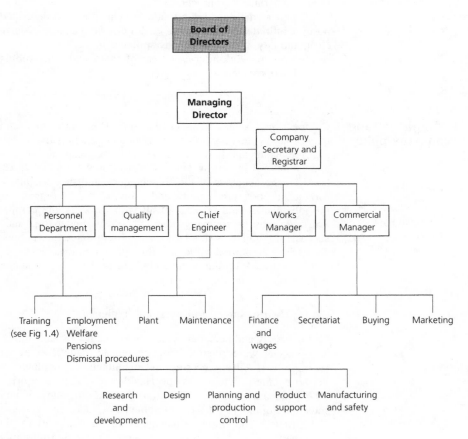

Figure 2.3 *Management structure*

This structure not only represents the lines of communication by which the senior management can ensure that decisions are passed down the line, it represents a route by which messages and requests are sent back up to the various levels of management. These channels of communication are part of company policy and, to bypass them, can lead to confusion and friction between the parties concerned.

Wherever possible, always use the standard forms provided when communicating within your company. This will result in your requests being treated seriously. Such forms may range from the stores requisition forms that you fill in daily, to job application forms and internal promotion application forms. Always follow laid down procedures.

External lines of communication are equally important so that the company can communicate with its customers and suppliers. Market research, public relations and advertising are essential to the success of a company and depend upon the use of suitable means of communication. This is why many companies employ firms of consultants specializing in these fields.

Verbal communications can take place via the telephone on a 'one to one' basis or via meetings when information has to be given to a number of people at the same time. The advantage of verbal communication is that an instant response can be received and a discussion can take place. The disadvantage of verbal communication is its lack of integrity. Messages can be forgotten, they can be repeated inaccurately, or they can be misinterpreted. All verbal messages should be backed up by written confirmation.

For accuracy, send a letter, fax, e-mail or a written memorandum in the first place. All firms of any standing use pro-forma documents such as letter paper with printed headings, official memorandum forms, official order forms, official invoice forms and despatch notes, and many other pre-printed documents. This ensures consistency of communication policy and saves time since only the details and an approved signature need to be added.

Nowadays electronics has speeded up internal and external communications and many firms are heading towards so-called 'paperless offices'. Increasingly, communications will be sent digitally. Files saved on disk instead of on paper remove the need for bulky filing cabinets.

2.4.3 Recording and filing

The need for keeping a training log and the need for using the standard forms supplied by your company has already been introduced. Nowadays most companies need their quality control system to be BS EN 9000 approved. This is because most of their customers will be so approved and will only be able to purchase their supplies from companies who are similarly approved. To trace the progress of all goods from supplier to customer records must be kept and filed. The principles of quality control will be outlined in Chapter 3.

It is no use completing forms and keeping records unless they are properly filed. The success of any filing system depends upon the ease with which any documents can be retrieved on demand. If any file is removed from a filing system, a card must be inserted in its place stating who has borrowed the file and when. The file must be returned as soon as possible so that it does not become lost.

2.5 Creating and maintaining effective working relationships with other people

As has been stated previously, you cannot work in isolation. Sooner or later you have to relate to other people. In fact, most working situations rely upon teamwork.

2.5.1 Positive attitudes

At work you should always try to adopt a positive and constructive attitude to other people. This can be difficult when you are tired or the person you are relating to is off-hand, aggressive, demanding, and asking for the near impossible. However, they are often under pressure themselves and allowances have to be made. Sometimes people are just out to annoy and provoke a confrontation. Try not to become involved. It is better to walk away from a quarrel than let it get out of hand. Always try to cool the aggressor down.

Sooner or later you are bound to come up against someone with whom you cannot get on. This may be a workmate, or an instructor. Often, there is no apparent reason for this problem, it is simply a clash of incompatible personalities. If you cannot resolve the matter amicably yourself, don't leave the situation to deteriorate, but seek advice from the appropriate member of staff such as your supervisor or manager. He or she may be able to solve the problem even if it may involve you being moved to another section. Remember that, during your training, your personal attitudes and your ability to work as a team member is as much under scrutiny as the engineering products that you produce.

2.5.2 Teamwork

Quite often you will have to work as a member of a team. This requires quite different skills in interpersonal relationships than when you are working on your own or under the guidance of your instructor. For example, consider the lifting of a large and heavy packing case when mechanical lifting gear is not available. Like any team, the lifting party has to have a team leader (captain). That person must have the respect and confidence of all the other members of the team because of his or her experience and expertise. The team should be picked from people who it is known can work together amicably and constructively. One oddball going his or her own way at a crucial moment could cause an accident and injury to other members of the team.

Although the team leader is solely responsible for the safe and satisfactory completion of the task, he or she should be sensible enough to consider comments and contributions from other members of the team. If you are a member of such a team and you think you have spotted a potential hazard in the job to be done, then it is your duty to draw it to the attention of the team leader. Eventually, however, discussion has to cease and the job has to be done. At this point the team leader has to make up his or her mind about how the job is to be done.

The team leader should not take an active part in the exercise, but should stand back where he or she can see everything that is going on. So, in the event of a potentially hazardous situation developing, the team leader is free to step in and correct the situation in order to prevent an accident.

2.5.3 Personal property

During a working lifetime most engineers acquire an extensive set of personal tools. Some may be bought and some may be made personally. You will be mightily unpopular in any workshop if you borrow any of these tools without the owner's consent. The same applies to overalls or any other personal belongings. Although we have considered company policy, each and every workshop has a code of conduct all of its own. This is not written down, it is not company policy, it is a code of behaviour that has grown up over the years amongst the people working in that shop. Woe betide anyone who disregards this code of conduct. However, respect it, obey it, and you will find that your relationships with your workmates and supervisors will be much more pleasant. You will receive more useful help and wise advice and will establish worthwhile friendships that can stand you in good stead throughout your working life.

Exercises

2.1 *Effective working relationships*
(a) You are engaged in an intricate machining operation when a colleague asks for your assistance. Explain how you would deal with this situation.
(b) You are having difficulty in understanding an engineering drawing and you want advice. Your instructor is engaged in conversation with the training manager. Explain what you should do in this situation.
(c) Your supervisor has directed you to help with a team activity in another department. Explain how you would introduce yourself to the team leader and how you would try to relate to the other members of the team.

2.2 *Dress, presentation and behaviour*
(a) Describe the dress code at your place of work or your training centre and explain why the dress code should be adhered to.
(b) Explain THREE possible consequences of 'fooling about' in an engineering workshop.
(c) Explain why you, as an engineering trainee, should:
  (i)   adopt a short, neat hair style;
  (ii) not wear dirty overalls;
  (iii) write up your logbook carefully and neatly, keep it in a plastic folder, and make sure it is available on demand for examination by your supervisor.

2.3 *Instructions*
(a) Draw an organization chart to show the chain of command in your training centre or in a company with which you are familiar.
(b) Upon receiving a verbal instruction, describe what you would do to ensure that you have understood it correctly.

(c) If a written instruction is unclear or badly printed, describe what you would do to avoid making a mistake in carrying out the instruction.

2.4 *How to ask for help*

(a) Describe a situation where your instructor might have sent you to another person, such as a more senior colleague, for advice. Explain who that person might be in your training centre or company.

(b) To avoid bothering your instructor when he or she is busy, describe:
  (i) the sort of practical assistance you might seek from a colleague;
  (ii) the sort of information you might seek from a colleague.

(c) State whom you would approach for advice, and why you have chosen that person, in the following circumstances:
  (i) clarification of instructions or unclear advice from a colleague;
  (ii) safe working practice concerning a new material that has been introduced into the workshop;
  (iii) assistance in completing forms;
  (iv) reporting personal injuries and accidents;
  (v) discussing personal problems.

(d) Give ONE example of the *correct approach* to another person when seeking that person's help or advice, and ONE *inappropriate approach* to another person when seeking that person's help or advice.

2.5 *How to give help when asked*

(a) List FIVE important criteria that you must remember when giving help or advice to another person.

(b) Describe THREE situations when you should refuse to offer help or advice.

(c) Explain how you would try to make such a refusal without giving offence.

2.6 *Reporting deficiencies in tools, equipment and materials*

(a) Give FIVE reasons why it is necessary to report deficiencies in tools, equipment and materials.

(b) Briefly describe the procedures used in your training centre or company for reporting defective tools, equipment and materials.

2.7 *Respect for other people's opinions and property*

(a) You may have to work with people whose values on work and life in general disagree with your own. Should you:
  (i) argue aggressively with them? OR
  (ii) respect their views despite your personal reservations?

(b) You are in a hurry and a long way from the stores. You know that your workmate has the equipment you need in his or her personal toolkit. Describe the correct procedure for borrowing and returning such equipment.

(c)   You are in a hurry to get home at the end of your shift. You are returning the tools you have been using to the stores. Should you clean them and check them or leave that to the stores personnel to save yourself time? Give reasons for your answer.

2.8   *Teamwork and co-operation*
(a)   Why is it necessary to take the time and trouble to gain some knowledge and understanding of what other people do in your training centre or company, both within your department and in other departments? How could this lead to improved co-operation and teamwork?
(b)   How do some companies expand their trainees' and apprentices' insight into the work of other departments in the organization?
(c)   Give reasons for your answers to the following. When working as a team:
   (i)   should you take part in discussions concerning the work to be done?
   (ii)   should you ask for clarification of matters you do not understand?
   (iii)   from whom should you take instructions?

2.9   *Difficulties in working relationships*
(a)   State FIVE possible *causes* of difficulty that may arise in your relationships with your workmates and more senior staff.
(b)   With whom should you discuss such problems in the first place?
(c)   Describe the procedures that exist for formally reporting such difficulties in your training centre or company if you can get no satisfaction from (b) above.

3 Handling engineering information

When you have read this chapter you should understand how to:

- Select information sources to undertake work tasks.
- Extract, interpret and evaluate engineering information.
- Record and process engineering information.

3.1 Selection of information sources

The need for clear communications that cannot be misinterpreted was introduced in Chapter 2. It is necessary therefore to select means of communication and information sources that ensure that the correct information is provided and used. Engineering drawings are used to transmit and receive information concerning components to be manufactured and assembled. Engineering drawings will be considered in detail in Chapter 5. However, some information has to be given in writing. For example:

- Manufacturing instructions such as the name of the parts to be made, the number required, any special finishes required and the date by which they are required.

- Technical data such as screw thread sizes, and manufacturers' recommended cutting speeds and feeds.

- Stock lists such as material sizes, standard 'bought-in parts', and standard cutting tools.

- Training logbooks.

Verbal instructions and telephone messages should be confirmed in writing or by fax. The latter is particularly useful if illustrations are involved. In industry and commerce all information must be produced in a way that is:

- Easy to understand with no risk of errors.

- Complete, with no essential details missing.

- Quick and easy to complete.

These goals are best achieved by the use of standardized forms. By providing much of the information in the form of boxes that can be ticked, even the interpretation of hand writing that is difficult to read is overcome.

Manufacturing organizations are concerned with making the goods required by their customers at a price their customers are prepared to pay, and in delivering those goods in the correct quantities at the correct time. This involves teamwork within the organizations and close liaison with their customers and suppliers, and can only be achieved by the selection of efficient communication and the efficient handling of engineering information.

3.2 Interpretation of information (graphical)

There are many ways in which information can be presented and it is essential to select the most appropriate method. This will depend upon such factors as:

- The information itself.
- The accuracy of interpretation required.
- The expertise of the audience to whom the information is to be presented.

Much of the information required for the manufacture of engineering products is numerical. This can be presented in the form of tables where precise information is required concerning an individual item. Sometimes, all that is required is a general overview of a situation that can be seen at a glance. In this case the numerical data is most clearly presented by means of graphs and diagrams. There are many different types of graph depending upon the relationship between the quantities involved and the numerical skills of the user group at which the graph is aimed. Let's look at some graphs in common use.

3.2.1 Line graphs

Figure 3.1(a) shows a graph for the relationship drill speed and drill diameter for a cutting speed of 15 m/min. In this instance it is in order to use a continuous curve flowing through the points plotted. This is because the points plotted on the graph are related by a mathematical expression and any value of drill speed or drill diameter calculated from that expression will lie on the curve.

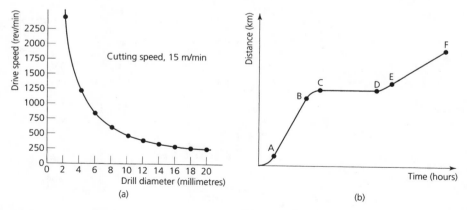

Figure 3.1 *Line graphs: (a) points connected by a smooth curve (point related mathematically); (b) points connected by straight lines*

This is not true in every instance as shown by Fig. 3.1(b). This graph connects time and distance travelled for a vehicle.

- From A to B the distance travelled is proportional to the time taken. That is, the straight line indicates that the vehicle is travelling with a constant speed.

- The curved bit at the beginning of the line shows that the vehicle was accelerating from a standing start. The curved bit at the end shows that the vehicle slowed down smoothly to a stop.

- From C to D there is no increase in distance with time. The vehicle is stationary.

- From E to F the vehicle recommences its journey at a reduced speed since the line slopes less steeply.

In this graph it is correct for the points to be connected by separate lines since each stage of the journey is unrelated to the previous stage or to the next stage. It would have been totally incorrect to draw a flowing curve through the points in this instance.

3.2.2 Histograms

Figure 3.2 shows the number of notifiable accidents which occur each year in a factory over a number of years. The points cannot be connected by a smooth, continuous curve as this would imply that the statistics follow some mathematical equation. Neither can they be connected by a series of straight lines. This would imply that, although the graph does not represent a mathematical equation, the number of accidents increased or decreased continuously and at a steady rate from one year to the next. In reality the number of accidents is scattered throughout the year in a random manner and the total for one year is independent of the total for the previous year or the next year. The correct way to present this information is by a histogram as shown.

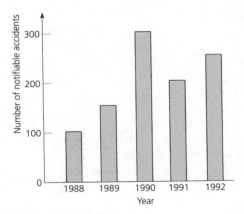

Figure 3.2 *Histogram*

3.2.3 Bar charts

These are frequently used for indicating the work in progress and they are used in production planning. An example is shown in Fig. 3.3.

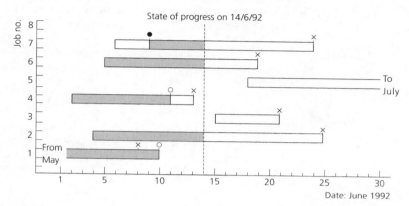

Figure 3.3 *Bar chart: × = scheduled completion date; ○ = actual completion date; ● = start delayed; shaded area = work completed to date*

3.2.4 Ideographs (pictograms)

These are frequently used for presenting statistical information to the general public. In Fig. 3.4 each symbol represents 1000 cars. Therefore in 1990, the number of cars using the visitors' car park at a company was 3000 (1000 cars for each of three symbols). Similarly, in 1991 the number of cars using the car park was 4000 and in 1992 the number had risen to 6000.

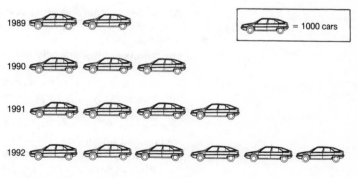

Number of cars using a car park each month

Figure 3.4 *Ideograph (pictogram): number of cars using a car park each month*

3.2.5   Pie charts

These are used to show how a total quantity is divided into its individual parts. Since a complete circle is 360°, and this represents the total, then a 60° sector would represent $60/360 = 1/6$ of the total. This is shown in Fig. 3.5(a). The total number of castings produced by a machine company's foundry divided up between the various machines manufactured can be represented by a pie chart as shown in Fig. 3.5(b).

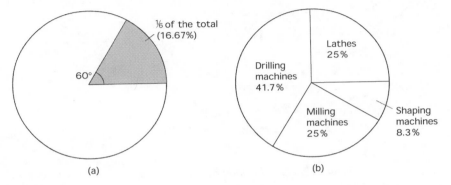

(a)

(b)

Figure 3.5 *Pie chart*

3.3   Interpretation of information (tables, charts and schedules)

3.3.1   Manufacturers' catalogues

Manufacturers' catalogues and technical manuals are an essential means of keeping up to date with suppliers' product lines. Also such catalogues and technical manuals usually include performance data and instructions for the correct and most efficient use for the products shown.

3.3.2   British and European Standards

At the start of the industrial revolution there was no standardization of components. Every nut and bolt was made as a fitted pair and was not interchangeable with any other nut and bolt. Imagine finding a box full of nuts and bolts of seemingly the same size and having to try every nut on every bolt until you found which nuts fitted which bolts. No wonder that screwed fasteners were the first manufactured goods to be standardized, although initially only on a national basis.

Modern industry requires a vast range of standardized materials and components to provide the interchangeability required for international trading and uniformity of quality. Initially this work was carried out by such organizations as the British Standards Institute (BSI) in the UK, by DIN in Germany, and by ANSI in America. Since 1947, the International Standards Organization (ISO) has been steadily harmonizing *national standards* and changing them into *international standards* in order to promote international trading in manufactured goods. The aims of standardization as defined by the BSI are:

- The provision of efficient communication amongst all interested parties. The promotion of economy in human effort, materials and energy in the production and exchange of goods through the mass production of standardized components and assemblies.

- The protection of consumer interests through adequate and consistent high quality of goods and consumer services.

- The promotion of international trade by the removal of barriers caused by differences in national practices.

3.3.3 Production schedules

These are usually in the form of bar charts or computer listings. The former will show the planned start and finish dates for various jobs and the machines onto which they are to be loaded. The actual progress of the jobs is superimposed on the ideal schedule so that any 'slippage' in production and the reason can be seen at a glance so that remedial action can be taken and, if necessary, the customer advised of possible delay. An example was shown in Fig. 3.3. Computer listings of production schedules and stock balances are updated regularly (on a daily basis) so that the sales staff of a company know what components and assemblies are in stock, and how soon new stock should be available if a particular item has sold out.

3.3.4 Product specifications

In addition to scheduling the work that is to be done, it is also necessary to issue full instructions to the works concerning the product to be made. That is, a *production specification* must be issued. For example, let's consider a car production line. It is set up to produce a continuous flow of a particular type of car. However, within that basic work pattern there are many variations. For example, some will have one colour and others will be different. Some will have one trim, others will have another. Some will have power steering, others will not, and so on. Therefore each car built will have a product specification, so that the customer will get the car he or she has chosen.

On a simpler basis is the *works order* issued in a batch production or in a jobbing workshop. This provides the information needed to manufacture a batch of components. An example of such a works order form is shown in Fig. 3.6.

The example shown provides the following information:

- It identifies the component to be made.

- It identifies the drawings to be used.

- It states the quantity of the product to be made.

- It specifies the material that is to be used.

- It specifies any special jigs, fixtures, tools and cutters that will be needed and their location in the stores.

ABC Engineering Co. Ltd		Job No.
Date issued	Date required	
Component		
Drawing numbers		
Quantity		
Material size	Type	Quantity
Tooling		
Finish /Colour		
Date commenced	Date finished	Operator
Inspection report		Inspector
Special requirements		
Destination		Authorised by

Figure 3.6 *Typical works order form*

- It specifies any heat treatment and finishing process that may be required.
- It specifies the issue date for the order and the date by which it is required.
- It specifies the destination of the job (stores, inspection department, etc.).
- It includes any special variations required by a particular customer.
- It identifies the personnel employed in the manufacture and the inspection of the job.
- It carries the signature that gives the managerial authority for the work to be done.
- It provides room for the actual dates to be inserted when the job was commenced, and when it finished.

You will notice that all this information is entered on a standard form. This saves time in issuing the information. It is much easier to fill in the blanks than to have to write out all the information from scratch. It is also easy to see if a 'box' is blank. This would indicate that a vital piece of information is missing. It is also easier for the person doing the job to see exactly what is required since the same sort of information always appears in the same place on the form every time.

3.3.5 Reference tables and charts

There are a number of 'pocketbooks' published for the different branches of engineering. A typical 'pocketbook' for use in manufacturing workshops would contain tables of information such as:

- Conversion tables for fractional to decimal dimensions in inch units, and conversion tables for inch to metric dimensions.

- Conversion tables for fractional (inch), letter, number and metric twist drill sizes.

- Standard screw thread and threaded fastener data tables.

- Tables for spacing holes around pitch circles as an aid to marking out.

- Speeds and feeds for typical cutting tool and workpiece material combinations for different processes.

This list is by no means exhaustive but just a brief indication of the sort of useful data provided. In addition, many manufacturers produce wall charts of similar data as it affects their particular products. These are not only more convenient for the user than having to open and thumb through a book with oily hands, but they are also good publicity for the manufacturers who issue them.

3.3.6 Drawings and diagrams

Engineers use drawings and diagrams to communicate with each other and with the public at large. The type of drawing or diagram will depend upon the audience it is aimed at and their ability to correctly interpret such information. The creation and interpretation of engineering drawings is considered in detail in Chapter 5.

3.4 Evaluating engineering information

Keep alert for errors in the information given. Suppose you have made several batches of a component from stainless steel and suddenly the works order form specifies silver steel. Is this a genuine change or a clerical error? So, the manager has signed it, but he is a very busy person and he may have missed the error. Therefore check with your supervisor before starting the job. Better to be sure than sorry.

If standards are referred to check that the issue on the shop floor is up to date. Standard specifications and EU regulations change rapidly these days. Out of date editions should be withdrawn immediately and the latest edition issued. However, it is surprising how long an out of date copy can keep circulating before someone spots it and destroys it.

3.5 Recording and processing engineering information

The need for, and importance of, accurate record keeping is increasing all the time in nearly all the areas of company activity. Let's now look at some of the more important aspects that affect all employees.

3.5.1 Quality control

Quality control now affects nearly all the manufacturing companies both large and small. This is because a firm that wants to sell its goods to a BS EN 9000 approved firm must itself be approved and, in turn, obtain its supplies from approved sources. In the UK the British Standard for Quality Assurance is BS EN 9000. The definition of quality upon which this standard is based is in the sense of '*fitness for purpose*' and '*safe in use*', and that the product or service has been designed to meet the needs of the customer.

A detailed study of quality control and total quality management is beyond the scope of this book. However, if you are employed in the engineering industry it is almost inevitable that you are employed in a company that is BS EN 9000 approved and that this will influence your working practices. A key factor in this respect is '*traceability*'. Therefore BS EN 9000 is largely concerned with documentation procedures. All the products needed to fulfil a customer's requirements must be clearly identifiable throughout the organization. This is necessary in order that any part delivered to a customer can have its history traced from the source from which the raw material was purchased, through all the stages of manufacture and testing, until it is eventually delivered to the customer. This is shown diagrammatically in Fig. 3.7.

The need for this *traceability* might arise in the case of a dispute with a customer due to non-conformity with the product specification, for safety reasons if an accident occurs due to failure of the product, and for statutory and legal reasons. For these reasons, like everyone else involved, your contribution to the above chain of events has to be accurately recorded and the records kept indefinitely. Otherwise the company's goods may not be certified and acceptable to the customer.

3.5.2 Health and safety

This is discussed in detail in Chapter 1. Here, also, record keeping is essential. Some of the documents and data that need to be maintained are:

- the accident register;
- the regular inspection and certification of lifting tackle and pressure vessels (boilers and compressed air receivers);
- dates of fire drills and the time taken to evacuate the premises: records of visits to the premises by local authority fire and safety officers and their reports.

3.5.3 Legal and financial reasons

Registered companies need to keep legal records to comply with the Companies Act. They must publish their Memorandum and Articles of

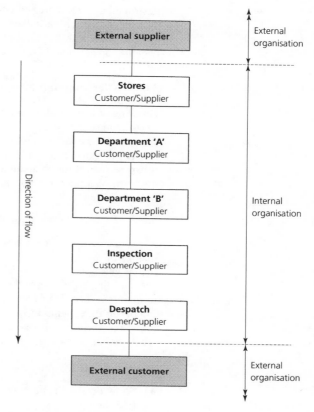

Figure 3.7 *Quality control chain (each stage is a customer of the previous stage and a supplier to the next stage, i.e. Department 'A' is a customer of the stores and a supplier to Department 'B')*

Association and lodge a copy at Companies House when the company is set up. They must keep accurate minutes of all meetings of the board of directors and make annual returns including a current list of directors and other information immediately following each annual general meeting (AGM) of the company.

Similarly it is important that a company keeps accurate and complete financial records so that it can keep its costs under control and ensure that a profit is made. It also needs these records to satisfy the accountants when they make their annual visit to audit the accounts and draw up the balance sheet as required by the directors and shareholders as well as the tax authorities.

3.6 Methods of record keeping

3.6.1 Computer files

Most records are nowadays kept on computer files in the form of magnetic disks, magnetic tapes and optical discs (compact discs). These are easily destroyed by fire, theft and computer viruses (bugs). For this reason such data should be regularly backed up so that, in an emergency, the data can be reinstated with the minimum of downtime and loss of business. Such backup copies should be kept in a burglar proof and fire proof safe.

3.6.2   Microfilm and microfiche

Paper records are bulky and easily lost and destroyed. Forms and technical drawings can be easily copied onto microfilm or microfiche systems. These can store large quantities of information photographically in a small space. Such material can be conveniently catalogued and, when required, it can be read through a suitable viewer or enlarged to its original size in the form of a photographic print.

3.6.3   Registers and logbooks

Registers are used for various purposes such as recording the maintenance history of machine tools, the testing and inspection of equipment such as lifting gear, pressure vessels and fire extinguishers, accidents to employees, and fire drills. Lorry drivers and sales representatives keep logbooks to maintain records of their journeys. For young trainees, one of the most important documents to be kept is your *training logbook*. The format of logbooks varies from one training establishment to another. No matter what format is chosen, your logbook should:

- Record the training you have undergone.

- Show details of the exercises you have undertaken and how you carried them out.

- Show how successfully you have completed each exercise.

- Show your instructor's comments on your performance and his or her signature verifying the entry.

3.7   Communications (miscellaneous)

Safety and hazard notices

There is a saying that *in an emergency people panic in their own language*. Therefore, all safety notices and operating instructions for potentially hazardous plant and processes should be printed in as many languages as there are employees from different ethnic backgrounds. Wherever possible internationally recognized hazard signs should be used.

Safety and hazard signs

All signs must comply with the Safety Signs Regulations 1980. These are recognized internationally and combine geometrical shape, colour and a pictorial symbol to put across the message. Some examples can be found in Section 1.7.2.

Colour coding

This is another means of communication that overcomes language barriers. Table 3.1 shows the colour codes for the contents of gas cylinders. A cylinder that is coloured wholly red or maroon or has a red band round it near the top contains a flammable gas. In the case of red cylinders the name of the gas should also be stated on the cylinder. Maroon coloured cylinders contain only acetylene gas for welding. A cylinder having a yellow band round the top contains a poisonous gas.

TABLE 3.1 *Colour codes for cylinder contents*

Gas	Ground colour of cylinder	Colour of bands
Acetylene	Maroon	None
Air	Grey	None
Ammonia	Black	Red and yellow
Argon	Blue	None
Carbon monoxide	Red (+ name)	Yellow
Coal gas	Red (+ name)	None
Helium	Medium brown	None
Hydrogen	Red (+ name)	None
Methane	Red (+ name)	None
Nitrogen	Dark grey	Black
Oxygen	Black	None

The identification colours for electric cables are shown in Table 3.2. Note that earth conductors are nowadays likely to be referred to as *circuit protective conductors*.

TABLE 3.2 *Colour codes for electrical cables*

Service	Cable		Colour
Single phase Flexible	Live		Brown
	Neutral		Blue
	Earth		Green/yellow
Single phase Non-flexible	Live		Red
	Neutral		Black
	Earth		Green/yellow
Three phase Non-flexible	Line (live)	colour denotes phase	Red White Blue
	Neutral		Black
	Earth		Green/yellow

Finally, pipe runs and electrical conduits are colour coded according to their contents as listed in Table 3.3. The method of application of the colour code is shown in Fig. 3.8.

TABLE 3.3 *Colour codes for pipe contents*

Colour	Contents
White	Compressed air
Black	Drainage
Dark grey	Refrigeration and chemicals
Signal red	Fire (hydrant and sprinkler supplies)
Crimson or aluminium	Steam and central heating
French blue	Water
Georgian green	Sea, river and untreated water
Brilliant green	Cold water services from storage tanks
Light orange	Electricity
Eau-de-Nil	Domestic hot water
Light brown	Oil
Canary yellow	Gas

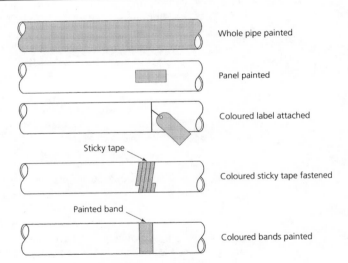

Figure 3.8 *Colour codes for contents of pipes*

Posters

Posters are also used to put over safety messages. They may be humorous or dramatic. The picture reinforces the caption so that the message is clear even for people who cannot read the words for some reason. Such posters should be displayed at strategic points adjacent to the hazard they represent. They should be changed frequently so as to attract attention.

Exercises   **3.1** *Information required to undertake work tasks*

(a)   You have just received the works order form for the next component you are to make. List the essential information you would expect to find on such a form.

(b)   As well as the works order form, what additional and essential document do you need before you can start the task?

3.2 *Interpretation of numerical information*

(a)   Graphs are often used for showing numerical relationships. Sketch suitable graphs to represent the following situations.

(i)   The relationship between the diameter and cross-sectional area of mild steel rods of 2, 4, 6, 8, 10 and 12 millimetres diameter.

(ii)   The relationship between time and total power in watts for an office that has eight fluorescent electric lights. Each light has a power rating of 80 watts. The lights are turned on, one at a time, at ten minute intervals until they are all on.

(iii) A firm has the following notable accident record:
1994   15 accidents
1995   24 accidents
1996   12 accidents
1997   7 accidents.

(b)   With the aid of simple examples explain when you would use the following types of graphical representation.

(i)   Ideograph (pictogram)

(ii)   Pie chart.

3.3 *Extraction and interpretation of engineering information*

(a)   The parts list of a general arrangement drawing specifies the use of a manufacturer's standard drill bush with a bore of 6 mm and an O/D of 12 mm. State where you would look for details of such bushes and list the information you would need to give to the stores so that they could purchase such a bush.

(b)   What do the following initial letters stand for: BSI, ISO, EN? (Note you may find two uses of the initials EN.) To what do the specifications BS 970 and BS 308 refer?

(c)   Explain briefly, with the aid of an example, what is meant by a *production schedule*.

(d)   Give an example of a *product specification* for any product with which you are familiar.

(e)   Table 3.4 shows an abstract from some screw thread tables. What is the pitch of an M10 thread and what tapping size drill is required for tapping an internal M10 screw thread?

3.4 *Evaluation of the accuracy and appropriateness of engineering information*

(a)   Give TWO reasons for cross-checking the accuracy of any reference books that might be lying around in your workshop.

(b)   To whom should you refer for guidance as to the accuracy and relevance of reference material available in your workshop?

TABLE 3.4 *Exercise 3.3(e)*

150 metric threads (coarse series)	Minor dia. (mm)	Tensile stress area (mm²)	Tapping drill (mm)	ISO Hexagon (mm)
M0.8 × 0.2	0.608	0.31	0.68	–
M1.0 × 0.25	0.675	0.46	0.82	2.5
M1.2 × 0.25	0.875	0.73	1.0	3.0
M1.4 × 0.30	1.014	0.98	1.2	3.0
M1.6 × 0.35	1.151	1.27	1.35	3.2
M1.8 × 0.35	1.351	1.70	1.55	–
M2.0 × 0.40	1.490	2.1	1.70	4.0
M2.2 × 0.45	1.628	2.5	1.90	–
M2.5 × 0.45	1.928	3.4	2.20	5.0
M3.0 × 0.5	2.367	5.0	2.65	5.5
M3.5 × 0.6	2.743	6.8	3.10	–
M4.0 × 0.7	3.120	8.8	3.50	7.0
M4.5 × 0.75	3.558	11.5	4.0	–
M5.0 × 0.8	3.995	14.2	4.50	8.0
M6.0 × 1.0	4.747	20.1	5.3	10.0
M8.0 × 1.25	6.438	36.6	7.1	13.0
M10.0 × 1.50	8.128	58.0	8.8	17.0
M12.0 × 1.75	9.819	84.3	10.70	19.0
M16.0 × 2.00	13.510	157.0	14.5	24.0

3.5 *Recording and processing engineering information*
  (a) State FOUR reasons for, and the importance of, accurate record keeping in a modern factory environment.
  (b) State whether it is a legal requirement to keep a log of notable accidents and, if so, who has the authority to demand access to such a log.
  (c) Describe briefly how quality control is maintained in your company, or your training centre, and what records are required.

3.6 *Methods of record keeping*
  (a) Computer files have superseded many manual filing systems. Why should backup copies of files be kept, and how can these be kept?
  (b) State the purposes for which the following methods of record keeping are used.
    (i) Logbooks (other than your training logbook).
    (ii) Forms and schedules.
    (iii) Photographic (pictorial and dye-line).
    (iv) Drawings and diagrams.
  (c) Why is it important to keep a training logbook, and why should it be kept carefully, away from dirt and oil, so that it is always clean, neat and tidy?

4 Engineering materials and heat treatment

When you have read this chapter you should understand:

- How to define the basic properties of engineering materials.
- How to correctly identify and select a range of engineering metals and alloys.
- How to correctly identify and select a range of non-metallic materials suitable for engineering applications.
- Safe working practices as applicable to heat treatment processes.
- The principles and purposes of heat treatment.
- The through hardening of plain carbon steels.
- The carburizing and case-hardening of low carbon steels.
- How to temper hardened steels.
- How to anneal and normalize steels.
- The basic heat treatment of non-ferrous metals and alloys.
- The principles, advantages and limitations of heat treatment furnaces.
- The temperature control of heat treatment furnaces.
- The advantages, limitations and applications of quenching media.

4.1 States of matter

Almost all matter can exist in three physical states by changing its temperature in appropriate conditions. These states are solids, liquids and gases.

- Ice is *solid* water and exists below 0°C.

- Water is a *liquid* above 0°C and below 100°C.

- Steam is water *vapour* above 100°C and becomes a *gas* as its temperature is raised further (superheated).

Metals such as brass, copper or steel are solid (frozen) at room temperatures but become liquid (molten) if heated to a sufficiently high temperature. If they are heated to a high enough temperature they will turn into a gas. On cooling, they will first turn back to a liquid and then back to a solid at room temperature. Providing no chemical change takes place (oxidation of the metal through contact with air at high temperatures) we can change substances backwards and forwards through the three states by heating and cooling as often as we like.

There are exceptions, for example when a thermosetting plastic has been heated during the moulding process it undergoes a chemical change called 'curing'. Once 'cured' it can never again be softened nor turned into a liquid by heating. It can be destroyed by overheating. Another example is the non-metallic element iodine. When heated this *sublimes* directly from a solid to a vapour without becoming a liquid.

With the exception of mercury all metals are solid at normal working temperatures. Metals can be melted into liquids by heating them sufficiently. In the liquid state they can be cast to shape in moulds.

4.2 Properties of materials

To compare and identify engineering materials, it is important to understand the meaning of their more common properties. For example, it is no good saying one material is stronger or harder than another material unless we know what is meant by the terms 'strength' and 'hardness'.

4.2.1 Strength properties

Tensile strength

This is the ability of a material to withstand a stretching load without breaking. This is shown in Fig. 4.1(a). The load is trying to stretch the

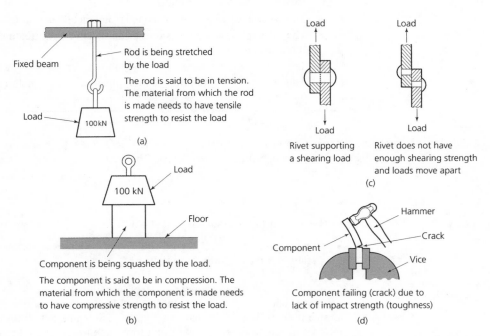

Figure 4.1 *Mechanical properties – strength: (a) tensile strength; (b) compression strength; (c) shear strength; (d) impact strength*

rod therefore the rod is said to be in a *state of tension*. It is being subjected to a tensile load. To resist this load without breaking, the material from which the rod is made needs to have sufficient *tensile strength*.

Compressive strength

This is the ability of a material to withstand a squeezing load without breaking. This is shown in Fig. 4.1(b). The load is trying to squash (crush or compress) the material from which the component is made, therefore the component is said to be in a *state of compression*. It is being subjected to a compressive load. To resist this load without breaking, the material from which it is made needs to have sufficient *compressive strength*.

Shear strength

This is the ability of a material to withstand an *offset* load without break-ing (shearing). This is shown in Fig. 4.1(c). The loads are trying to pull the joint apart and the rivet is trying to resist them. The loads are not in line, but are offset. The rivet is subjected to a shear load. The material from which it is made must have sufficient *shear strength* or the rivet will fail as shown, and the loads will move apart. The rivet is said to have *sheared*. The same effect would have occurred if the loads had been pushing instead of pulling.

Note: Riveted joints should be designed so that the load always acts in shear across the shank of the rivet as shown. It must never pull on the heads of the rivet. The heads are intended only to keep the rivet in place.

Toughness

The ability of a material to withstand an impact load. This is shown in Fig. 4.1(d). The impact loading is causing the metal to crack. To resist this impact loading without breaking, the material from which it is made needs to have sufficient *toughness*. Strength and toughness must not be confused. Strength refers to tensile strength – the ability to withstand an axial pulling load. For example, when you buy a rod of high carbon steel (e.g. silver steel) it is in the soft condition and it is strong and tough. It has a relatively high tensile strength and its toughness will enable it to withstand relatively high impact loading before it cracks.

If this metal is quench-hardened (Section 4.16) its *tensile strength* will have greatly *increased*, it will also have become very *brittle*. In this hard and brittle condition it will now break with only a light tap with a ham-mer – it can *no longer resist impact loads* – it has *lost its toughness*.

Brittleness

We have just mentioned brittleness. This property is the opposite of tough-ness. It is the ability to shatter when subject to impact. For example, the way a glass window behaves when struck by a cricket ball.

Rigidity

This property is also referred to as stiffness. This is the ability of a metal to retain its original shape under load. That is, to resist plastic or elastic deformation. Cast iron is an example of a rigid material. Because it is rigid and because it can be cast into intricate shapes, it is a good material for use in making the beds and columns for machine tools.

4.2.2 Forming properties

Elasticity

This property enables a material to change shape under load and to return to its original size and shape when the load is removed. Components such as springs are made from elastic materials as shown in Fig. 4.2(a). Note that springs will only return to their original length providing they are not overloaded.

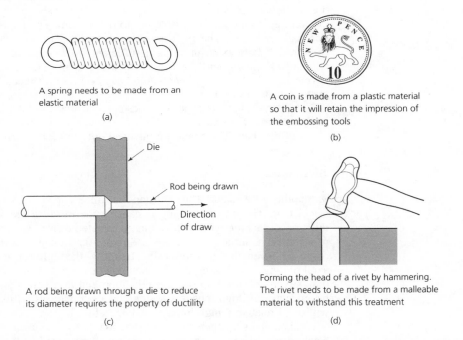

A spring needs to be made from an elastic material

(a)

A coin is made from a plastic material so that it will retain the impression of the embossing tools

(b)

A rod being drawn through a die to reduce its diameter requires the property of ductility

(c)

Forming the head of a rivet by hammering. The rivet needs to be made from a malleable material to withstand this treatment

(d)

Figure 4.2 *Mechanical properties – flow: (a) elasticity; (b) plasticity; (c) ductility; (d) malleability*

Plasticity

This property enables a material to deform under load and to retain its new shape when the load is removed. This is shown in Fig. 4.2(b). The coin is made from a copper alloy that is relatively soft and plastic. It takes the impression of the dies when compressed between them, and retains that impression when the dies are opened. When the deforming force is tensile as when wire drawing, the property of plasticity is given the special name *ductility*. When the deforming force is compressive, for example when coining, the property of plasticity is given the special name *malleability*.

Ductility

As stated above, this property enables a material to deform in a plastic manner when subjected to a tensile (stretching) force. For example, when wire drawing as shown in Fig. 4.2(c). Also, the bracket shown in Fig. 4.2(c) requires a ductile material. The outer surface of the material stretches as it bends and is in a state of tension. At the same time the material must remain bent when the bending force is removed so it must be plastic. A *ductile* material combines *tensile strength* and *plasticity*. Note that even the most ductile of metals still show a degree of elasticity. Therefore, when bending the bracket to shape, it must be bent through slightly more than a right angle. This 'overbend' allows for any slight 'springback'.

Malleability

As stated above, this property enables a material to deform in a plastic manner when subjected to a compressive (squeezing) force. For example, when forging or when rivet heading as shown in Fig. 4.2(d). The material must retain its shape when the compressive force is removed so it must be plastic. A *malleable* material combines *compressive strength* and *plasticity*.

Hardness

This is the ability of a material to resist scratching and indentation. Figure 4.3 shows a hard steel ball being pressed into the surface of two pieces of material using the same standard load. When pressed into a hard material, the ball makes only a shallow indentation. When pressed into a soft material, under the same test conditions, the ball sinks into the material further and makes a deeper impression. This is the basic principle of all standard hardness tests.

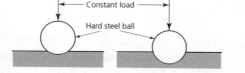

When pressed into a hard material the ball only makes a **shallow** indentation

Constant load

Hard steel ball

When pressed into a soft material the ball makes a **deep** indentation

Figure 4.3 *Hardness*

4.2.3 Heat properties

Heat conductivity

This is the ability of a material to conduct heat. Metals are good conductors of heat and non-metals are poor conductors of heat. Figure 4.4(a)

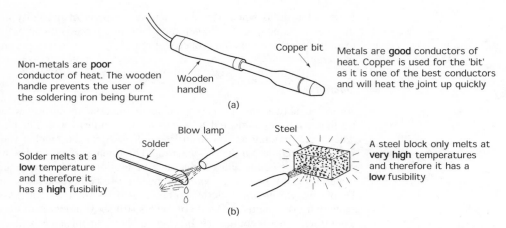

Figure 4.4 *Heat properties: (a) heat conductivity; (b) fusibility*

shows an electrically heated soldering iron. The bit is made of copper because this is the best of the common metals for conducting heat. It conducts the heat from the heating element to the joint to be soldered. Copper also has an affinity for soft solder so it can be easily 'tinned'. The handle is made of wood or plastic as these materials are easily shaped and are poor conductors of heat. They are heat-insulating materials. They keep cool and are pleasant to handle.

Refractoriness

You must not mix up poor heat conductivity with good refractory properties. *Refractory* materials are largely unaffected by heat. The firebricks used in furnaces are refractory materials. They do not burn or melt at the operating temperature of the furnace. They are also good heat-insulating materials. However, the plastic or wooden handle of the soldering iron shown in Fig. 4.4(a) had good heat-insulating properties but these are not refractory materials since plastics and wood are destroyed by high temperatures.

Fusibility

This is the ease with which materials melt. Soft solders melt at relatively low temperatures; other materials melt at much higher temperatures. Figure 4.3(b) shows the effect of turning a gas blowpipe onto a stick of soft solder. The solder quickly melts. The same flame turned onto a block of steel makes the steel hot (possibly red-hot) but does not melt it.

- The soft solder *melts at a relatively low temperature* because it has *high fusibility*.

- The steel *will not melt* in the flame of the blowpipe because it has *low fusibility* and will melt only at a very *high temperature*.

4.2.4 Corrosion resistance

This is the ability of a material to withstand chemical or electrochemical attack. A combination of such everyday things as air and water will chemically attack plain carbon steels and form a layer of rust on its exposed surfaces. Stainless steels are alloys of iron together with carbon, nickel and chromium; they will resist corrosion. Many non-ferrous metals are corrosion resistant which is why we use copper for waterpipes, and zinc or lead for roofing sheets and flashings.

4.2.5 Hot and cold working

Metals can be cast to shape by melting them and pouring them into moulds. Metals can also be cut to shape by using hand tools and machine tools. However, there is the alternative of *working* them to shape. This is how a blacksmith shapes metal by hammering it to shape on the anvil. Metals that have been shaped by working (also called 'flow forming') are said to be *wrought*.

Metals may be worked hot or cold. In either case the crystalline structure of the metal is distorted by the working process and the metal becomes harder, stronger and less ductile.

- In *cold-working* metals the crystalline structure (grain) becomes distorted due to the processing and remains distorted when the processing has finished. This leaves the metal harder, stronger and less ductile. Unfortunately, further cold working could cause the metal to crack.

- In *hot-working* metals the grain also becomes distorted but the metal is sufficiently hot for the grains to reform as fast as the distortion occurs, leaving the metal soft and ductile. Some grain refinement will occur so that the metal should be stronger than at the start of the process. The metal is easier to work at high temperatures and less force is required to form it. This is why the blacksmith gets his metal red-hot before forging it to shape with a hammer.

- *Recrystallization* is the term used when the distorted grains reform when they are heated. The temperature at which this happens depends upon the type of metal or alloy and how severely it has been previously processed by cold working.

- *Cold working* is the flow forming of metal *below* the temperature of recrystallization. For example, cold heading rivets.

- *Hot working* is the flow forming of metals *above* the temperature of recrystallization. For example, rolling red-hot ingots into girders in a steel mill.

Figure 4.5 shows examples of hot and cold working, and Tables 4.1 and 4.2 summarize the advantages and limitations of hot- and cold-working processes.

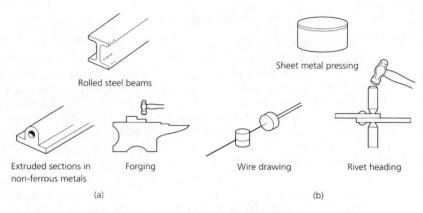

Rolled steel beams

Extruded sections in
non-ferrous metals

Forging

Sheet metal pressing

Wire drawing

Rivet heading

(a)

(b)

Figure 4.5 *Examples of (a) hot-working and (b) cold-working processes*

TABLE 4.1 *Hot-working processes*

Advantages	Limitations
1. Low cost 2. Grain refinement from cast structure 3. Materials are left in the fully annealed condition and are suitable for cold working (heading, bending, etc.) 4. Scale gives some protection against corrosion during storage 5. Availability as sections (girders) and forgings as well as the more usual bars, rods, sheets, strip and butt-welded tube	1. Poor surface finish – rough and scaly 2. Due to shrinkage on cooling the dimensional accuracy of hot-worked components is of a low order 3. Due to distortion on cooling and to the processes involved, hot working generally leads to geometrical inaccuracy 4. Fully annealed condition of the material coupled with a relatively coarse grain leads to a poor finish when machined 5. Low strength and rigidity for metal considered 6. Damage to tooling from abrasive scale on metal surface

TABLE 4.2 *Cold-working processes*

Advantages	Limitations

1. Good surface finish
2. Relatively high dimensional accuracy
3. Relatively high geometrical accuracy
4. Work hardening caused during the cold-working processes:
  (a) increases strength and rigidity
  (b) improves the machining characteristics of the metal so that a good finish is more easily achieved
	1. Higher cost than for hot-worked materials. It is only a finishing process for material previously hot worked. Therefore, the processing cost is added to the hot-worked cost
	2. Materials lack ductility due to work hardening and are less suitable for bending, etc.
	3. Clean surface is easily corroded
	4. Availability limited to rods and bars also sheets and strip, solid drawn tubes

4.3 Classification of materials

Almost every known substance has found its way into the engineering workshop at some time or other. Neither this chapter nor in fact the whole of this book could hold all the facts about all the materials used by engineers. Therefore, to keep things simple, first these materials are grouped into similar types and then the properties and uses of some examples from each group will be considered. These main groups are shown in Fig. 4.6.

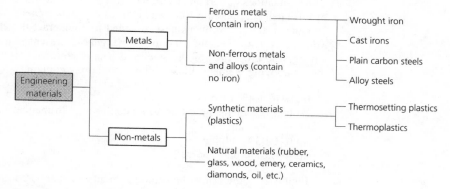

Figure 4.6 *Classification of engineering materials*

4.3.1 Metals

For the purposes of this book, we can consider metals as substances that have a lustrous sheen when cut, are good conductors of heat, and are good conductors of electricity. Some examples are aluminium, copper and iron. Sometimes metals are mixed with non-metals. For example, cast irons and plain carbon steels are mixtures of iron and carbon with traces of other elements. Sometimes metals are mixed with other metals to form *alloys*. For example, brass is an alloy of copper and zinc.

4.3.2 Non-metals

These can be elements, compounds of elements and mixtures of compounds. They include wood, rubber, plastics, ceramics and glass. Some materials are compounds of metals and non-metals. For example, naturally occurring abrasive grits, such as emery and corundum contain between 70% and 90% of aluminium oxide (a compound of aluminium and oxygen). Aluminium oxide (also known as alumina) is used in firebricks for furnace linings.

Organic compounds are based on the element *carbon* chemically combined with other substances. Some examples of organic materials are natural materials such as wood and some rubbers, and synthetic materials such as plastics.

4.4 Ferrous metals (plain carbon steels)

Ferrous metals and alloys are based on the metal *iron*. They are called ferrous metals because the Latin name for iron is *ferrum*. Iron is a soft grey metal and is rarely found in the pure state outside a laboratory. For engineering purposes the metal iron is usually associated with the non-metal carbon.

4.4.1 Plain carbon steels

Plain carbon steels, as their name implies, consist mainly of iron with small quantities of carbon. There will also be traces of impurities left over from when the metallic iron was extracted for its mineral ore. A small amount of the metal manganese is added to counteract the effects of the impurities. However, the amount of manganese present is insufficient to change the properties of the steel and it is, therefore, not considered to be an alloying element. Plain carbon steels may contain:

0.1% to 1.4% carbon
up to 1.0% manganese (not to be confused with magnesium)
up to 0.3% silicon
up to 0.05% sulphur
up to 0.05% phosphorus

Figure 4.7 shows how the carbon content of a plain carbon steel affects the properties of the steel. For convenience we can group plain carbon steels into three categories:

- low carbon steels (below 0.3% carbon);

- medium carbon steels (0.3% to 0.8% carbon);

- high carbon steels (between 0.8% and 1.4% carbon).

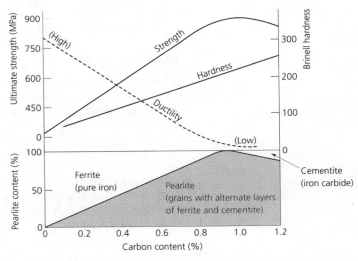

Figure 4.7 *The effect of carbon content on the properties of plain carbon steels*

4.4.2 Low carbon steels

These are also referred to as mild steels. If the carbon content is kept between 0.1% and 0.15% the steel is often referred to as 'dead mild' steel. This steel is very ductile and very soft, and can be pressed into complicated shapes for car body panels at room temperature without cracking. It is not used for machined components since its softness would cause it to tear and leave a poor surface finish. It is slightly weaker than the next group of low carbon steels to be considered.

If the carbon content is between 0.15% and 0.3% the steel is stronger, but slightly less soft and ductile. It is often referred to as 'mild' steel. It can be forged, rolled and drawn both in the hot and in the cold condition. It is easily machined with high-speed steel cutting tools. Because of its ease of manufacture and the very large quantities produced, mild steels are the cheapest and most plentiful of the steel products. Hot worked mild steel is available as structural sections (girders, reinforcing rods and mesh for concrete), forgings, sheet, strip, plate, rods, bars and seam-welded tubes. Cold worked mild steel – also known as bright drawn mild steel (BDMS) – is available as bright drawn bars and rods; solid drawn tubes; sheet and strip, and formed wire goods.

Some low carbon steels contain additives such as lead or sulphur to make them 'free-cutting'. The greatly improved machining properties imparted by these additives are achieved only at the expense of the strength and toughness of the steel.

4.4.3 Medium carbon steels

There are two groups of medium carbon steels:

- 0.3% to 0.5% carbon. These can be heat treated to make them tough and strong.

- 0.5% to 0.8% carbon. These can be heat treated to make them fairly hard yet retain a degree of toughness (impact resistance).

Medium carbon steels are harder, stronger and tougher than low carbon steels. They are also more expensive. They cannot be bent or formed in the cold condition to the same extent as low carbon steels without cracking. However, medium carbon steels hot forge well, but close temperature control is required to prevent:

- 'Burning' at high temperatures over 1150°C, as this leads to embrittlement. The metal cannot be reclaimed and the forging has to be scrapped.

- Cracking when forging is continued below 700°C. Cracking is due to work hardening as the steel is in the 'cold' condition from a forging point of view.

Medium carbon steels with a carbon content in the 0.3 to 0.5% range are used for such products as drop-hammer die blocks, laminated springs, wire ropes, screwdriver blades, spanners, hammer heads and heavy duty forgings.

Medium carbon steels with a carbon content in the 0.5 to 0.8% range are used for such products as wood saws, cold chisels, forged blanks for connecting rods, crankshafts, gears and other stressed components such as high-tensile pipes and tubes.

4.4.4 High carbon steels

These are harder, less ductile and more expensive than both mild and medium carbon steels. They are also less tough and are mostly used for springs, cutting tools and forming dies. High carbon steels work-harden readily and, for this reason, they are not recommended for cold working. However, they forge well providing the temperature is controlled at between 700°C and 900°C. There are three groups of high carbon steels:

- 0.8% to 1.0% carbon where both toughness and hardness are required. For example, sheet metal pressing tools where the number of components to be produced does not warrant the cost of expensive alloy steels. Also, cold chisels for fine work, some hand tools, shear blades, coil springs and high-tensile wire (piano wire).

- 1.0% to 1.2% carbon for sufficient hardness for most metal cutting tools, for example wood drills, screw-cutting taps and screw-cutting dies.

- 1.2% to 1.4% carbon where extreme hardness is required for woodworking tools and knives where a very keen cutting edge is required.

For all of these applications the steel has to undergo heat treatment to enhance its properties. Heat treatment processes are considered later in this chapter.

4.5 Ferrous metals (alloy steels)

These are essentially plain carbon steels to which other metals (*alloying elements*) have been added in sufficient quantities to materially alter the properties of the steel. The most common alloying elements are:

- *Nickel*, to refine the grain and strengthen the steel.

- *Chromium*, to improve the response of the steel to heat treatment; also to improve the corrosion resistance of the steel.

- *Molybdenum*, to reduce temper brittleness during heat treatment, welding, and operation at sustained high temperatures.

- *Manganese*, improves the strength and wear resistance of steels. Steels containing a high percentage of manganese (14%) are highly wear resistant and these steels are used for such applications as bulldozer blades and plough blades.

- *Tungsten* and *cobalt*, improve the ability of a steel to remain hard at high temperatures and are used extensively in cutting tool materials.

Alloy steels are used where great strength is required, corrosion resistance is required, or where the ability to remain hard at high temperatures is required. In this book we only need to consider high-speed steels for cutting tools, and stainless steels where corrosion resistance is required.

4.5.1 High-speed steels

High-speed steels are a group of alloy steels containing metallic elements such as tungsten and cobalt. They are used to make tools suitable for cutting metals. These cutting tools are for use with machine tools where the heat generated by the cutting process would soon soften high carbon steel tools. High-speed steels can operate continuously at 700°C, whereas high carbon steel starts to soften at 220°C. Table 4.3 lists the composition and uses of some typical high-speed steels.

TABLE 4.3 *Typical high-speed steels*

Type of steel	Composition* (%)						Hardness (VNP)	Uses
	C	Cr	W	V	Mo	Co		
18% tungsten	0.68	4.0	19.0	1.5	–	–	800–850	Low-quality alloy, not much used
30% tungsten	0.75	4.7	22.0	1.4	–	–	850–950	General-purpose cutting tools for jobbing work shops
6% cobalt	0.8	5.0	19.0	1.5	0.5	6.0	800–900	Heavy-duty cutting tools
Super HSS 12% cobalt	0.8	5.0	21.0	1.5	0.5	11.5	850–950	Heavy-duty cutting tools for machining high-tensile materials

*C = Carbon, Cr = chromium, W = tungsten, V = vanadium, Mo = molybdenum, Co = cobalt.

4.5.2 Stainless steels

These are also alloy steels. They contain a high proportion of chromium to provide corrosion resistance. Various grades of stainless steel and

TABLE 4.4 Typical stainless steels

Type of steel	Composition					Mechanical properties				Heat treatment	Applications
	C	Mn	Cr	Ni	Si	R_m	R_e	A	H_B		
403S17 Ferritic	0.04	0.45	14.0	0.50	0.80	510	340	31	–	Condition soft. Cannot be hardened except by cold work	Soft and ductile; can be used for fabrications, pressings, drawn components, spun components. Domestic utensils
420S45 Martensitic	0.30	1.0	13.0	1.0	0.80	1470	–	–	450	Quench from 950–1000°C. Temper 400–450°C. Temper 150–180°C	Corrosion-resistant springs for food processing and chemical plant. Corrosion-resistant cutlery and edge tools
						1670	61	–	534		
							278	50	170		
302S25 Austenitic	0.1	1.0	18.0	8.50	0.80	896	803	30	–	Condition soft solution treatment from 1050°C	18/8 stainless steel widely used for fabrications and domestic and decorative purposes

their applications are listed in Table 4.4. Because it is ductile and so easily formed 18/8 stainless steel (BS 302S25) is the most widely used alloy.

4.6 Ferrous metals (cast irons)

These are also ferrous metals containing iron and carbon. They do not require the expensive refinement processes of steel making and provide a relatively low cost engineering material that can be easily cast into complex shapes at much lower temperatures than those associated with cast steel. There are four main groups of cast iron, these are:

- Grey cast iron.

- Spheroidal graphite cast iron.

- Malleable cast iron.

- Alloy cast ion.

In this book we are only concerned with *grey cast iron*. Unlike steels, where the carbon content is deliberately restricted so that all of it can combine with the iron, in cast irons there is so much carbon present (about 3%) that not all of it can combine with the iron and some of the carbon is left over. This surplus carbon appears as flakes of graphite between the crystals of metallic iron.

Graphite is the type of carbon that is used to make pencil leads and it is these flakes of graphite that give cast irons their characteristic grey colour when fractured, its 'dirtiness' when machined or filed, and its weakness when it is subjected to a tensile load. The graphite also promotes good machining characteristics by acting as an internal lubricant and causes the chips (swarf) to break up into easily disposable granules. The cavities containing the flakes of graphite have a damping effect upon vibrations – cast iron is *anti-resonant* – and this property makes it particularly suitable for machine tool frames and beds. The graphite also tends to make the slideways self-lubricating.

Most important of all, cast irons have a low melting point compared with steels. Grey cast irons melt between 1130°C and 1250°C depending upon the composition. Cast irons are very fluid when molten which enables them to flow into and fill the most complex of moulds. Also, they expand slightly as they solidify and this enables them to take up the finest detail in the moulds. However, once solidified they contract like any other metal as they cool.

4.7 Abbreviations

Table 4.5 lists some of the abbreviations used for ferrous metals. They may be found on storage racks in the stores and on engineering drawings. Such abbreviations are very imprecise and refer mainly to groups of materials that can vary widely in composition and properties within the

TABLE 4.5 *Abbreviations for ferrous metals*

Abbreviation	Metal
CI	Cast iron (usually 'grey' cast iron)
SGCI	Spheroidal graphite cast iron
MS	Mild steel (low-carbon steel)
BDMS	Bright drawn mild steel
HRPO	Hot-rolled pickled and oiled mild steel
CRCA	Cold-rolled close annealed mild steel
GFS	Ground flat stock (gauge plate)
LCS	Low-carbon steel
SS	Silver steel (centreless ground high-carbon steel)
HSS	High-speed steel
Bright bar	Same as BDMS
Black bar	Hot-rolled steel still coated with scale

group. It is better to specify a material precisely using a British Standard coding.

4.8 British standards for wrought steels

During World War II all wrought steels were standardized in BS 970, and the steels were given EN numbers. The initials EN stood for either *emergency number* or for *economy number*, the exact meaning having become lost in the mists of time. This was a random system of numbering in which EN8 was a medium carbon steel, EN32 a case hardening low carbon steel and EN24 a high tensile nickel chrome alloy steel. Despite the fact that the BSI issued memoranda to all major suppliers and users of wrought steel that the old system should be discontinued as soon as possible after 1972 to avoid confusion, these outdated specifications are still used.

Between 1970 and 1972, BS 970 was reissued using number and letter codes that more accurately described the composition and properties of the steels listed. This code is built up as follows.

The first three symbols are a number code indicating the type of steel.

- 000 to 199   Carbon and carbon manganese steels. The numbers indicate the manganese content × 100.
- 200 to 240   Free cutting steels, with the second and third numbers indicating the sulphur content × 100.
- 250   Silicon valve steels.
- 300 to 499   Stainless steels.
- 500 to 999   Alloy steels.

The fourth symbol is a letter code and is applied as follows.

- A   The steel is supplied to a chemical composition determined by chemical analysis of a batch sample.

- H   The steel is supplied to a hardenability specification. This is the maximum hardness that can be obtained for a specimen of a specified diameter.

- M   The steel is supplied to a mechanical property specification.

- S   The material is a stainless steel.

The fifth and sixth symbols are a number code indicating the average carbon content for a given steel. The code is carbon content × 100.

Therefore a steel that is specified as BS 970.040A10 is interpreted as:

- BS 970   indicates the standard being applied.

- 040   lies between 000 and 199 and indicates that we are dealing with a plain carbon steel containing some manganese.

- 040   also indicates that the steel contains 0.40% manganese since 0.40 × 100 = 040.

- A   indicates that the composition has been determined by batch analysis.

- 10   indicates that the steel contains 0.1% carbon since 0.1 × 100 = 10.

This revised BS 970 is currently issued in four parts:

Part 1   General inspection and testing procedures and specific requirements for carbon, carbon manganese, alloy and stainless steels.

Part 2   Requirements for steels for manufacture of hot formed springs.

Part 3   Bright bars for general engineering purposes.

Part 4   Valve steels.

The revised BS 970 is now being phased out and replaced by a new family of standards covering all aspects of steel making and supply. These range between BS EN 10001 and BS EN 10237 inclusive. The initials EN now indicate that these standards are the English language versions of European standards (EN = European number). These new standards are outside the scope of this book.

4.9 Non-ferrous metals and alloys

Non-ferrous metals and alloys refer to the multitude of metals and alloys that do not contain iron or, if any iron is present, it is only a minute trace. The most widely used non-ferrous metals and alloys are:

- Aluminium and its alloys.

- Copper and its alloys.

- Zinc-based die-casting alloys.

- Titanium and its alloys used in the aerospace engineering including airframe and engine components.

In this book we are only interested in the first two groups.

4.9.1 Aluminium and its alloys

Aluminium is the lightest of the commonly used metals. Its electrical and thermal conductivity properties are very good, being second only to copper. It also has good corrosion resistance and is cheaper than copper. Unfortunately, it is relatively mechanically weak in the pure state and is difficult to solder and weld. Special techniques and materials are required for these processes. Pure aluminium is available as foil, sheet, rod, wire and sections (both drawn and extruded). It is also the basis of a wide range of alloys. These can be classified as:

- Wrought alloys (not heat-treatable).

- Wrought alloys (heat-treatable).

- Casting alloys (not heat-treatable).

- Casting alloys (heat-treatable).

The composition and uses of some typical examples of each group of aluminium alloys are listed in Table 4.6.

4.9.2 Copper and its alloys

Copper has already been introduced as a corrosion resistant metal with excellent electrical and thermal conductivity properties. It is also relatively strong compared with aluminium and very easy to join by soldering or brazing. It is very much heavier than aluminium and also more costly. Copper is available as cold drawn rods, bars, wire and tubes, cold rolled sheet and strip, extruded sections, castings and powder for sintered components. So-called 'pure copper' is available in the following grades.

Cathode copper

This is used for the production of copper alloys. As its name implies, cathode copper is manufactured by an electrolytic refining process.

High conductivity copper

This is better than 99.9% pure and is used for electrical conductors and heat exchangers.

Tough pitch copper

This is a general purpose, commercial grade copper containing some residual copper oxide from the refining process. It is this copper oxide content

TABLE 4.6 *Typical aluminium alloys*

	Composition (%)						Category	Applications
Copper	Silicon	Iron	Manganese	Magnesium	Other elements			
0.1 max.	0.5 max.	0.7 max.	0.1 max.	–	–		Wrought Not heat-treatable	Fabricated assemblies. Electrical conductors. Food and brewing processing plant. Architectural decoration
0.15 max.	0.6 max.	0.75 max.	1.0 max.	4.5–5.5	0.5 chromium		Wrought Not heat-treatable	High-strength shipbuilding and engineering products. Good corrosion resistance
1.6	10.0	–	–	–	–		Cast Not heat-treatable	General purpose alloy for moderately stressed pressure die-castings
–	10.0–13.0	–	–	–	–		Cast Not heat-treatable	One of the most widely used alloys. Suitable for sand, gravity and pressure die-castings. Excellent foundry characteristics for large marine, automative and general engineering castings

(continued overleaf)

TABLE 4.6 (continued)

Composition (%)						Category	Applications
Copper	Silicon	Iron	Manganese	Magnesium	Other elements		
4.2	0.7	0.7	0.7	0.7	0.3 titanium (optional)	Wrought Heat-treatable	Traditional 'Duralumin' general machining alloy. Widely used for stressed components in aircraft and elsewhere
–	0.5	–	–	0.6	–	Wrought Heat-treatable	Corrosion-resistant alloy for lightly stressed components such as glazing bars, window sections and automotive body components
1.8	2.5	1.0	–	0.2	0.15 titanium 1.2 nickel	Cast Heat-treatable	Suitable for sand and gravity die-casting. High rigidity with moderate strength and shock resistance. A general purpose alloy
–	–	–	–	10.5	0.2 titanium	Cast Heat-treatable	A strong, ductile and highly corrosion-resistant alloy used for aircraft and marine castings both large and small

that increases its strength and toughness but reduces its electrical conductivity and ductility. It is suitable for roofing sheets, chemical plant, general presswork, decorative metalwork and applications where special properties are not required.

Phosphorous deoxidized, non-arsenical copper

This is a welding quality copper. Removal of the dissolved oxygen content prevents gassing and porosity. Also the lack of dissolved and combined oxygen improves the ductility and malleability of the metal. It is used in fabrications, castings, cold impact extrusion and severe presswork.

Arsenical tough pitch and phosphorous deoxidized copper

The addition of traces of the metal arsenic improves the strength of the metal at high temperatures. Arsenical coppers are used for boiler and firebox plates, flue tubes and general plumbing.

The main groups of copper-based alloys are:

- High copper content alloys (e.g. cadmium copper, silver copper, etc.).

- Brass alloys (copper and zinc).

- Tin bronze alloys (copper and tin).

- Aluminium bronze alloys (copper and aluminium).

- Cupro-nickel alloys (copper and nickel).

In this book we are interested only in the brass alloys and the tin bronze alloys.

Brass alloys

Brass alloys of copper and zinc tend to give rather weak and porous castings. The brasses depend largely upon hot and/or cold working to consolidate the metal and improve its mechanical properties. The brass alloys can be hardened only by cold working (work hardening). They can be softened by heat treatment (the annealing process). The composition and uses of the more commonly available brass alloys are given in Table 4.7.

Tin bronze alloys

These are alloys of copper and tin together with a *de-oxidizer*. The de-oxidizer is essential to prevent the tin content from oxidizing at high temperatures during casting and hot working. Oxidation is the chemical combination of the tin content with the oxygen in the atmosphere, and it results in the bronze being weakened and becoming hard, brittle and 'scratchy'. Two de-oxidizers are commonly used:

- A small amount of phosphorus in the *phosphor bronze* alloys.

- A small amount of zinc in the *gun metal* alloys.

TABLE 4.7 *Typical brass alloys*

Name	Composition (%)			Applications
	Copper	Zinc	Other elements	
Cartridge brass	70	30	–	Most ductile of the copper–zinc alloys. Widely used in sheet metal pressing for severe deep drawing operations. Originally developed for making cartridge cases, hence its name
Standard brass	65	35	–	Cheaper than cartridge brass and rather less ductile. Suitable for most engineering processes
Basis brass	63	37	–	The cheapest of the cold-working brasses. It lacks ductility and is only capable of withstanding simple forming operations
Muntz metal	60	40	–	Not suitable for cold working, but hot works well. Relatively cheap due to its high zinc content, it is widely used for extrusion and hot-stamping processes
Free-cutting brass	58	39	3% lead	Not suitable for cold working, but excellent for hot working and high-speed machining of low-strength components
Admiralty brass	70	29	1% tin	This is virtually cartridge brass plus a little tin to prevent corrosion in the presence of salt water
Naval brass	62	36	1% tin	This is virtually Muntz metal plus a little tin to prevent corrosion in the presence of salt water

The composition and uses of some typical tin bronze alloys are listed in Table 4.8. Unlike the brasses, which are largely used in the wrought condition (rod, sheet, etc.), only low tin content bronzes can be worked and most bronze components are in the form of castings. The tin bronze alloys are more expensive than the brass alloys but they are stronger and give sound, pressure-tight castings that are widely used for steam and hydraulic valve bodies and mechanisms. They are highly resistant to corrosion.

TABLE 4.8 *Typical tin–bronze alloys*

Name	Composition (%)					Application
	Copper	Zinc	Phosphorus	Tin	Lead	
Low-tin bronze	96	–	0.1–0.25	3.9–3.75	–	This alloy can be severely cold worked to harden it so that it can be used for springs where good elastic properties must be combined with corrosion resistance, fatigues resistance and electrical conductivity, e.g. contact blades

TABLE 4.8 *(continued)*

Name	Composition (%)					Application
	Copper	Zinc	Phosphorus	Tin	Lead	
Drawn phosphor-bronze	94	–	0.1–0.5	5.9–5.5	–	This alloy is used in the work-hardened condition for turned components requiring strength and corrosion resistance, such as valve spindles
Cast phosphor-bronze	rem.	–	0.03–0.25	10	–	Usually cast into rods and tubes for making bearing bushes and worm wheels. It has excellent anti-friction properties
Admiralty gunmetal	88	2	–	10	–	This alloy is suitable for sand casting where fine-grained, pressure-tight components such as pump and valve bodies are required
Leaded-gunmetal (free-cutting)	85	5	–	5	5	Also known as 'red brass', this alloy is used for the same purposes as standard, Admiralty gunmetal. It is rather less strong but has improved pressure tightness and machine properties
Leaded (plastic) bronze	74	–	–	2	24	This alloy is used for lightly loaded bearings where alignment is difficult. Due to its softness, bearings made from this alloy 'bed in' easily

4.10 Workshop tests for the identification of metals

Materials represent a substantial investment in any manufacturing company. It is essential that all materials are carefully stored so that they are not damaged or allowed to deteriorate before use. Ferrous metals must be stored in a warm, dry environment so that rusting cannot occur. This is particularly the case when storing bright drawn sections and bright rolled sheet. Rusting would quickly destroy the finish and cause such materials to be unfit for use. Materials must also be carefully labelled or coded so that they can be quickly and accurately identified. Mistakes, resulting in the use of the incorrect material, can be very costly through waste. It can also cause serious accidents if a weak metal is used in mistake for a strong one for highly stressed components.

The similarity in appearance between many metals of different physical properties makes it essential that some form of permanent identification should be marked on them, e.g. colour coding. However, mix-ups do occur from time to time and also bar 'ends' are often used up for 'one-off' jobs. Table 4.9 gives some simple workshop tests of identification.

4.11 Non-metals (natural)

Non-metals are widely used in engineering today. Some of the materials occur naturally. For example:

TABLE 4.9 *Workshop identification tests*

These are not foolproof and require some experience

Metal	Appearance	Hammer cold	Type of chip	'Spark test' on grinding wheel
Mild steel ('black')	Smooth scale with blue/black sheen	Flattens easily	Smooth, curly ribbon-like	Stream of yellow white sparks, varying in length: slightly 'fiery'
Mild steel ('bright')	Smooth, scale-free, silver grey surface	Flattens easily	Smooth, curly ribbon-like	Stream of yellow white sparks, varying in length: slightly 'fiery'
Medium-carbon steel	Smooth scale, black sheen	Fairly difficult to flatten	Chip curls more tightly and discolours light brown	Yellow sparks, shorter than m/s, and finer and more feathery
High-carbon steel	Rougher scale, black	Difficult to flatten	Chip curls even more tightly and discolours dark blue	Sparks less bright, starting near grinding wheel, and more feathery with secondary branching (distinctive acrid smell)
High-speed steel	Rougher scale, black with reddish tint	Very difficult to flatten. Tends to crack easily	Long ribbon-like chip. Distinctive smell. Over-heats tool easily	Faint red streak ending in fork (distinctive acrid smell)
Cast iron	Grey and sandy	Crumbles	Granular, grey in colour	Faint red spark, ending in bushy yellow sparks (distinctive acrid smell)
Copper	Distinctive 'red' colour	Flattens very easily	Ribbon-like, with razor edge	Should not be ground – no sparking
Aluminium	Silvery when polished. Pale grey when oxidized. Very light in weight compared with other metals	Flattens very easily	Ribbon-like chip	Should not be ground – no sparking

- *Rubber* is used for anti-vibration mountings, coolant and compressed air hoses, transmission belts, truck wheel tyres.

- *Glass* is used for spirit level vials (the tube that contains the bubble), lenses for optical instruments.

- *Emery and corundum* (aluminium oxides) are used for abrasive wheels, belts and sheets, and as grinding pastes. Nowadays it is usually produced artificially to control the quality.

- *Wood* for making casting patterns.
- *Ceramics* for cutting tool tips and electrical insulators.

4.12 Non-metals (synthetic)

These are popularly known as *plastics*. When we were considering the properties of materials, a plastic material is said to be one that deforms to a new shape under an applied load and retains its new shape when the load is removed. Yet, the range of synthetic materials we call plastics are often tough and leathery, or hard and brittle, or elastic. They are called plastics because, during the moulding operation by which they are formed, they are reduced to a plastic condition by heating them to about twice the temperature of boiling water.

There are many families of 'plastic' materials with widely differing properties. However, they all have certain properties in common.

- *Electrical insulation.* All plastic materials are, to a greater or lesser extent, good electrical insulators (they are also good heat insulators). However, their usefulness as insulators is limited by their inability to withstand high temperatures and their relative softness compared with ceramics. They are mainly used for insulating wires and cables and for moulded switch gear and instrument components and cases.

- *Strength/weight ratio.* Plastic materials vary considerably in strength. All plastics are much less dense than metals and this results in a favourable strength/weight ratio. The high strength plastics and reinforced plastics compare favourably with the aluminium alloys and are often used for stressed components in aircraft construction.

- *Degradation.* Plastics do not corrode like metals. They are all inert to most inorganic chemicals. They can be used in environments that are chemically hostile to even the most corrosion resistant metals. They are superior to natural rubber in their resistance to attack by oils and greases. However, all plastics degrade at high temperatures and many are degraded by the ultraviolet content of sunlight. Plastics that have to be exposed to sunlight (window frames and roof guttering) usually contain a pigment that filters out the ultraviolet rays. Some thermoplastics can be dissolved by suitable solvents.

- *Safety*. Plastics can give off very dangerous toxic fumes when heated. Note the number of people who have died from inhaling the smoke from plastic furniture padding in house fires! Solvents used in the processing of plastics are often highly toxic and should not be inhaled but used in well-ventilated surroundings. Make sure you know the likely dangers before starting work on plastic materials and always follow the safe working practices laid down by the safety management.

Plastic materials can be grouped into two distinct families. These are the *thermosetting plastics* and the *thermoplastics*. Typical examples of each of these families will now be considered. Note that thermosetting plastics are often referred to simply as 'thermosets'.

4.12.1 Thermosetting plastics

These undergo a chemical change called 'curing' during hot moulding process. Once this chemical change has taken place, the plastic material from which the moulding is made can never again be softened and reduced to a plastic condition by reheating.

Thermosetting resins are unsuitable for use by themselves and they are usually mixed with other substances (additives) to improve their mechanical properties, improve their moulding properties, make them more economical to use, and provide the required colour for the finished product. A typical moulding material could consist of:

- Resin   38% by weight
- Filler   58% by weight
- Pigment   3% by weight
- Mould release agent 0.5% by weight
- Catalyst   0.3% by weight
- Accelerator   0.2% by weight

The pigment gives colour to the finished product. The mould release agent stops the moulding sticking to the mould. It also acts as an internal lubricant and helps the plasticized material to flow to the shape of the mould. The catalyst promotes the curing process and the accelerator speeds up the curing process and reduces the time the moulds have to be kept closed, thus improving productivity.

Fillers are much cheaper than the resin itself and this is important in keeping down the cost of the moulding. Fillers also have a considerable influence on the properties of the mouldings produced from a given thermosetting resin. They improve the impact strength (toughness) and reduce shrinkage during moulding. Typical fillers are:

- *Shredded paper* and *shredded cloth* give good strength and reasonable electrical insulation properties at a low cost.
- *Mica granules* give good strength and heat resistance (asbestos is no longer used).
- *Aluminium powder* gives good mechanical strength and wear resistance.
- *Wood flour (fine sawdust)* and *calcium carbonate (ground limestone)* provide high bulk at a very low cost but with relatively low strength.
- *Glass fibre (chopped)* gives good strength and excellent electrical insulation properties.

Some typical examples of thermosetting plastics and their uses are given in Table 4.10.

4.12.2 Thermoplastics

These can be softened as often as they are reheated. They are not so rigid as the thermosetting plastics but they tend to be tougher. Additives (other

TABLE 4.10   *Some typical thermosetting plastic materials*

Material	Characteristics
Phenolic resins and powders	These are used for dark-coloured parts because the basic resin tends to become discoloured. These are heat-curing materials
Amino (containing nitrogen) resins and powders	These are colourless and can be coloured if required; they can be strengthened by using paper-pulp fillers, and used in thin sections
Polyester resins	Polyester chains can be cross-linked by using a monomer such as styrene; these resins are used in the production of glass-fibre laminates
Epoxy resins	These are also used in the production of glass-fibre laminates

TABLE 4.11   *Some typical thermoplastic materials*

Type	Material	Characteristics
Cellulose plastics	Nitrocellulose	Materials of the 'celluloid' type are tough and water resistant. They are available in all forms except moulding powders. They cannot be moulded because of their flammability
	Cellulose acetate	This is much less flammable than the above. It is used for tool handles and electrical goods
Vinyl plastics	Polythene	This is a simple material that is weak, easy to mould, and has good electrical properties. It is used for insulation and for packaging
	Polypropylene	This is rather more complicated than polythene and has better strength
	Polystyrene	Polystyrene is cheap, and can be easily moulded. It has a good strength but it is rigid and brittle and crazes and yellows with age
	Polyvinyl chloride (PVC)	This is tough, rubbery, and almost non-inflammable. It is cheap and can be easily manipulated: it has good electrical properties
Acrylics (made from an acrylic acid)	Polymethyl methacrylate	Materials of the 'Perspex' type have excellent light transmission, are tough and non-splintering, and can be easily bent and shaped
Polyamides (short carbon chains that are connected by amide groups – NHCO)	Nylon	This is used as a fibre or as a wax-like moulding material. It is fluid at moulding temperature, tough, and has a low coefficient of friction
Fluorine plastics	Polytetrafluoroethylene (PTFE)	Is a wax-like moulding material; it has an extremely low coefficient of friction. It is very expensive
Polyesters (when an alcohol combines with an acid, an 'ester' is produced)	Polyethylene terephthalate	This is available as a film or as 'Terylene'. The film is an excellent electrical insulator

than a colourant and an internal lubricant) are not normally used with thermoplastics. Some typical examples of thermoplastics and their uses are given in Table 4.11.

4.13 Forms of supply

There is an almost unlimited range to the forms of supply in which engineering materials can be supplied to a manufacturer or to a fabricator. Figure 4.8 shows some of these forms of supply.

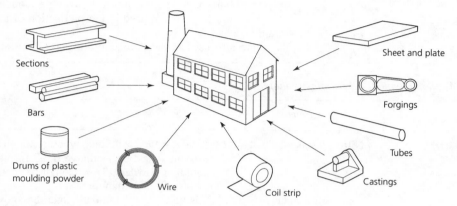

Sections

Bars

Drums of plastic moulding powder

Wire

Coil strip

Castings

Sheet and plate

Forgings

Tubes

Figure 4.8 *Forms of supply*

- *Sections* such as steel angles, channel sections, H-section beams and joists and T-sections in a wide range of sizes and lengths. They are usually hot-rolled with a heavily scaled finish. Such sections are mostly used in the steel fabrication and civil engineering and construction industries. Bright-drawn steel angle sections are available in the smallest sizes. Non-ferrous metal sections are normally extruded to close tolerances and have a bright finish. Both standard sections and sections to customers' own requirements are made this way. The sizes available are very much smaller than for steel sections.

- *Bars* may be 'flats', which are available in rectangular sections, 'squares', or 'rounds', which have a cylindrical section and this term applies to the larger sizes. In the smaller size they are usually referred to as 'rods'. They are available in hot-rolled (black) or cold-drawn (bright) finishes. Hexagon section bars for making nuts and bolts are always cold-drawn.

- *Plastics* may be supplied in powder or granular form for moulding into various shapes. They may also be supplied semi-finished in rounds, flats, squares, tubes, and sheet. They may also come in sections to manufacturers' own requirements such as curtain rails and insulation blocks ready for cutting off to length. Reinforced plastics such as 'Tufnol' are also available in standard sections and mouldings.

- *Wire* is available bright-drawn or hot-rolled depending upon its size and the use to which it is going to be put. Bright-drawn, high carbon steel wire (piano wire) is used for making springs. Copper wire is used for electrical conductors. The smaller the diameter of any wire the greater the length that can be made in one piece.

- *Coil strip* is used for cold stamping and pressing where continuous automatic feed to the presses is required. It is available in a range of thicknesses and finishes. Steel strip is available in such finishes as bright-rolled (BR), hot-rolled, pickled and oiled (HRPO) and cold-rolled, closed-annealed (CRCA). It can be sheared on continuous rotary shears to the customer's specification where accurate control of the width is required. Alternatively it can be left with a 'mill-edge' where the flats' surfaces are bright-rolled and the edges are left rounded and in the hot-rolled state. Non-ferrous strip is usually bright-rolled and sheared to width. The rolling process tends to work harden the strip which is sold in various 'tempers' according to the amount of cold working it has received since annealing. For example, dead-soft, soft, quarter-hard, half-hard, etc.

- *Castings* can be made in most metals and alloys but the moulding process will vary depending upon the type of metal, the size of the casting, the accuracy of the casting and the quantities involved. There are no 'standard' castings. They are made to the customer's own patterns or, in the case of die-casting, in the customer's own dies.

- *Tubes* and *pipes* can be made in ferrous and non-ferrous metals and alloys and in plastic. Tubes refer to the smaller sizes and pipes to the larger sizes. Steel pipes may be cold-drawn or hot-drawn without seams for the highest pressures. They may also be rolled from strip with a butt-welded seam running along the length of the pipe or tube where lower pressures are involved, or they are used only for sheathing (electrical conduit is made like this). Plastic tube may be rigid or flexible.

- *Forgings* may be manufactured by forming the red-hot metal with standard tools by a 'blacksmith' when only small quantities are required. The size may range from horseshoes, farm implements, and decorative wrought-iron work made by hand, to turbine shafts and ships' propeller shafts forged under huge hydraulic presses. Where large quantities of forging of the same type are required, these are drop-forged. The red-hot steel is forged in dies which impart the finished shape to the forging. Light alloy (aluminium alloy) forgings are used by the aircraft industry. Because of the low melting temperature of such alloys compared with steel, they have to be forged at a lower temperature. This requires a greater forging pressure and care must be taken that cracking does not occur.

- *Sheet and plate* starts off as very wide coiled strip and is then passed through a series of rollers to flatten it. It is sheared to length by 'flying shears' that cut it whilst the flattened strip is moving. The terminology is somewhat vague and depends upon the metal thickness. Generally, 'sheet' can be worked with hand tools and ranges from foil (very thin sheet) to about 1.5 mm thick. Then comes 'thin plate' up to about 6 mm thick. After that it becomes thick plate. Both thin and thick plate have to be cut and formed using power driven tools. Sheet is available in both cold- and hot-rolled finishes, whereas plate is available only as hot-rolled. For the sizes of any standard metallic products, see BS 6722: 1986 (amended 1992).

4.14 Heat treatment processes (introduction)

Heat treatment processes as a means of modifying the properties of metals have already been mentioned earlier in this chapter. Table 4.12 summarizes and defines the more common heat treatment processes. Because of the wide range of non-ferrous metals and alloys that exist, the heat treatment processes for non-ferrous metals vary widely and all such processes are quite different to the processes used for the heat treatment of plain carbon steels. However, some of the more important processes for the heat treatment of copper-based and aluminium-based alloys will be included in this chapter.

TABLE 4.12 *Heat treatment definitions*

Term	Meaning
Annealed	The condition of a metal that has been heated above a specified temperature, depending upon its composition, and then cooled down in the furnace itself or by burying it in ashes or lime. This annealing process makes the metal very soft and ductile. Annealing usually precedes flow-forming operations such as sheet metal pressing and wire and tube drawing
Normalised	The condition of a metal that has been heated above a specified temperature, depending upon its composition, and then cooled down in free air. Although the cooling is slow, it is not as slow as for annealing so the metal is less soft and ductile. This condition is not suitable for flow forming but more suitable for machining. Normalizing is often used to stress relieve castings and forgings after rough machining
Quench hardened	The condition of a metal that has been heated above a specified temperature, depending upon its composition, and then cooled down very rapidly by immersing it in cold water or cold oil. Rapid cooling is called **quenching** and the water or oil is called the **quenching bath**. This rapid cooling from elevated temperatures makes the metal very hard. Only medium- and high-carbon steels can be hardened in this way
Tempered	Quench-hardened steels are brittle as well as hard. To make them suitable for cutting tools they have to be reheated to a specified temperature between 200 and 300°C and again quenched. This makes them slightly less hard but very much tougher. Metals in this condition are said to be *tempered*

4.15 Heat treatment processes (safety)

General safety was introduced in Chapter 1. However, heat treatment can involve large pieces of metal at high temperatures and powerful furnaces. Therefore it is now necessary to consider some safety practices relating specifically to heat treatment processes, before discussing the processes involved.

4.15.1 Protective clothing

Ordinary workshop overalls do not offer sufficient protection alone. Many are made from flammable cloths. Further, synthetic cloths made from nylon or rayon fibres, or mixtures of natural and synthetic fibres, can melt and stick to your skin at the temperatures met with in heat treatment. This worsens any burn you may receive. Overalls used in heat treatment shops should be made from a flame resistant or a flame retardant material and be labelled accordingly. In addition a leather apron should be worn to prevent your overalls coming into contact with hot workpieces and hot equipment.

4.15.2 Gloves

Gloves should be worn to protect your hands. These should be made from leather or other heat resistant materials and should have gauntlets to protect your wrists and the ends of the sleeves of your overalls. Leather gloves offer protection up to 350°C.

4.15.3 Headwear, goggles and visors

Headwear, goggles and visors, such as those described in Chapter 1, should be worn when there is any chance of danger to your eyes, the skin of your face, and your hair and scalp. Such dangers can come from:

- splashes from the molten salts when using salt bath furnaces;
- splashes from hot liquids when quenching;
- the accidental ignition of oil quenching baths due to overheating;
- radiated heat from large furnaces when their doors are opened;
- accidental 'flashbacks' when lighting up furnaces.

4.15.4 Safety shoes and boots

The safety shoes and boots as recommended for wearing in workshops were introduced in Chapter 1. They are also most suitable for use in heat treatment shops. They not only protect you from cuts and crushing from heavy falling objects, being made of strong leather they also protect against burns from hot objects. Your first instinctive reaction to accidentally picking up anything hot is to let go quickly and drop it. This is when the toe protection of industrial safety shoes earns its keep. In addition, it is advisable that leather spats are worn. These protect your lower legs and ankles from splashes of molten salts or spillage of hot quenching fluids. Spats are particularly important if you wear safety shoes rather than safety boots.

4.15.5 Safety equipment

Heat treatment can cover a whole range of processes and sizes of workpieces from hardening a simple tool made from a piece of silver steel using a gas blowpipe to heat it and a bucket of cold water to quench it in, to the production treatment of large components. They all have the same basic problem. That is, very hot metal has to be handled. There are very many methods of handling hot workpieces depending upon their size, the quantity involved, type of furnace being used and the process. Here are a few examples of how the hot components can be handled:

- Small components can be handled individually using tongs.

- Quantities of small components can be handled on trays or in baskets. These trays and baskets are usually made from a heat resistant metal such as the nickel alloy called *inconel*. The baskets can be handled in or out of salt bath furnaces and in or out of the quenching bath using a hoist.

- Large components and trays of smaller components can be handled in or out of muffle type furnaces on rollers. Long handled hooks and rakes are used to push the components into the furnace or to pull them out when hot.

4.15.6 Safety notices

Whilst metal is red-hot it is obviously in a dangerous condition. However, most accidents occur when the metal has cooled down to just below red heat. Although no longer glowing, it is still hot enough to cause serious burns and to start fires if flammable substances come into contact with it. Hot workpieces must never be stored in gangways and warning notices must be used as shown in Fig. 4.9. Such notices must satisfy the legal requirements of the Health and Safety Executive.

4.15.7 Fire

Quenching baths using a quenching oil must have an airtight lid. In the event of the oil overheating and igniting, the lid can be closed and the lack of air puts the fire out. Quenching tanks should always have sufficient reserve capacity so that the oil does not overheat. If the oil is allowed to overheat:

- The oil will not cool the work quickly enough to harden it.

- The oil may catch fire.

Only quenching oil with a high flash point and freedom from fuming should be used. *Lubricating oil must never be used.* A suitable fire extinguisher, or several fire extinguishers if a large quenching tank is used, should be positioned conveniently near to the bath in case of an emergency. The type of extinguisher should be suitable for use on oil fires.

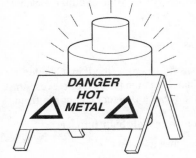

Figure 4.9 *Safety notices must be placed by hot objects*

Furnaces and blowpipes must not be lit or closed down without proper instruction and permission. Incorrect setting of the controls and incorrect lighting-up procedures can lead to serious explosions. All personnel working in heat treatment shops must be alert to the possibility of fires.

- They must be conversant with and trained in the correct fire drill.
- Fire drills must be practised regularly to ensure everyone knows what to do.
- They must know where the nearest alarm is and how to operate it.
- They must know where the nearest telephone is and how to summon the fire brigade.
- They must know where the exits are and how to evacuate the premises. Fire exits must be left clear of obstructions.
- They must know where to assemble so that a roll-call can be taken.
- They must know the correct fire-fighting procedures so that the fire can be contained until the professional brigade arrives, only providing this can be done safely.
- When an outbreak of fire is discovered the correct fire drill must be put into action immediately.

4.16 The heat treatment of plain carbon steels

Plain carbon steels are subjected to heat treatment processes for the following reasons:

- To improve the properties of the material as a whole, for example by imparting hardness to prevent wear or softness and grain refinement to improve its machining properties.
- To remove undesirable properties acquired during previous processing – for example, hardness and brittleness imparted by cold working.

The heat treatment processes we are now going to consider in order to modify the properties of plain carbon steels are:

- Through (quench) hardening.
- Tempering.
- Annealing.
- Normalizing.
- Case hardening.

4.16.1 Through-hardening

Basically the process by which we 'through-harden' (also referred to as *quench hardening*) consists of heating a suitable steel to a critical temperature that is dependent upon the carbon content of the steel and cooling it quickly (quenching it) in water or quenching oil. The hardness attained will depend upon:

- The carbon content of the steel (the higher the carbon content the harder the steel).

- The rate of cooling (the faster the cooling the harder the steel).

For example, to harden a chisel made from 8% carbon steel, the temperature to which the steel is heated should be between 800°C and 830°C. That is, the steel should glow 'cherry red' in colour. It is then quenched by cooling it in cold water. Any increase in temperature will make no difference to the hardness of the chisel. It will only result in 'grain growth' and weakening of the steel. Grain growth means that the hotter the steel becomes and the longer it is kept at excessively high temperatures the bigger the grains in the metal will grow by merging together.

As previously stated, the steel has to be heated to within a critical temperature range if it is to be correctly hardened. The temperature range for hardening plain carbon steels is shown in Fig. 4.10.

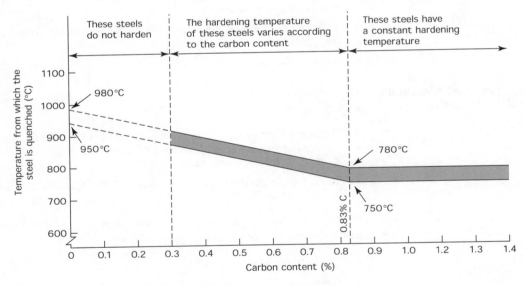

Figure 4.10 *Hardening temperatures for plain carbon steels*

Figure 4.10 shows that the hardening temperatures for plain carbon steels lie in a narrow band depending upon the carbon content of the steel. If the hardening temperature for any given steel is not achieved, it will not harden. If it is exceeded no increase in hardness is achieved but grain growth will occur and the steel will be weakened.

It has already been stated that the more quickly a component is cooled the harder it becomes for any given carbon content. However, some care is required because the faster you cool the workpiece, the more likely it is to crack and distort. Therefore the workpiece should never be cooled more quickly than is required to give the desired degree of hardness (*critical cooling rate*). The most common substances used for quenching (*quenching media*) are:

- *Brine* (a solution of sodium chloride and water) is the most rapid quenching bath – it will give the greatest hardness and is the most likely to cause cracking.

- *Water* is less severe and is the most widely used quenching bath for plain carbon steels.

- *Oil* is the least severe of the liquid quenching media. Only plain carbon steels of the highest carbon content will harden in oil, and then only in relatively small sections. Oil quenching is mostly used with alloy die steels and tool steels.

- *Air blast* is the least severe of any of the quenching media used. It can be applied only to heavily alloyed steels of small section such as high-speed steel tool bits.

Table 4.13 summarizes the effect of carbon content and rate of cooling for a range of plain carbon steels.

TABLE 4.13 *Effect of carbon content and rate of cooling on hardness*

Type of steel	Carbon content (%)	Effect of heating and quenching (rapid cooling)
Low carbon	Below 0.25	Negligible
Medium carbon	0.3–0.5	Becomes tougher
	0.5–0.9	Becomes hard
High carbon	0.9–1.3	Becomes very hard

Carbon content (%)	Quenching bath	Required treatment
0.30–0.50	Oil	Toughening
0.50–0.90	Oil	Toughening
0.50–0.90	Water	Hardening
0.90–1.30	Water	Hardening

Notes:
1. Below 0.5% carbon content, steels are not hardened as cutting tools, so water hardening has not been included.
2. Above 0.9% carbon content, any attempt to harden the steel in water could lead to cracking.

4.16.2 Quenching, distortion and cracking

Quenching and distortion

When quenching hot metal, some thought must be given to the way the work is lowered into the bath to avoid distortion and to get the most effective quenching. For example, when hardening a chisel, the shank of the chisel is held with tongs and the chisel is dipped vertically into the quenching bath.

- This results in the cutting end of the steel entering the bath first and attaining maximum hardness whilst the quenching medium is at its minimum temperature.

- The shank is masked to some extent by the tongs and this results in reduced hardness. This does not matter in this example as we want the shank to be tough rather than hard so that it does not shatter when struck with a hammer.

- The chisel should be stirred around in the bath so that it is constantly coming into contact with fresh and cold water. It also prevents steam pockets being generated round the chisel that would slow up the cooling rate and prevent maximum hardness being achieved.

- Dipping a long slender workpiece like a chisel vertically into the bath prevents distortion. This is shown in Fig. 4.11. This figure also shows

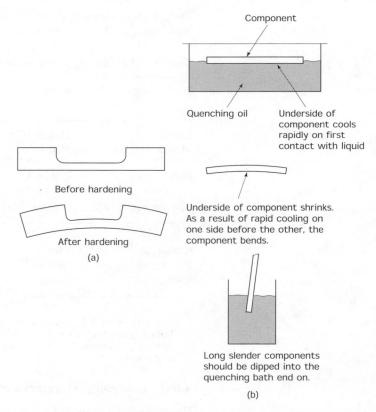

Figure 4.11 *Causes of distortion: (a) distortion caused by an unbalanced shape being hardened; (b) how to quench long, slender components to avoid distortion*

what happens if the component is quenched flat and also how the shape of the component itself can cause uneven cooling and distortion.

Cracking

Figure 4.12 shows some typical causes of cracking occurring during and as a result of heat treatment. Careful design and the correct selection of materials can result in fewer problems in the hardening shop.

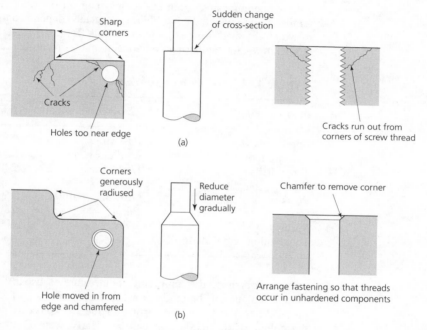

Figure 4.12 *Causes of cracking: (a) incorrect engineering that promotes cracking; (b) correct engineering to reduce cracking*

- Avoid sharp corners and sudden changes of section.

- Do not position holes, slots and other features near the edge of the workpiece.

- Do not include screw threads in a hardened component. Apart from the chance of cracking occurring, once hardened you cannot run a die down the thread to ease it if it has become distorted during the hardening process.

- For complex shapes, which are always liable to cracking and distortion during hardening, always use an alloy steel that has been formulated so that minimum distortion and shrinkage (movement) will occur during heat treatment. Such steels are oil or air hardened and this also reduces the chance of cracking.

4.16.3 Tempering

When you heat and quench a plain carbon steel as described previously, you not only harden the steel, you also make it *very brittle*. In this condition it is unsuitable for immediate use. For instance, a chisel would shatter if you hit it with a hammer. After hardening we have to carry out another process known as *tempering*. This greatly reduces the brittleness and increases the toughness. However, the tempering process also reduces the hardness to some extent.

Tempering consists of reheating the hardened steel workpiece to a suitable temperature and again quenching it in oil or water. The tempering temperature to which the workpiece is reheated depends only upon the use to which the workpiece is going to be put. Table 4.14 lists some suitable temperatures for tempering components made from plain carbon steels.

TABLE 4.14 *Tempering temperatures*

Component	Temper colour	Temperature (°C)
Edge tools	Pale straw	220
Turning tools	Medium straw	230
Twist drills	Dark straw	240
Taps	Brown	250
Press tools	Brownish-purple	260
Cold chisels	Purple	280
Springs	Blue	300
Toughening (crankshafts)	–	450–600

In a workshop, the tempering temperature is usually judged by the 'temper colour' of the oxide film that forms on the surface of the workpiece. After hardening, the surface of the workpiece is polished so that the colour of the oxide film can be clearly seen. Figure 4.13 shows a chisel being tempered. The chisel is not uniformly heated. As shown, the shank is heated in the flame and the temper colours are allowed to 'run down' the chisel until the cutting edge reaches the required colour. When the cutting edge is the required temper colour, the chisel is immediately

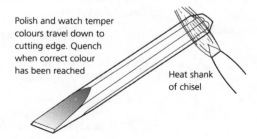

Polish and watch temper colours travel down to cutting edge. Quench when correct colour has been reached

Heat shank of chisel

Figure 4.13 *Tempering a cold chisel*

'dipped' vertically into the quenching bath again. This gives the cutting edge the correct temper but leaves the shank softer and tougher so that it can withstand being struck with a hammer.

Complex and large components and batches of components should be tempered in a furnace with atmosphere and temperature control to ensure consistent results.

4.16.4   Annealing

Annealing processes are used to soften steels that are already hard. This hardness may be imparted in two ways.

- *Quench hardening.* This has previously been described in Section 4.15.

- *Work hardening.* This occurs when the metal has been cold worked (see Section 4.2.5). It becomes hard and brittle at the point where cold working occurs as this causes the grain structure to deform. For example, if a strip of metal is held in a vice, bending the metal back and forth causes it to work harden at the point of bending. It will eventually become sufficiently hard and brittle to break off at that point.

Full annealing

The temperatures for full annealing are the same as for hardening. To *anneal* (soften the workpiece), you allow the hot metal to cool down as slowly as possible. Small components can be buried in crushed limestone or in ashes. Larger components and batches of smaller components will have been heated in furnaces. When the correct temperature has been reached, the component is 'soaked' at this temperature so that the temperature becomes uniform throughout its mass. The furnace is then shut down, the flue dampers are closed and the furnace is sealed so that it cools down as slowly as possible with the work inside it.

Although such slow cooling results in some grain growth and weakening of the metal, it will impart maximum ductility. This results in the metal being in the correct condition for cold forming. However, because of its extreme softness and grain growth the metal will tend to tear and leave a poor surface finish if it is machined. Components to be machined should be *normalized* as described in Section 4.16.5.

Stress-relief annealing

This process is reserved for steels with a carbon content below 0.4%. Such steels will not satisfactorily quench harden but, as they are relatively ductile, they will be frequently cold worked and become work hardened. Since the grain structure will have become severely distorted by the cold working, the crystals will begin to reform and the metal will begin to soften (theoretically) at 500°C. In practice, the metal is rarely so severely stressed as to trigger *recrystallization* at such a low temperature. Stress-relief annealing is usually carried out between 630°C and 700°C to speed up the process and prevent excessive grain growth. Stress-relief annealing is also known as:

- *Process annealing* since the work hardening of the metal results from cold-working (forming) processes.
- *Inter-stage annealing* since the process is often carried out between the stages of a process when extensive cold working is required. For example, when deep drawing sheet metal in a press.

The degree of stress-relief annealing and the rate of cooling will depend not only upon the previous processing the steel received before annealing, but also upon the processing it is to receive *after* annealing. If further cold working is to take place, the maximum softness and ductility is required. This is achieved by prolonged heating and very slow cooling to encourage grain growth. However, if grain refinement, strength and toughness are more important, then heating and cooling should be more rapid.

4.16.5 Normalizing

Plain carbon steels are normalized by heating them to the temperatures shown in Fig. 4.14. This time we want a finer grain structure in the steel. To achieve this, we have to heat the metal up more quickly and cool it more quickly. The workpiece is taken out of the furnace when its normalizing temperature has been achieved and allowed to cool down in the free air of the heat treatment shop. The air should be able to circulate freely round the workpiece. However, the workpiece must be sited so that it is free from cold draughts. Warning notices that the steel is dangerously hot must be placed around it.

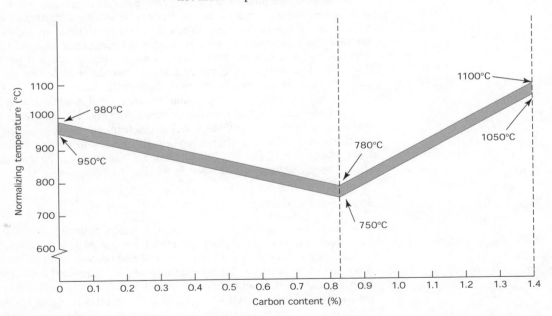

Figure 4.14 *Normalizing temperatures for plain carbon steels*

Castings and forgings are produced by high temperature processes. As they cool down and shrink they often develop high internal stresses. Machining tends to partially release these stresses and over a period of time the machined components 'move' or distort and become inaccurate. At one time, large castings and forgings were rough machined and left out of doors to 'weather' over a period of a year or more. The continual changes in temperature released all the stresses and the components became 'stabilized' ready for finish machining. No further movement then took place.

Keeping such a large amount of valuable stock tied up over a long period of time is no longer economically viable and weathering has given way to *normalizing*. The normalizing process is now frequently used for stress relieving between the rough machining of castings and forgings and the finish machining of such workpieces. This is done to stabilize such workpieces and to avoid 'movement' or distortion subsequent to machining. When normalizing is used for the stabilization of castings and forgings, it is sometimes referred to as 'artificial weathering'.

4.16.6 Case hardening

Often, components need to be hard and wear resistant on the surface, yet have a tough and strong core to resist shock loads. These two properties do not normally exist in a single steel but are achieved by a process called *case hardening*. This is a process by which carbon is added to the surface layers of low carbon steels or low alloy steels to a carefully regulated depth. This addition of carbon is called *carburizing*. After carburizing the component is put through successive heat treatment processes to harden the case and refine the core. This process has two distinct steps as shown in Fig. 4.15. First, the workpiece is heated to between 900°C and 950°C in contact with the carburizing compound until the additional carbon has

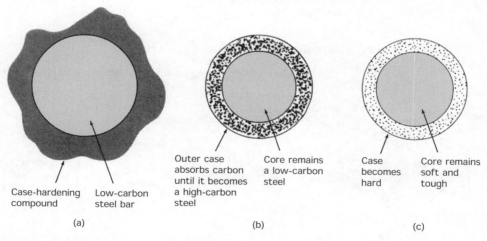

Case-hardening compound Low-carbon steel bar

(a)

Outer case absorbs carbon until it becomes a high-carbon steel   Core remains a low-carbon steel

(b)

Case becomes hard   Core remains soft and tough

(c)

Figure 4.15 *Case hardening: (a) carburizing; (b) after carburizing; (c) after quenching a component from a temperature above 780°C*

been absorbed to the required depth. Second, the workpiece is removed from the carburizing compound, reheated to between 780°C and 820°C and dipped off (quenched) in cold water.

Carburizing

This depends upon the fact that very low carbon (0.1%) steels will absorb carbon when heated to between 900°C and 950°C. Various carbonaceous materials are used in the carburizing process.

- *Solid media* such as bone charcoal or charred leather, together with an energizer such as sodium and/or barium carbonate. The energizer makes up to 40% of the total composition.

- *Molten salts* such as sodium cyanide, together with sodium carbonate and/or barium carbonate and sodium or barium chloride. Since cyanide is a deadly poison such salts must be handled with great care and the cyanide makes up only between 20 and 50% of the total. Stringent safety precautions must be taken in its use. The components to be carburized are immersed in the molten salts.

- *Gaseous media* based upon natural gas (methane) are increasingly used. Methane is a hydrocarbon gas containing organic carbon compounds that are readily absorbed into the steel. The methane gas is frequently enriched by the vapours that are given off when mineral oils are 'cracked' by heating them in contact with the metal platinum which acts as a catalyst.

It is a common fallacy that carburizing hardens the steel. *It does not*, it adds carbon only to the surface of the steel and leaves the steel in a fully annealed (soft) condition. It is the subsequent heat treatment that hardens the steel.

Superficial hardening

This produces a shallow case on simple components as shown in Fig. 4.16.

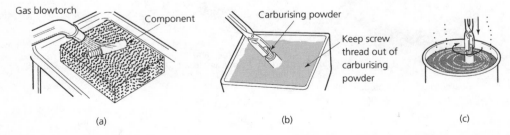

Figure 4.16 *Superficial hardening: (a) heat to bright red in brazing hearth; (b) plunge red-hot component into carburizing powder (repeat to give desired depth of case; (c) reheat to cherry red and quench in water*

- The component is raised to red heat using a gas torch and brazing hearth.

- The red-hot component is then plunged into a case-hardening powder. This consists of carbon rich compounds plus an energizer as previously described.

- The component absorbs the powder onto its surface. This 'carburizes' the surface of the metal and increases its carbon content.

- The heating and dipping can be repeated several times to increase the depth of carbon infusion.

- Finally, the component is again heated to red heat and plunged immediately into cold water. If the case-hardening powder has done its job, there should be a loud 'crack' and any surplus powder breaks away from the surface of the metal.

- The surface of the metal should now have a mottled appearance and it should be hard. The component is now case hardened.

- Because this technique results in only a fairly shallow case, it is referred to as 'superficial hardening'. The case is not deep enough for finishing by grinding processes, although polishing is permissible.

- Bright-drawn steels do not absorb carbon readily unless the drawn surface is removed by machining. Wherever possible use a case-hardening quality steel which is formulated and processed to suit this treatment.

Deep case hardening

Where a deep case is required so that components can be finished by grinding (e.g. surface grinding or cylindrical grinding) the following procedure is required.

- The component is 'pack-carburized' by burying it in the carburizing compound in a steel box, sealed with an airtight lid.

- The box is heated in a furnace for several hours depending upon the depth of case required. The carburizing temperature is about 950°C as shown in Fig. 4.17.

- The box is removed from the furnace and allowed to cool down. The component is removed from the box and cleaned so as to remove any residual powder from its surface.

- The component will be soft and have a coarse grain structure because of the long time for which it has been heated at a high temperature, and its subsequent slow cooling.

- The core of the component will have a carbon content of less than 0.3%. The low carbon steel core of the component is toughened by refining its grain. To do this, the component is heated to 870°C as shown at A in Fig. 4.17 and then quenched in oil.

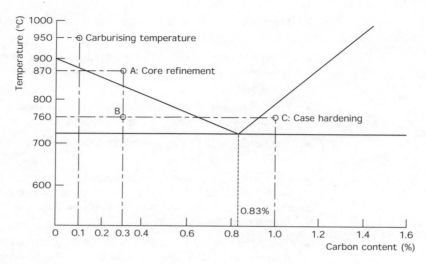

Figure 4.17 *Case-hardening temperatures*

- Since this temperature is well below the carburizing temperature which caused the grain growth and because of the rapid cooling the core will now have a fine grain.

- This rapid cooling will also have the effect of hardening the case. Unfortunately the case will have a coarse grain since it was heated to above its correct hardening temperature as shown at B in Fig. 4.17.

- To refine the grain of the case and reharden it, the component is heated to 760°C, as shown at C in Fig. 4.17, and quenched in water. This is the correct hardening procedure for a 1.0% carbon steel which is what the surface of the component has become. This temperature is too low to affect the fine grain of the core.

- Finally the component can be tempered if required.

Localized case hardening

It is often undesirable to case harden a component all over. For example, it is undesirable to case harden screw threads. Not only would they be extremely brittle, but any distortion occurring during carburizing and hardening could be corrected only by expensive thread grinding operations. Various means are available for avoiding local infusion of carbon during the carburizing process.

- Heavily copper plating those areas to be left soft. The layer of copper prevents intimate contact between the component and the carburizing medium. Copper plating cannot be used for salt-bath carburizing as the molten salts dissolve the copper.

- Encasing the areas to be left soft in fire-clay. This technique is mostly used when pack carburizing.

- Leaving surplus metal where a soft area is required. This is machined off between carburizing and hardening (dipping off). An example is shown in Fig. 4.18. Although more expensive because of the extra handling involved, it is the most sure and effective way of leaving local soft features.

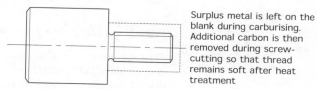

Surplus metal is left on the blank during carburising. Additional carbon is then removed during screw-cutting so that thread remains soft after heat treatment

Figure 4.18 *Localized case hardening*

4.17 The heat treatment of non-ferrous metals and alloys

None of the non-ferrous metals and only a very few non-ferrous alloys can be quench hardened like plain carbon steels. The majority of non-ferrous metals can only be hardened by cold-working processes. Alternatively they can be manufactured from cold-rolled (spring temper) sheet or strip, or they can be manufactured from cold-drawn wire. Work-hardened non-ferrous metals can be annealed by a recrystallization process that is similar to the process of annealing for plain carbon steels. The main difference is that non-ferrous metals do not have to be cooled slowly. They can be quenched after heating and this has the advantage that the rapid cooling causes the metal to shrink suddenly and this removes the oxide film. In the case of copper and its alloys this is even more effective if the metal is pickled in a weak solution of sulphuric acid whilst still warm. (*Safety*. If an acid bath is used, protective clothing and eye protection such as goggles or, better still, a visor *must* be worn.) Suitable annealing temperatures are:

- Aluminium   500°C to 550°C   (pure metal)
- Copper   650°C to 750°C   (pure metal)
- Cold-working brass   600°C to 650°C   (simple alloy of copper and zinc)

Heat treatable aluminium alloys ('duralumin' is such an alloy) require somewhat different treatment. They can be softened by *solution treatment* and hardened by *natural ageing* or they can be hardened artificially by *precipitation treatment*. The alloy 'duralumin' contains traces of copper, magnesium, manganese and zinc; aluminium makes up the remainder of the alloy.

4.17.1 Solution treatment

To soften duralumin type aluminium alloys, they are raised to a temperature of about 500°C (depending upon the alloy). At this temperature the alloying elements can form a solid solution in the aluminium. The alloy is quenched from this temperature to preserve the solution at room temperature. Gradually, the solid solution will break down with age and the alloy will become harder and more brittle. Therefore solution treatment must be carried out immediately before the alloy is to be processed. The breakdown of the solution can be delayed by refrigeration at between $-6°C$ and $-10°C$. Conversely it can be speeded up by raising the temperature.

4.17.2 Precipitation treatment

The natural hardening mentioned above is called *age hardening*. This is the result of hard particles of aluminium−copper compounds precipitating out of the solid solution. This hardens and strengthens the alloy but makes it less ductile and more brittle. Precipitation hardening can be accelerated by heating the alloy to about 150°C to 170°C for several hours. This process is referred to as *artificial ageing* or *precipitation hardening*. The times and temperatures vary for each alloy and the alloy manufacturer's heat treatment specifications must be carefully observed, especially for critical components such as those used in the aircraft industry.

4.18 Heat treatment furnaces

The requirements of heat treatment furnaces are as follows:

- *Uniform heating of the work*. This is necessary in order to prevent distortion of the work due to unequal expansion, and also to ensure uniform hardness.

- *Accurate temperature control*. We have previously discussed the critical nature of heat treatment temperatures. Therefore, not only must the furnace be capable of operating over a wide range of temperatures, it must be easily adjustable to the required process temperature.

- *Temperature stability*. Not only is it essential that the temperature is accurately adjustable but, once set, the furnace must remain at the required temperature. This is achieved by ensuring that the mass of the heated furnace lining (refractory) is very much greater than the mass of the work (charge). It can also be achieved by automatic temperature control, or by both.

- *Atmosphere control*. If the work is heated in the presence of air, the oxygen in the air attacks the surface of the metal to form metal oxides (scale). This not only disfigures the surface of the metal, it can also change the composition of the metal at its surface. For example, in the case of steels, the oxygen can also combine with the carbon at the surface of the metal. Reducing the carbon content results in the metal surface becoming less hard and/or tough.

- To provide atmosphere control, the air in the furnace is replaced with some form of inert gas which will not react with the workpiece material. Alternatively the work may be totally immersed in hot, molten salts.

- *Economical use of fuels*. This is essential if heat treatment costs are to be kept to a minimum. If the furnaces can be run continuously on a shift work basis considerable economies can be made. The fuel required to keep firing up furnaces from cold is much greater than that required for continuous running. Thus it is more economical for small workshops to contract their heat treatment out to specialist firms who have sufficient volume of work to keep their furnaces in continuous use.

- *Low maintenance costs*. The furnace is lined with a heat resistant material such as firebrick. Since the furnace must be taken out of commission each time this lining is renewed, it should be designed to last as long as possible.

4.18.1 Open-hearth furnace

Figure 4.19 shows the simplest form of furnace. This is little different to heating a component on a brazing hearth except that the furnace arch reflects heat back onto the component and provides rather more uniform heating. In this furnace a gas or oil burner plays directly onto the charge. Heat is also reflected onto the work from the furnace lining as previously mentioned. The advantages and limitations of this type of furnace are as follows:

Advantages

- Low initial cost.

- Simplicity in use and maintenance.

- Fuel economy since it heats up quickly.

Limitations

- Uneven heating.

- Poor temperature control.

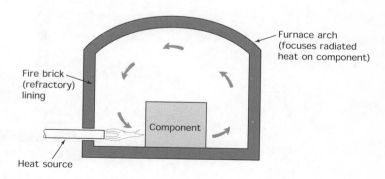

Figure 4.19 *Gas-heated open hearth furnace*

- Poor temperature stability.

- Complete lack of atmosphere control resulting in heavy scaling and flue gas contamination of the work.

4.18.2 Semi-muffle furnace

Figure 4.20 shows a semi-muffle furnace. This is an improvement upon the open-hearth furnace previously described. The flame from the burner does not play directly onto the charge, but passes under the hearth to provide 'bottom heat'. This results in more uniform heating. The advantages and limitations of this type of furnace are as follows:

Advantages

- Comparatively low initial cost.

- Simplicity in use and maintenance.

- Fuel economy.

- Fairly rapid heating.

- Heating is more uniform than for the open-hearth type of furnace.

- Limited atmosphere control can be achieved by varying the gas–air mixture through a system of dampers. The flue outlets are situated just inside the furnace door so that any atmospheric oxygen that may leak past the door is swept up the flue before it can add to the scaling of the work.

- Reasonable temperature control.

- Reasonable atmosphere stability due to the greater mass of the furnace lining compared with the open-hearth type furnace.

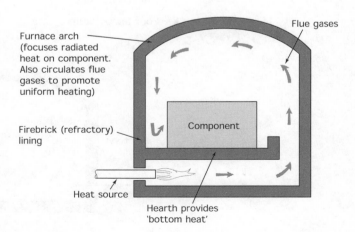

Figure 4.20 *Gas-heated semi-muffle furnace*

Limitations

- Heating is still comparatively uneven compared with more sophisticated furnace types.

- Atmosphere control is somewhat limited. Although oxidation can be reduced by careful control of the gas–air mixture, some scaling will still take place and there will still be flue gas contamination of the work.

4.18.3 Muffle furnace (gas heated)

Figure 4.21 shows a full muffle furnace. You can see from the figure that the work is heated in a separate compartment called a *muffle*. The work is completely isolated from the flame and the products of combustion. The advantages and limitations for this type of furnace are as follows:

Advantages

- Uniform heating.

- Reasonable temperature control.

- Good temperature stability due to the mass of refractory material forming the muffle and the furnace lining compared with the mass of the work.

- Full atmosphere control is possible. Any sort of atmosphere can be maintained within the muffle since no combustion air is required in the muffle chamber.

Limitations

- Higher initial cost.

- Maintenance more complex and costly.

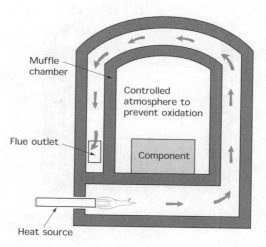

Figure 4.21 *Gas-heated muffle furnace*

- Greater heat losses and slow initial heating result in lower fuel economy unless the furnace can be operated continuously.

4.18.4 Muffle furnace (electric resistance)

Figure 4.22 shows a typical electric resistance muffle furnace. The electric heating elements are similar to those found in domestic electric ovens. They are independent of the atmosphere in which they operate. Therefore they can be placed within the muffle chamber itself, resulting in a higher operating efficiency compared with the gas heated muffle furnace, which more than offsets the higher energy cost for electricity compared with gas. The advantages and limitations of this type of furnace are as follows:

Advantages

- Uniform heating of the work.
- Accurate temperature control.
- Ease of fitting automatic control instrumentation.
- High temperature stability.
- Full atmosphere control.
- Comparatively easy maintenance.

Limitations

- Higher energy source costs.
- Lower maximum operating temperatures, as above 950°C to 1000°C the life of the resistance elements is low.

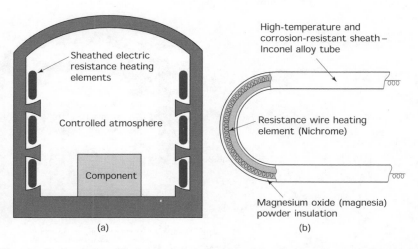

(a)   (b)

Figure 4.22 *Electrically heated muffle furnace: (a) the electric resistance furnace; (b) heating element*

4.19 Temperature measurement

The importance of temperature measurement and control during heat treatment processes has already been discussed in this chapter. For the high temperatures met with in heat treatment furnaces one or other of the temperature measuring devices known as *pyrometers* is required.

4.19.1 Thermocouple pyrometer

This is the most widely used temperature measuring device for heat treatment purposes. Figure 4.23(a) shows the principle of the thermocouple pyrometer. If the junction of two wires made from dissimilar metals (such as a copper wire and an iron wire) form part of a closed electric circuit and the junction is heated, a small electric current will flow. The presence of this current can be indicated by a sensitive galvanometer. Increasing the temperature difference between the hot and cold junctions increases the current in the circuit. If the galvanometer is calibrated in degrees of temperature, we have a temperature measuring device called a pyrometer.

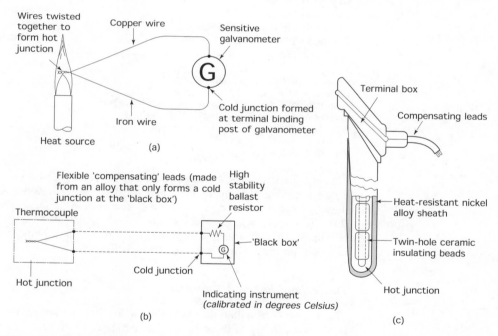

Figure 4.23 *The thermocouple pyrometer: (a) principle of operation; (b) pyrometer circuit; (c) thermocouple probe*

Figure 4.23(b) shows how these principles can be applied to a practical thermocouple pyrometer. The component parts of this instrument are:

- the thermocouple probe (hot junction);
- the indicating instrument (milli-ammeter);

- the 'ballast' or 'swamp' resistor;
- the compensating leads.

The *thermocouple probe* consists of a junction of two wires of dissimilar metals contained within a tube of refractory metal or of porcelain. Porcelain beads are used to insulate the two wires and locate them in the sheath as shown in Fig. 4.23(c). Table 4.15 lists the more usual hot junction material combinations, together with their temperature ranges and sensitivities.

TABLE 4.15 *Thermocouple combinations*

Thermocouple	Sensitivity (millivolts/°C)	Temperature range (°C)
Copper–constantan	0.054	−220 to + 300
Iron–constantan	0.054	−220 to + 750
Chromel–alumel	0.041	−200 to + 1200
Platinum–platinum/rhodium	0.0095	0 to + 1450

Notes:
Constantan = 60% copper, 40% nickel.
Chromel = 90% nickel, 10% chromium.
Alumel = 95% nickel, 2% aluminium, 3% manganese.
Platinum/rhodium = 90% platinum, 10% rhodium.

The indicating instrument

This is a sensitive milli-ammeter calibrated in degrees celsius (°C) so that a direct reading of temperature can be made. A common error is to set this instrument to read *zero* when the system is cold. In fact it should be set to read the *atmospheric temperature* at the point of installation. The terminals of this instrument form the cold junction and should be placed in a cool position where they are screened from the heat of the furnace.

The 'ballast' or 'swamp' resistor

This is contained within the case of the indicating instrument. Its purpose is to give stability to the system. The resistance of electrical conductors increases as their temperature increases, and the conductors that make up a pyrometer circuit are no exception. The variation in resistance with temperature would seriously affect the calibration of the instrument if the ballast resistor were not present. This resistor is made from manganin wire. Manganin is an alloy whose resistance is virtually unaffected by heat. By making the resistance of the ballast resistor very large compared with the resistance of the rest of the circuit, it *swamps* the effects of any changes in resistance that may occur in the rest of the circuit and renders them unimportant.

Compensating leads

These are used to connect the thermocouple probe to the indicating instrument. They are made of a special alloy so that they form a cold junction with the terminals of the indicating instrument but not with the terminals of the probe. To avoid changes in calibration, the compensating leads must not be changed in length, nor must alternative conductors be used. The thermocouple, compensating leads and the indicating instrument must always be kept together as a set.

4.19.2   The radiation pyrometer

This device is used to measure the temperature:

- Of large hot components that have been removed from the furnace.
- Where the furnace temperature is so high it would damage the thermocouple probe.
- Where the hot component is inaccessible.
- Where the temperature of the component in the furnace needs to be measured rather than the temperature of the furnace atmosphere itself.

The principle of this type of pyrometer is shown in Fig. 4.24. Instead of the thermocouple probe being inserted into the furnace atmosphere, the radiant heat from the furnace or the component being heated in the furnace is focused onto the thermocouple by a parabolic mirror.

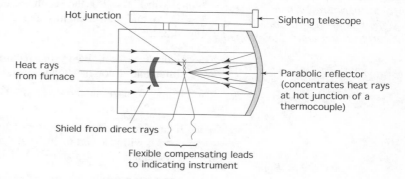

Figure 4.24   *The radiation pyrometer*

Remember that as the temperature of a work reaches the furnace temperature, the rate at which the temperature of the work increases slows down. It is difficult to assess just when, if ever, the component reaches furnace temperature. Certainly, the soaking time involved would give rise to excessive grain growth. Furnaces are frequently operated above the required process temperature, and the work is withdrawn from the furnace when it has reached its correct temperature as measured by a radiation pyrometer.

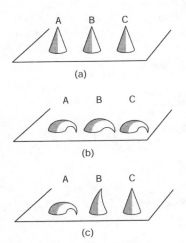

Figure 4.25 *Use of Seger cones: (a) temperature too low – no cones soften; (b) temperature too high – all the cones soften; (c) temperature correct – cone A softens and droops, cone B just starts to droop, cone C unaffected*

4.19.3   Temperature assessment

The devices and techniques described above give precise temperature measurement. There are simpler ways of assessing the *approximate* temperature; some of these will now be described.

Paints and crayons

These are applied to the surface of the component to be heat treated. The mark left on the surface by their application changes in colour and appearance when the desired temperature has been reached. The paints and crayons are available in a range of compositions to suit the temperature required. They have the advantage of indicating the temperature of the component at the point of application. It has been stated previously that the temperature of the charge does not necessarily reflect the temperature in the furnace. They can also be used to indicate the pre-heating temperature of components to be joined by welding. Another application is to mark the blades of gas turbines (jet engines) so, when undergoing routine maintenance, it can be seen if the blades have been overheated and therefore weakened.

Ceramic cones

These are also known as 'Seger' cones and may be conical or pyramidal in shape. The latter have a triangular base. The 'cones' are made with various compositions so that they soften at different temperatures. It is usual to choose three cones, one slightly below the required temperature (cone A in Fig. 4.25), the second at the required temperature (cone B in Fig. 4.25), and a third slightly above the required temperature (cone C in Fig. 4.25).

- If the furnace is below the required temperature none of the cones soften and droop as shown in Fig. 4.25(a).

- If the furnace is too hot, all the cones will droop as shown in Fig. 4.25(b).

- If the furnace is at the correct temperature, cone A will droop a lot, cone B will just start to droop at the tip, and cone C will be unaffected. This situation is shown in Fig. 4.25(c).

4.20   Atmosphere control

When natural gas is burnt in a furnace, excess air is usually present to ensure complete and efficient combustion. The resulting *products of combustion* (flue gases) contain oxygen, carbon dioxide, sulphur, nitrogen and water vapour. These all react to a greater or lesser degree with the surface of the workpiece whilst it is in the furnace. They will produce heavy scaling and, in the case of steel, surface decarburization and softening. The situation is not so serious in the case of a muffle furnace as the fuel is burnt in a separate chamber and cannot come into contact with the work. However, the oxygen and water vapour in the air are still present in the muffle chamber and will cause some scaling and decarburization of the work.

Little can be done to offset this effect in simple furnaces. However, in muffle furnaces air in the muffle chamber can be replaced by alternative atmospheres, depending upon the process being performed and the metal being treated. This is known as *atmosphere control*. These controlled atmospheres can be based upon natural gas (methane) and LPG gases such as propane and butane. For special applications, ammonia gas and 'cracked' ammonia gas are used.

Exercises   **4.1**   *Material properties*

(a)   Name the properties required by the materials used in the following applications:
  (i)   A metal-cutting tool.
  (ii)   A forged crane hook.
  (iii)   A motor car radiator.
  (iv)   A motor car road wheel axle.
  (v)   The conductors in an electric cable.
  (vi)   A crane sling.
  (vii)   The sheathing of an electric cable.
  (viii)   A kitchen sink.
  (ix)   A garden hosepipe.
  (x)   Concrete for a machine foundation.
  (xi)   Lathe tailstock.

(b)   Giving reasons for your choice, name a suitable plain carbon steel and state its heat treatment condition for each of the following applications.
  (i)   Cold chisel.
  (ii)   Engineer's file.
  (iii)   Vehicle leaf spring.
  (iv)   Sheet steel for pressing out car body panels.
  (v)   Rod for making small turned parts on an automatic lathe.

4.2   *Material applications and classification*

(a)   Copy out and complete Table 4.16.

TABLE 4.16   *Exercise 4.2(a)*

Material	Typical application
Cast iron	
High-speed steel	
Duralumin	
Stainless steel (austenitic)	
Gunmetal	
Phosphor bronze	

(continued overleaf)

TABLE 4.16   *(continued)*

Material	Typical application
70/30 Brass	
60/40 Brass	
Free-cutting brass	
Tufnol	
Nylon	
PTFE	
Perspex	
Polystyrene	
PVC	
Glass fibre-reinforced polyester	
Epoxy resin	
Urea–formaldehyde	

(b)   Copy out and complete Table 4.17 by explaining briefly the meaning of the following terms:

TABLE 4.17   *Exercise 4.2(b)*

Term	Meaning	Example
Ferrous metal		
Non-ferrous metal		
Thermoplastic		
Thermosetting plastic		
Synthetic material		
Natural material		
Metallic		
Non-metallic		
Alloy		

4.3   *Forms of supply, identification, and specification*

(a)   Table 4.18 lists a number of material applications. Copy out and complete the table by naming the 'form of supply' in which you would expect to receive the material for each application.

(b)   (i)   State the meaning of the following abbreviations as applied to plain carbon steels: MS, BDMS, HRPO, CRCA.

(ii)   What do the terms 'quarter-hard', 'half-hard', etc., refer to when ordering non-ferrous sheet metal and rolled strip?

(c)   Describe the methods of material identification used in the raw material stores at your place of work or your training workshop.

(d)   The following specifications are based upon the current edition of BS 970. Explain their meaning.

TABLE 4.18   *Exercise 4.3(a)*

Applications	Form of supply
Car body panels	
Lathe bed	
Turned parts	
Plastic mouldings	
Structural steel work	
The two main raw materials for GRP boat hull mouldings	
Plastic window frames	
Connecting rods for high-power motor cycle engines	

(i)	080 A15
(ii)	080 M 15
(iii)	230 M 07
(iv)	230 M 07 (leaded)
(v)	080 M 40
(vi)	605 M 36
(vii)	708 M 40
(viii)	817 M 40

4.4   *Heat treatment safety*

(a)   Briefly describe the type of clothing and protective devices you should wear when carrying out heat treatment processes.

(b)   Sketch THREE warning signs you would expect to find in a heat treatment shop.

4.5   *Reasons for heat treatment*

(a)   State the main TWO purposes for the heat treatment of metallic materials.

(b)   Explain why a coppersmith would anneal a blank cut from a sheet of copper before beating it to shape, and why would he/she need to re-anneal the metal from time to time as forming proceeds.

4.6   *Hardening plain carbon steels*

(a)   What two factors does the hardness of a plain carbon steel depend upon when through-hardening?

(b)   Explain why steels have to be tempered after hardening and how the degree of temper is controlled when this is done over a brazing hearth in the workshop.

(c)   When through-hardening, what is the effect of:
   (i)   overheating the steel;
   (ii)   underheating the steel.

(d)   When through-hardening, explain how the hot metal should be quenched and what precautions must be taken to avoid cracking and distortion.

4.7 *Local hardening*

(a) With the aid of sketches show how a simple component can be superficially case hardened at the brazing hearth in a workshop.

(b) List the operations for case hardening the component shown in Fig. 4.26 so that the threads are left soft.

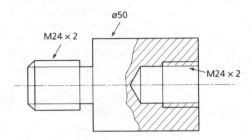

Figure 4.26 *Exercise 4.7(b)*

(c) Name an example of:
  (i) a solid case-hardening compound;
  (ii) a gaseous case-hardening compound;
  and give an example where each would be used.

4.8 *Annealing and normalizing*

(a) Describe the essential differences between annealing and normalizing plain carbon steels.

(b) Describe the essential differences between full annealing and subcritical annealing as applied to plain carbon steels.

(c) Describe the essential differences between the annealing of plain carbon steels and the annealing of non-ferrous metals (other than the heat treatable aluminium alloys).

(d) Describe how 'duralumin' is softened. What is the name of the process used, and what is the name of the natural process by which this aluminium alloy gradually becomes hard again?

4.9 *Heat treatment equipment*

(a) List the main requirements of a heat treatment furnace.

(b) With the aid of sketches describe any heat treatment furnace with which you are familiar. Draw particular attention to its main features. List the main advantages and limitations for the furnace type chosen.

(c) Describe the precautions that must be taken when starting up and shutting down furnaces.

(d) Describe the need for, and a method of, atmosphere control in heat treatment furnaces.

(e) Describe a method of temperature measurement suitable for a furnace used for the occasional hardening of high carbon steel components.

5   Engineering drawing

When you have read this chapter you should understand how to:

- Interpret (read) drawings in first and third angle projection.
- Sketch and dimension mechanical components in first and third angle projection.
- Sketch mechanical components in isometric and oblique projection.

5.1   Engineering drawing (introduction)

Figure 5.1(a) shows a drawing of a simple clamp. This is a pictorial drawing. It is very easy to see what has been drawn, even to people who have not been taught how to read an engineering drawing. Unfortunately such drawings have only a limited use in engineering. If you try to put

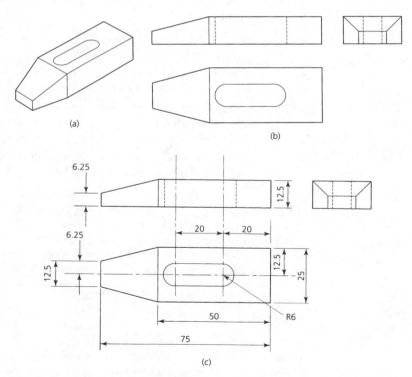

Figure 5.1   *Clamp: (a) pictorial drawing; (b) orthographic drawing; (c) fully dimensioned in millimetres*

all the information that is required to make the clamp onto this drawing it would become very cluttered and difficult to interpret. Therefore we use a system called *orthographic drawing* when we make engineering drawings.

An example of an orthographic drawing of our clamp is shown in Fig. 5.1(b). We now have a collection of drawings each one looking at the clamp from a different direction. This enables us to show every feature of the clamp that can be seen and also some things that cannot be seen (hidden details). Features that cannot be seen are indicated by broken lines. Finally we can add the sizes (dimensions) that we need in order to make the clamp. These are shown in Fig. 5.1(c). A drawing that has all the information required to make a component part, such as Fig. 5.1(c), is called a *detail drawing*, but more of that later.

5.2 First angle orthographic drawing

There are two systems of orthographic drawing used by engineers:

- First angle or English projection.
- Third angle or American projection.

In this section we are going to look at *first angle* projection. We are again going to use the clamp you first met in Fig. 5.1(a). We look at the clamp from various directions.

- Look down on the top of the clamp and draw what you see as shown in Fig. 5.2(a). This is called a *plan view*.
- Look at the end of the clamp and draw what you see as shown in Fig. 5.2(a). This is called an *end view*.
- Look at the side of the clamp and draw what you see as shown in Fig. 5.2(a). Although this is a side view, it is given a special name. It is called an *elevation*.
- You can now assemble these views together in the correct order as shown in Fig. 5.2(b) to produce a *first angle orthographic drawing* of the clamp.

As well as the things that can be seen from the outside of the clamp, we also included some 'hidden detail' in the end view and elevation. Hidden detail indicates a slot through the clamp in this example. The slot is shown by using *broken lines*. We did this because if we had shown the slot as an oval in the plan view it could have meant one of two things:

- A slot passing right through the clamp.
- A slot recessed part way into the clamp.

It *could not* have been an oval-shaped lump on top of the clamp as this would have shown up in the end view and in the elevation.

Sometimes only two views are used when the plan and elevation are the same. For example, a cylindrical component such as a shaft. Figure 5.3

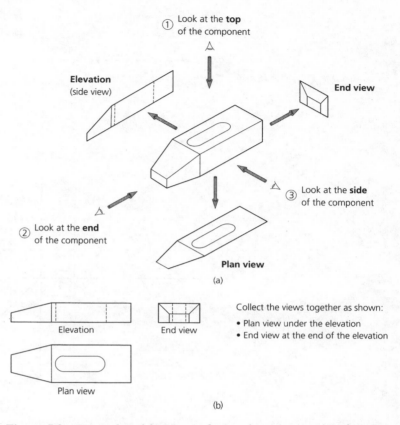

① Look at the **top**
of the component

Elevation
(side view)

End view

② Look at the **end**
of the component

③ Look at the **side**
of the component

Plan view

(a)

Elevation

End view

Collect the views together as shown:

• Plan view under the elevation
• End view at the end of the elevation

Plan view

(b)

Figure 5.2 *Principles of drawing in first angle projection: (a) plan view, end view, and elevation (side view); (b) collected views together make up an orthographic drawing*

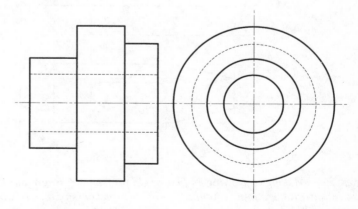

Figure 5.3 *First angle drawing of a cylindrical component: the elevation and plan views are the same and need only be drawn once*

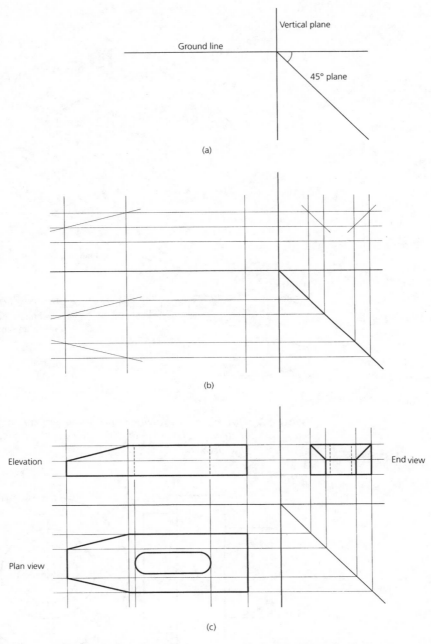

Figure 5.4 *Making a drawing in first angle projection: (a) ground line and planes; (b) initial construction lines; (c) line in the outline (outline is twice the thickness of the construction lines)*

shows that an elevation and an end view provide all the information we require.

Finally let's see how a first angle orthographic drawing is constructed.

- First draw the ground lines and a plane at 45° as shown in Fig. 5.4(a).

- Then start to draw in the construction lines faintly using lines that are half the thickness of the final outline. Figure 5.4(b) shows the construction lines in place.

- Then follow each construction line round all the views in order to avoid confusion.

- Finally, we 'line in' the outline so that it stands out boldly as shown in Fig. 5.4(c).

5.3 Third angle orthographic drawing

To draw the clamp in third angle (American) orthographic projection, you merely have to rearrange the relative positions of the views. Each view now appears at the same side or end of the component from which you are looking at it. This is shown in Fig. 5.5(a). That is:

- Look down on the clamp and draw the plan view above the side view or elevation.

- Look at the left-hand end of the clamp and draw the end view at the same end.

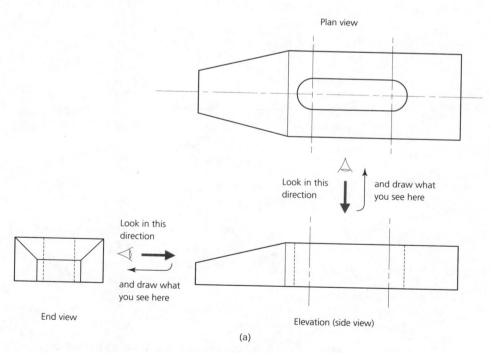

Figure 5.5   (a) Principles of drawing in third angle projection; (b) projection symbol

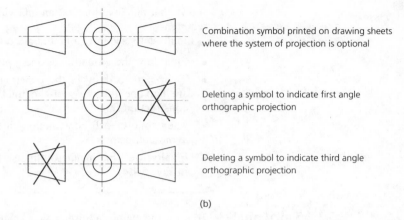

(b)

Figure 5.5 *(continued)*

So what is the advantage of third angle projection? Consider the general arrangement drawing for an airliner drawn to a fairly large scale so that fine detail can be shown. In first angle projection, the end view looking at the nose of the aircraft would be drawn somewhere beyond the tail. An end view looking at the tail of the aircraft would be drawn somewhere beyond the nose. It is much more convenient to draw the end view of the nose of the aircraft at the nose end of the elevation. Also, it is more

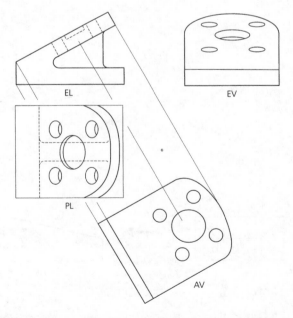

Figure 5.6 *Auxiliary view: EL = elevation; EV = end view; PL = plan; AV = auxiliary view*

convenient to draw an end view of the tail of an aircraft next to the tail of the elevation.

To avoid confusion, always state the projection used on the drawing. Sometimes the projection used is stated in words, more usually it is indicated by the use of a standard symbol. Figure 5.5(b) shows the combined projection symbol and how it is used.

So far we have only considered features that are conveniently arranged at right angles to each other so that their true shape is shown in the plan, elevation or the end view. This is not always the case and sometimes we have to include an *auxiliary view*. This technique is important in the production of working drawings so that the positions of features on the surface that is inclined not only appear undistorted but can also be dimensioned. Figure 5.6 shows a bracket with an inclined face. When it is drawn in first angle projection, it can be seen that the end view showing the inclined surface and its features is heavily distorted. However, these features appear correct in size and in shape in the auxiliary view (AV) which is projected at right angles (perpendicular) to the inclined face.

5.4 Conventions

An engineering drawing is only a means of recording the intentions of the designer and communicating those intentions to the manufacturer. It is not a work of art and, apart from the time spent in its preparation, it has no intrinsic value. If a better and cheaper method of communication could be discovered, then the engineering drawing would no longer be used. We are already part way along this road with CAD where the drawings are stored digitally on magnetic or optical disks and can be transmitted between companies by the internet. However, hard copy, in the form of a printed drawing, still has to be produced for the craftsperson or the technician to work to.

As an aid to producing engineering sketches and drawings quickly and cheaply we use *standard conventions*. These are recognized internationally and are used as a form of drawing 'shorthand' for the more frequently used details.

In the UK we use the British Standard for Engineering Drawing Practice as published by the British Standards Institute (BSI). This standard is based upon the recommendations of the International Standards Organization (ISO) and, therefore, its conventions and guidelines, and drawings produced using such conventions and guidelines are accepted internationally.

5.4.1 Types of line

Figure 5.7 shows the types of line recommended by BS 308, together with some typical applications. The following points should be noted in the use of these lines.

- *Dashed* lines should consist of dashes of consistent length and spacing, approximately to the proportions shown in the figure.

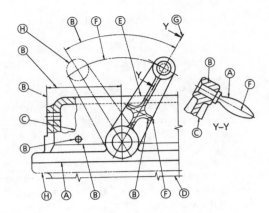

Figure 5.7 *Types of line and their applications*

Line		Description	Application
A	————	Continuous thick	Visible outlines and edges
B	————	Continuous thin	Dimension, projection and leader lines, hatching, outlines of revolved sections, short centre lines, imaginary intersections
C	⌒⌒⌒	Continuous thin irregular	Limits of partial or interrupted views and sections, if the limit is not an axis
D	⌁⌁	Continuous thin straight with zigzags	
E	- - - - - -	Dashed thin	Hidden outlines and edges
F	— — — —	Chain thin	Centre lines, lines of symmetry, trajectories and loci, pitch lines and pitch circles
G	⌐ —	Chain thin, thick at ends and changes of direction	Cutting planes
H	— — ·· — —	Chain thin double	Outlines and edges of adjacent parts, outlines and edges of alternative and extreme positions of movable parts, initial outlines prior to forming, bend lines on developed blanks or patterns

- *Thin chain lines* should consist of long dashes alternating with short dashes. The proportions should be generally as shown in the figure, but the lengths and spacing may be increased for very long lines.

- *Thick chain lines* should have similar lengths and spacing as for thin chain lines.

- *General.* All chain lines should start and finish with a long dash. When thin chain lines are used as centre lines, they should cross one another at solid portions of the line. Centre lines should extend only a short distance beyond the feature unless required for dimensioning or other purposes. They should not extend through the spaces between the views and should not terminate at another line of the drawing. Where angles are formed in chain lines, long dashes should meet at the corners and should be thickened as shown. Arcs should join at tangent points. Dashed lines should also meet at corners and tangent points with dashes.

5.4.2 Abbreviations for written statements

Table 5.1 lists the standard abbreviations for written statements as used on engineering drawings. Some examples of their use are shown in Fig. 5.8. Some further examples will be given when we discuss the dimensioning of drawings.

TABLE 5.1 *Abbreviations for written statements*

Term	Abbreviation	Term	Abbreviation
Across flats	A/F	Hexagon head	HEX HD
British Standard	BS	Material	MATL
Centres	CRS	Number	NO.
Centre line	CL *or* ℄	Pitch circle diameter	PCD
Chamfered	CHAM	Radius (in a note)	RAD
Cheese head	CH HD	Radius (preceding a dimension)	R
Countersunk	CSK		
Countersunk head	CSK HD	Screwed	SCR
Counterbore	C'BORE	Specification	SPEC
Diameter (in a note)	DIA	Spherical diameter or radius	SPHERE Ø *or* R
Diameter (preceding a dimension)	Ø	Spotface	S'FACE
Drawing	DRG	Standard	STD
Figure	FIG.	Undercut	U'CUT
Hexagon	HEX		

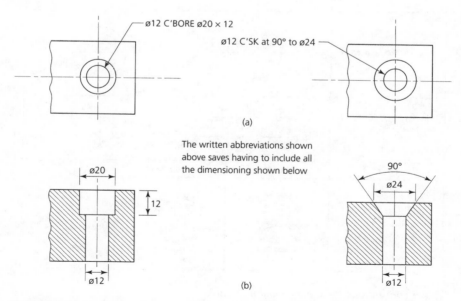

(a)

The written abbreviations shown above saves having to include all the dimensioning shown below

(b)

Figure 5.8 *Examples of the use of standard abbreviations: (a) counterbored hole; (b) countersunk hole*

5.4.3 Conventions

Figure 5.9 shows some typical conventions used in engineering drawings. It is not possible, in the scope of this book, to provide the full set of conventions or to provide detailed explanations of the use. For this it is necessary to consult texts specializing in engineering drawing together with British Standard 308. The full standard is expensive but you should find the special abridged edition, BS PP7308: 1986: Engineering Drawing Practice for Schools and Colleges, adequate for your needs. This edition is published at a very affordable price.

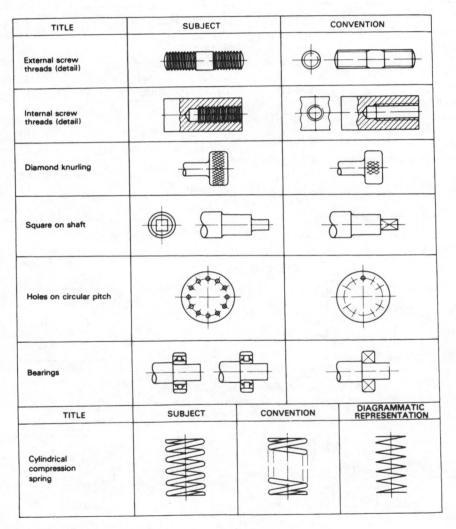

Figure 5.9 *Typical conventions for some common features*

5.5 Redundant views

It has been stated and shown earlier that where a component is symmetrical you do not always require all the views to provide the information required for manufacture. A ball looks the same from all directions, and to represent it by three circles arranged as a plan view, an elevation and an end view would just be a waste of time. All that is required is one circle and a note that the component is spherical. The views that

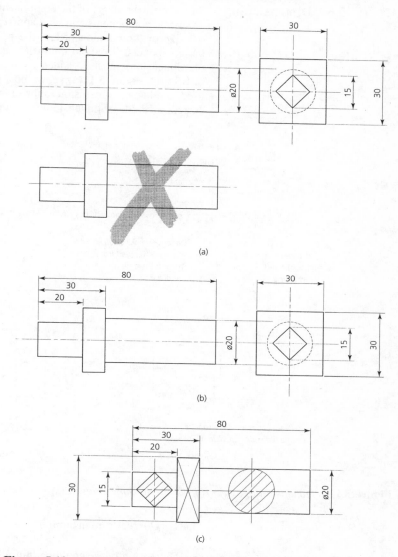

Figure 5.10 *Redundant views: (a) first angle working drawing of a symmetrical component (plan view redundant); (b) symmetrical component reduced to two views; (c) working drawing reduced to a single view by using revolved sections and BS convention for the square flange*

can be discarded without loss of information are called *redundant views*. Figure 5.10 shows how drawing time can be saved and the drawing simplified by eliminating the redundant views when drawing symmetrical components.

5.6 Dimensioning

So far, only the shape of the component has been considered. However, in order that components can be manufactured, the drawing must also show the size of the component and the position and size of any features on the component. To avoid confusion and the chance of misinterpretation, the dimensions must be added to the drawing in the manner laid down in BS 308. Figure 5.11(a) shows how projection and dimension lines are used to relate the dimension to the drawing, whilst Fig. 5.11(b) shows the correct methods of dimensioning a drawing.

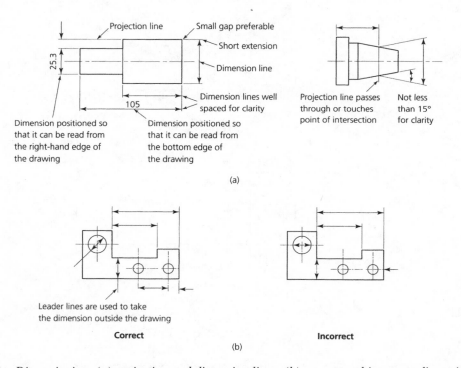

Figure 5.11 *Dimensioning: (a) projection and dimension lines; (b) correct and incorrect dimensioning*

5.6.1 Correct dimensioning

- Dimension lines should be thin full lines not more than half the thickness of the component outline.

- Wherever possible, dimension lines should be placed outside the outline of the drawing.

- The dimension line arrowhead must touch but not cross the projection line.

- Dimension lines should be well spaced so that the numerical value of the dimension can be clearly read and so that they do not obscure the outline of the drawing.

5.6.2 Incorrect dimensioning

- Centre lines and extension lines must *not* be used as dimension lines.
- Wherever possible dimension line arrowheads must not touch the outline directly but should touch the projection lines that extend from the outline.
- If the use of a dimension line within the outline is unavoidable, then try to use a leader line to take the dimension itself outside the outline.

5.6.3 Dimensioning diameters and radii

Figure 5.12(a) shows how circles and shaft ends (circles) should be dimensioned. It is preferable to use those techniques that take the dimension

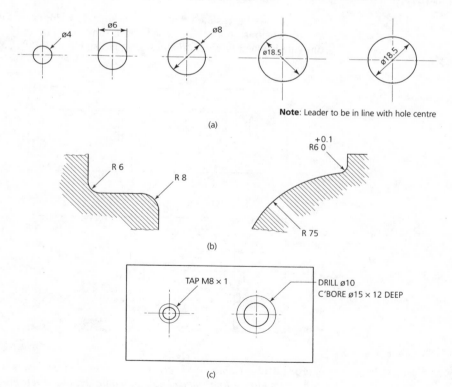

Figure 5.12 *Dimensioning – diameters and radii: (a) dimensioning holes; (b) dimensioning the radii of arcs which need not have their centres located; (c) use of notes to save full dimensioning*

outside the circle, unless the circle is so large that the dimension will neither be cramped nor will it obscure some vital feature. Note the use of the symbol Ø to denote a diameter.

Figure 5.12(b) shows how radii should be dimensioned. Note that the radii of arcs of circles need not have their centres located if the start and finish points are known.

Figure 5.12(c) shows how notes may be used to avoid the need for the full dimensioning of certain features of a drawing.

Leader lines

These indicate where notes or dimensions are intended to apply and end in either arrowheads or dots.

- *Arrowheads* are used where the leader line touches the outline of a component or feature.

- *Dots* are used where the leader line finishes within the outline of the component or feature to which it refers.

5.6.4 Auxiliary dimensions

It has already been stated that, to avoid mistakes, duplicated or unnecessary dimensions should not appear on a drawing. The only exception to this rule is when *auxiliary dimensions* are used to avoid the calculation of,

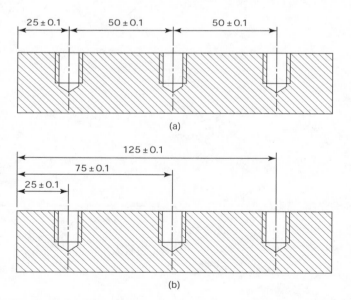

Figure 5.13 *Cumulative error: (a) string (incremental) dimensioning – cumulative tolerance equals sum of individual tolerances; (b) dimensioning from one common datum (absolute dimensioning) to eliminate cumulative effect (dimensions in millimetres)*

say, overall dimensions. Such auxiliary dimensions are placed in brackets as shown in Fig. 5.13. Auxiliary dimensions are also sometimes referred to as *non-functional* dimensions.

5.7 Toleranced dimensions

It is true to say that if ever a component was made exactly to size no one would ever know because it could not be measured exactly. Having calculated the ideal size for a dimension, the designer must then decide how much variation from that size he will tolerate. This variation between the smallest and the largest acceptable size is called the *tolerance*.

When toleranced dimensions are used, *cumulative errors* can occur wherever a feature is controlled by more than one toleranced dimension as shown in Fig. 5.13(a). It can be seen that chain dimensioning gives a build-up of tolerance that is greater than the designer intended. In this example the maximum tolerance for the right-hand hole centre is three times the individual tolerances. That is, the sum of the individual tolerances is $(\pm 0.1) + (\pm 0.1) + (\pm 0.1)$ mm $= \pm 0.3$ mm from the left-hand datum edge. This *cumulative* effect can be eliminated easily by dimensioning each feature individually from a common datum as shown in Fig. 5.13(b).

It is not usually necessary to tolerance every individual dimension, only the important ones. The rest can be given a *general tolerance* in the form of a note in the title block as shown in Fig. 5.14. This general statement may refer either to *open dimensions* or it may say *except where otherwise stated*. In the examples shown, the general tolerance is 0.5 mm

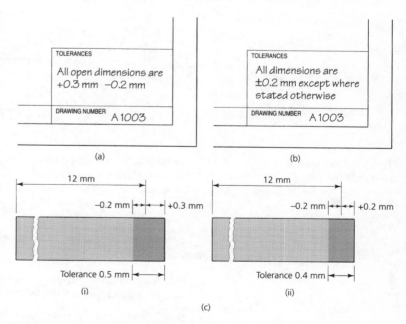

Figure 5.14 *General tolerances*

with the limits stated as $+0.3$ mm and -0.2 mm in the example shown in Fig. 5.15(a) and with limits stated as ± 0.2 mm in the example shown in Fig. 5.14(b). Both examples mean the same thing. Applied to an open dimension of 12 mm, the actual size is acceptable if it lies as shown in Fig. 5.14(c).

5.8 Sectioning

Sectioning is used to show the internal details of engineering components that cannot be shown clearly by other means. The stages of making a sectioned drawing are shown in Fig. 5.15. It should be realized that the steps (a), (b) and (c) are performed mentally in practice and only (d) is actually drawn.

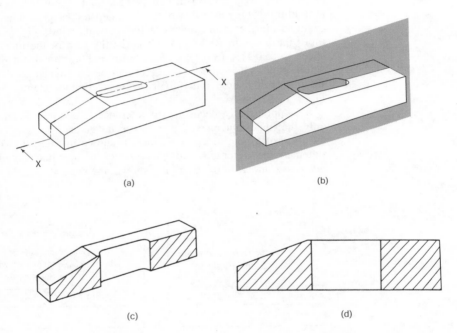

Figure 5.15 *Section drawing: (a) the clamp is to be sectioned along line X–X; (b) the cutting plane is positioned on the line X–X as shown; (c) that part of the clamp that lies in front of the cutting plane is removed leaving the sectioned component; (d) sectioned orthographic elevation of the clamp shown in (a) – note that section shading lines lie at 45° to the horizontal and are half the thickness of the outline*

The rules for producing and reading sectioned drawings can be summarized as follows.

- Drawings are only sectioned when it is impossible to show the internal details of a component in any other way.

- Bolts, studs, nuts, screws, keys, cotters and shafts are not usually sectioned even when the cutting plane passes through them.

- Ribs and webs are not sectioned when parallel to the cutting plane.

- The cutting plane must be indicated in the appropriate view.

- Hidden detail is not shown in sectioned views when it is already shown in another view.

- The section shading (hatching) is normally drawn at 45° to the outline of the drawing using thin, continuous lines that are half the thickness of the outline. If the outline contains an angle of 45° then the hatching angle can be changed to avoid confusion.

- Adjacent parts are hatched in opposite directions. To show more than two adjacent parts, the spacing between the hatched lines can be varied. A practical example of sectioning is shown in Fig. 5.16.

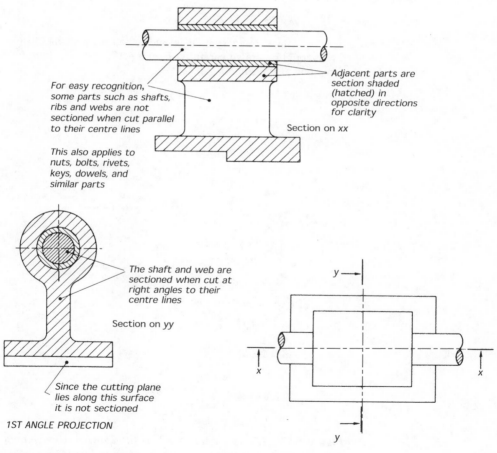

For easy recognition, some parts such as shafts, ribs and webs are not sectioned when cut parallel to their centre lines

This also applies to nuts, bolts, rivets, keys, dowels, and similar parts

Adjacent parts are section shaded (hatched) in opposite directions for clarity

Section on *xx*

The shaft and web are sectioned when cut at right angles to their centre lines

Section on *yy*

Since the cutting plane lies along this surface it is not sectioned

1ST ANGLE PROJECTION

Figure 5.16 *Practical sectioning*

5.9 Machining symbols

Machining symbols and instructions are used to:

- specify a particular surface finish;
- determine a machining process;
- define which surfaces are to be machined.

Figure 5.17(a) shows the standard machining symbol (BS 308) and the proportions in millimetres to which it should be drawn. When applied to views of a drawing, as shown in Fig. 5.17(b), the symbol should be drawn as follows (in this context '*normal*' means '*at right angles to*'):

- Normal to a surface.
- Normal to a projection line.
- Normal to an extension line.
- As a general note.

Because a machining symbol is interpreted as a precise instruction, its form should be drawn carefully. Figure 5.17(c) shows three fundamental variations of the symbol.

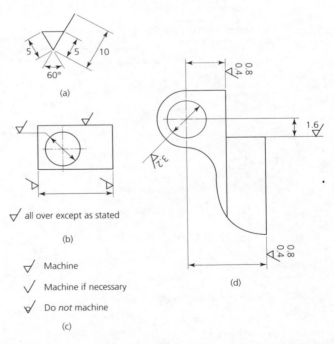

Figure 5.17 *The machining symbol: (a) drawing a machining symbol; (b) applying the machining symbol as an instruction; (c) machining symbols; (d) specifying surfaces texture on a casting – dimensions omitted for clarity*

These symbols must be used carefully; one incorrect symbol or incorrect application of a symbol can result in unnecessary manufacturing costs or even the scrapping of a component.

5.10 Types of engineering drawings

To save time in the drawing office, most companies adopt a standardized and pre-printed drawing sheet as shown in Fig. 5.18 if manual drawing is still used. The layout and content will vary from company to company but, generally, such sheets will provide the following information:

- The drawing number and title.
- The projection used (first angle or third angle).
- The scale.
- The general tolerance.
- The material specification.
- Warning notes.

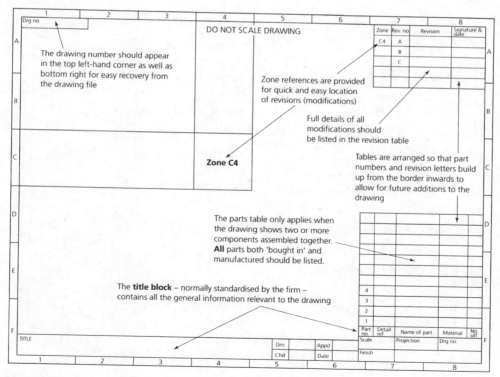

Figure 5.18 *Layout of drawing sheet*

- Any corrections or revisions, the date these were made, and the zone in which they occur.

- Special notes concerning, for example, heat treatment, decorative, corrosion resistant or other surface finishes.

If manual drawing is to be used then a pre-printed tracing sheet on tracing paper or plastic sheet will be used. The latter is more expensive but it is more durable if many copies of the drawing are required over an extended period of time. Modern drawing offices now use CAD systems. The standard layout is saved in the memory of the computer as a 'template' and can be called up by a keystroke whenever a drawing is to be made.

5.10.1 General arrangement drawings

An example of a *general arrangement* (GA) drawing is shown in Fig. 5.19. It shows all the components correctly assembled, and lists all the parts required. For those parts that will be 'bought in', it will state the maker and catalogue reference for the benefit of the purchasing department. For those parts to be made in the factory, the detail drawing numbers will be provided together with the material specification and the quantity of parts required. General arrangement drawings do not

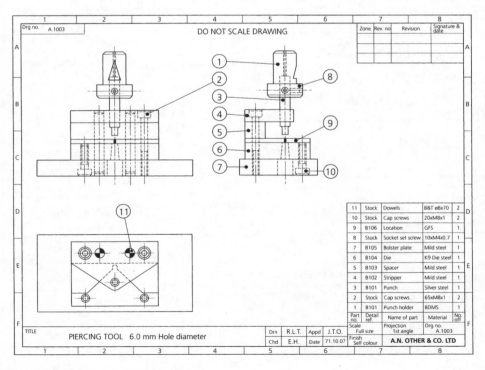

Figure 5.19 *General arrangement drawing*

normally carry dimensions except, occasionally, overall dimensions for reference only.

5.10.2 Detail drawings

Detail drawings provide all the details required to make a component, and an example is shown in Fig. 5.20. A detail drawing not only shows the shape of the component but also its size and the tolerances within which it must be manufactured. In this example it also states the materials to be used and the heat treatment of the punch. Similar detail drawings would be required for all the other components shown in the general arrangement drawing.

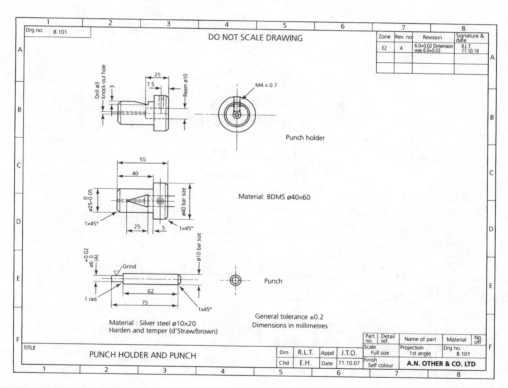

Figure 5.20   *Detail drawing*

5.10.3 Exploded (assembly) drawings

You will find these mainly in the service manuals for machines and similar devices. They show the components in the correct relationship to each other and the stock reference number for each component to facilitate the ordering of spare parts. An example is shown in Fig. 5.21.

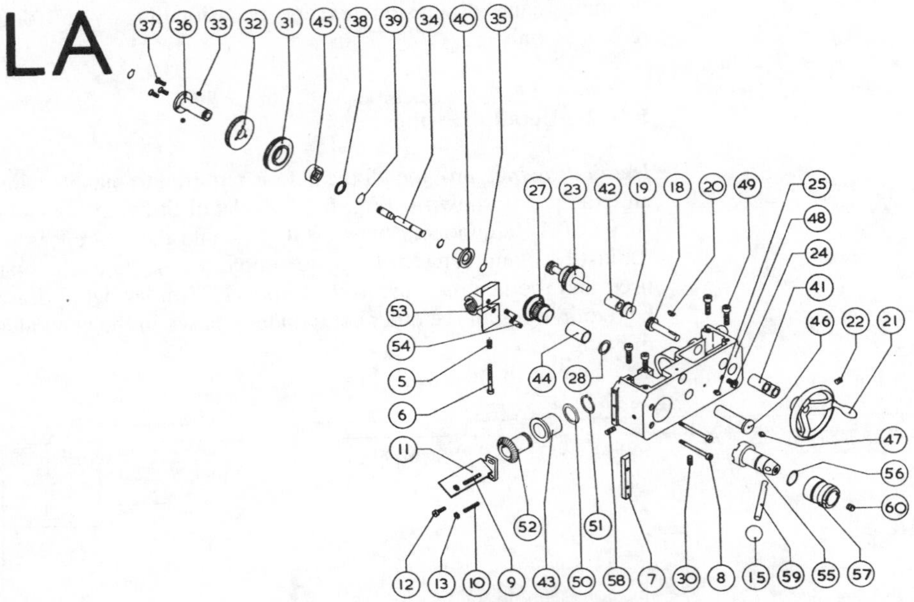

APRON ASSEMBLY

SECTION LA

APRON ASSEMBLY

Drg. Ref.	Part No.	Description	No. Off/Mc.
LA5	A4729	Spring—Leadscrew Nut	1
LA6		Cap Hd. Screw—Leadscrew Nut (2 B.A. x $1\frac{3}{4}$″)	1
LA7	A2082	Gib Strip—Leadscrew Nut	1
LA8	A9193	Ch. Hd. Screw—Strip Securing	2
LA9	A9194	Adjusting Screw—Gib Strip	1
LA10	A9195	Adjusting Screw—Gib Strip	1
LA11	A9196	Leadscrew Guard	1
LA12		Hex. Hd. Set Screw (2 B.A. x $\frac{1}{2}$″)	1
LA13		Hex. Locknut (2 B.A.)	2
LA15	80002	Ball Knob (KB5/100)	1
LA18	A9198	Hand Traverse Pinion	1
LA19	65004	Sealing Plug—Apron (AQ330/15)	1
LA20	70002	Woodruff Key (No. 404)	1
LA21	A2087	Handwheel Assembly	1
LA22		Socket Set Screw ($\frac{1}{4}$″ B.S.F. x $\frac{1}{4}$″) (Knurled Cup Point)	1
LA23	A9199	Rack Pinion Assembly	1
LA24	A2531	Oil Level Plug	1
LA25	65000	Oil Nipple (Tecalemit NC6055)	1
LA27	A9201	Bevel Gear Cluster Assembly (includes LA44)	1
LA28	A9202	Thrust Washer	1
LA30		Socket Set Screw ($\frac{1}{4}$″ B.S.F. x $\frac{1}{2}$″) (Knurled Cup Point)	1
LA31	A9204	Clutch Gear Assembly (includes LA45)	1
LA32	A9205	Drive Gear	1
LA33	73010	Ball—Clutch (5 mm ⌀)	2
LA34	A9206	Operating Spindle	1
LA35		Circlip (Anderton 1400—$\frac{3}{8}$″)	3
LA36	A9207	Drive Shaft	1
LA37		C's'k Hd. Socket Screw (2 B.A. x $\frac{3}{8}$″)	3
LA38	A9782	Washer—Drive Shaft	1
LA39		Circlip—Drive Shaft (Anderton 1400—$\frac{5}{8}$″)	1
LA40	A9208	Knob Operating Spindle	1
LA41	A9210	'Oilite' Bush	2
LA42	A9211	'Oilite' Bush	1
LA43	A9212/1	'Oilite' Bush—Flanged	1
LA44	A7595	'Oilite' Bush	1
LA45	A9220	Clutch Insert	1
LA46	A9203/1	Stud—Gear Cluster	1
LA47	65001	Oil Nipple (Tecalemit NC6057)	1
LA48	10025/1	Apron Assembly (includes LA41, LA42, LA43)	1
LA49		Cap Screw (M6 x 1 x 25 mm)	4
LA50	10217	Thrust Washer	1
LA51	10431	Circlip	1
LA52	A9200/1	Bevel Pinion	1
LA53	A1975/3	Leadscrew Nut – set	1
LA54	10508	Cam Peg	2
LA55	10528	Cam	1
LA56	65007	'O' Ring (BS/USA115)	1
LA57	10529	Eccentric Sleeve	1
LA58		Socket Set Screw ($\frac{5}{16}$″ B.S.F. x $\frac{5}{8}$″, Half Dog Point)	1
LA59	10530	Lever	1
LA60		Socket Set Screw (2 B.A. x $\frac{1}{4}$″, Cup Point)	1
LA61	10424	Guard Plate (not illustrated)	1

Figure 5.21 *Exploded view and parts list (source: Myford Ltd)*

5.11 Pictorial views

At the start of this chapter we introduced a pictorial drawing of a clamp. In fact it was in a style of drawing called isometric projection. It is now time to look at pictorial views in more detail starting with oblique projection.

5.11.1 Oblique projection

Figure 5.22 shows a simple component drawn in *oblique projection*. The component is positioned so that you can draw one face true to size and shape. The lines running 'into' the page are called *receding lines* and these are usually drawn at 45° to the front face as shown. To improve the proportions of the drawing and make it look more realistic, you draw the receding lines *half their true length*. For ease of drawing you should observe the following rules.

- Any curve or irregular face should be drawn true shape (front view). For example, a circle on a receding face would have to be constructed as an ellipse, whereas if it were positioned on the front face it could be drawn with compasses.

- Wherever possible, the longest side should be shown on the front, true view. This prevents violation of perspective and gives a more realistic appearance.

- For long circular objects such as shafts, the above two rules conflict. In this instance the circular section takes preference and should become the front view for ease of drawing, even though this results in the long axis receding.

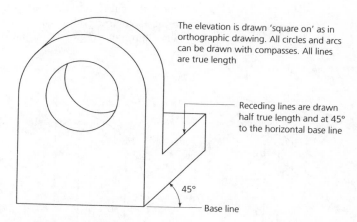

The elevation is drawn 'square on' as in orthographic drawing. All circles and arcs can be drawn with compasses. All lines are true length

Receding lines are drawn half true length and at 45° to the horizontal base line

45°

Base line

Figure 5.22 *Oblique drawing*

5.11.2 Isometric projection

The bracket shown in Fig. 5.23 is drawn in *isometric projection*. The isometric axes are drawn at 30° to the base line. To be strictly accurate you should draw these receding lines to isometric scale and only the

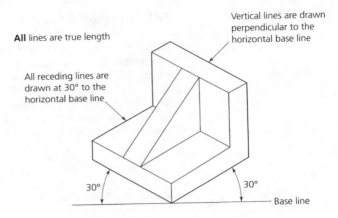

All lines are true length

Vertical lines are drawn
perpendicular to the
horizontal base line

All receding lines are
drawn at 30° to the
horizontal base line

30°   30°

Base line

Figure 5.23 *Isometric drawing*

vertical lines are drawn to true scale. However, for all practical purposes, all the lines are drawn *true length* to save time.

Although isometric drawing produces a more pleasing representation than oblique drawing, it has the disadvantage that no curved profiles such as arcs, circles, radii, etc., can be drawn with compasses. All curved lines have to be constructed. You can do this by erecting a grid over the feature in orthographic projection as shown in Fig. 5.24(a). You then draw a grid of equal size where it is to appear on the isometric drawing. The points where the circle cuts the grid in the orthographic drawing are transferred to the isometric grid as shown in Fig. 5.24(b). You then draw a smooth curve through the points on the isometric grid and the circle appears as an ellipse.

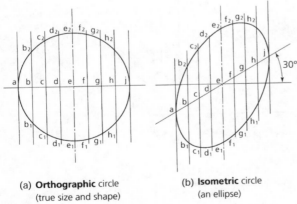

(a) **Orthographic** circle
(true size and shape)

(b) **Isometric** circle
(an ellipse)

1. Construct a grid over the true circle by dividing its centre line into an equal number of parts and erecting a perpendicular at each point.

2. Construct a similar grid on the isometric centre line.

3. Step off distances b_1–b–b_2, c_1–c–c_2, etc. on the isometric grid by transferring the corresponding distances from the true circle.

4. Draw a fair curve through the points plotted.

Figure 5.24 *Construction of isometric curves*

5.12   Sketching

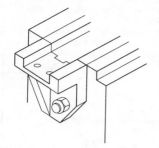

Figure 5.25   *Bracket*

The information given so far in this chapter should enable you, with practice, to correctly make and interpret formal engineering drawings. It is also important to be able to produce freehand sketches suitable for the manufacture of components. For example, the manufacture of replacement parts for maintenance purposes. The same rules apply as for formal drawings, except that you will be sketching freehand on any convenient, clean piece of paper.

5.12.1   Orthographic sketching

Figure 5.25 shows a bracket that has to be made and fitted to the end of a machine tool bed. Figure 5.26 shows the steps required to make a freehand orthographic sketch for the bracket. In fact it is a freehand detail drawing.

- Use a sheet of clean flat good quality paper of adequate size and an 'H' grade pencil. You also want a clean flat surface to draw on. A clipboard is handy.

- Paper feint ruled with squares is helpful as it gives you a guide for lines at right angles to each other.

- Now make outline sketches of the views you require using thin, faint lines.

- When you are satisfied with your initial sketches, draw in the outline more heavily and add any necessary details.

- When the basic sketch is complete check it for the omission of any essential details.

- Having completed the outline, you now have to add the dimensions. Use a rule or other instruments such as micrometer and vernier calipers to take the measurements you require and transfer them to the drawing. If the measurements are taken accurately and shown correctly on your sketch, your sketch does not have to be to scale. In any case a drawing should never be scaled since you cannot draw to the accuracy required for the manufacture of an engineering component.

- Make enlarged sketches of any small details that cannot be clearly shown in the main views.

- Although it is only a sketch for use once, it must incorporate all the rules, information and conventions discussed earlier in this chapter. Only then will the person making the component be able to make it correctly.

5.12.2   Pictorial sketching

Pictorial sketches can be in oblique projection or in isometric projection. Figure 5.27 shows you how to make a sketch in *oblique* projection.

1.   Sketch 'boxes' to contain the outline of the finished drawing.

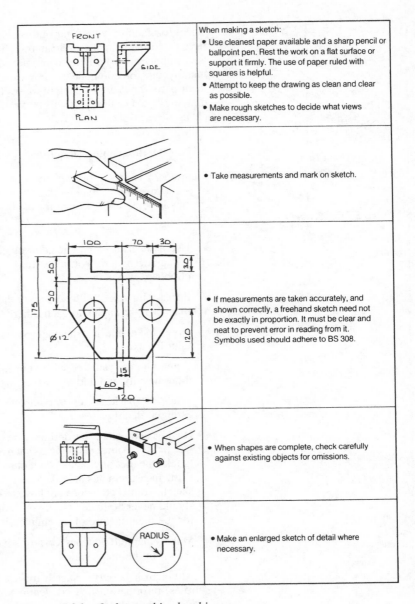

The following notes accompany the figure:

When making a sketch:
- Use cleanest paper available and a sharp pencil or ballpoint pen. Rest the work on a flat surface or support it firmly. The use of paper ruled with squares is helpful.
- Attempt to keep the drawing as clean and clear as possible.
- Make rough sketches to decide what views are necessary.

- Take measurements and mark on sketch.

- If measurements are taken accurately, and shown correctly, a freehand sketch need not be exactly in proportion. It must be clear and neat to prevent error in reading from it. Symbols used should adhere to BS 308.

- When shapes are complete, check carefully against existing objects for omissions.

- Make an enlarged sketch of detail where necessary.

Figure 5.26 *Orthographic sketching*

2. Lightly sketch in the details of the component or assembly being drawn.

3. Go over the outline more heavily to make it stand out.

4. Remove any construction lines that may cause confusion.

5. Add dimensions as required.

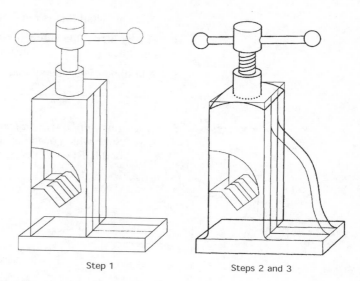

Step 1   Steps 2 and 3

Figure 5.27 *Pictorial sketching (oblique): Step 1 – general outlines (very faint); Steps – add details and line in*

Figure 5.28 shows you how to make a sketch of a two jaw chuck in *isometric* projection. The technique is similar to that used for the previous, oblique sketch. However, the initial outline 'boxes' are drawn in isometric projection.

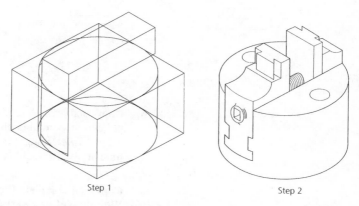

Step 1   Step 2

Figure 5.28 *Pictorial sketching (isometric): Step 1 – general outlines (very faint); Step 2 – add details and line in*

1. Sketch the outline boxes in isometric projection as shown.
2. Now sketch the curves using faint lines. Remember that in isometric projection these will be ellipses or parts of ellipses. A template may be helpful.

3. Add any detail that is required.

4. Finally line in the outline more heavily and remove any construction lines that may cause confusion.

5. Add dimensions as required.

Exercises **5.1** *First and third angle projection*
(a) State which of the examples shown in Fig. 5.29 are in FIRST or THIRD angle projection.

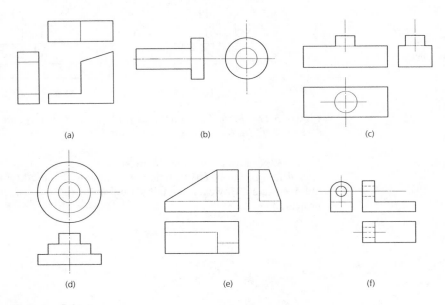

(a)   (b)   (c)

(d)   (e)   (f)

Figure 5.29 *Exercise 5.1(a)*

(b) Copy and complete the examples shown in Fig. 5.30. The projection symbol is placed below each example for your guidance. (*Note*: Sometimes complete views are missing, sometimes only lines and features.)

5.2 *Types of line*
(a) Copy and complete Fig. 5.31.
(b) With the aid of a sketch show what is meant by the terms:
   (i) dimension line;
   (ii) leader line;
   (iii) projection line.

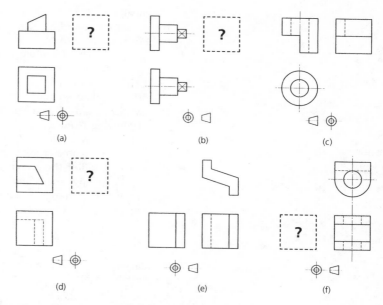

Figure 5.30   *Exercise 5.1(b)*

Line	Description	Application
————	Continuous bold	
———	Continuous fine	
~~		Limit of partial view
------------	Fine short dashes	
—·—·—		Centre lines
	Fine chain, bold at ends and changes of direction	Cutting planes

Figure 5.31   *Exercise 5.2(a)*

(c) With reference to exercise (b):
    (i)   state the type of line that should be used;
    (ii) indicate on your sketch where a short extension is required and where a small gap is required.

5.3 *Dimensioning*
  (a) With the aid of sketches show how a simple component can be dimensioned from:
    (i) a pair of mutually perpendicular datum edges (or surfaces);
    (ii) a datum line;
    (iii) a datum point.
  (b) With the aid of sketches show how you should dimension the following features:
    (i) a circle (show FOUR methods of dimensioning and use the diameter symbol);
    (ii) a radius (both convex and concave);
    (iii) an angle or chamfer.
  (c) Figure 5.32 shows a number of abbreviations found on engineering drawings. Copy and complete the figure.

Name	Abbreviation	Sketch
	S'FACE	
	C'BORE	
	C'SK	

Figure 5.32 *Exercise 5.3(c)*

5.4 *Conventions*
  (a) Give TWO reasons why standard conventions are used on engineering drawings.
  (b) Figure 5.33 relates to some commonly used drawing conventions. Copy and complete the figure.

5.5 *Sectioning*
Sketch a section through the component shown in Fig. 5.34 on the cutting planes XX and YY.

5.6 *Pictorial views*
  (a) Figure 5.35 shows a simple workpiece. Sketch it in:
    (i) oblique projection;
    (ii) isometric projection.
  (b) Figure 5.36 shows a component in isometric projection. Sketch it full size in:
    (i) *first angle* orthographic projection with the necessary dimensions so that your sketch can be used as a detail drawing for the manufacture of the component;

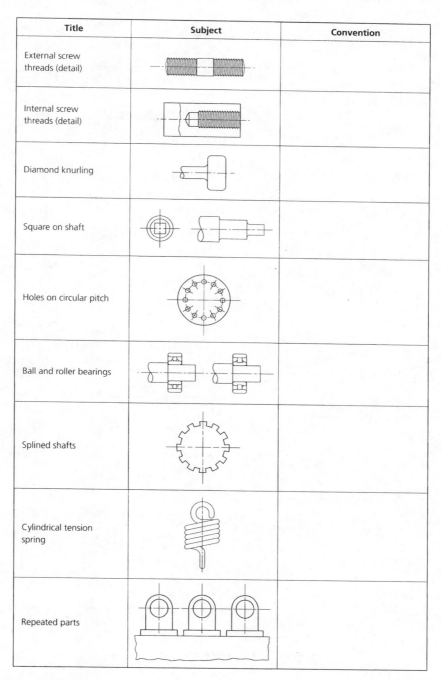

Title	Subject	Convention
External screw threads (detail)		
Internal screw threads (detail)		
Diamond knurling		
Square on shaft		
Holes on circular pitch		
Ball and roller bearings		
Splined shafts		
Cylindrical tension spring		
Repeated parts		

Figure 5.33 *Exercise 5.4(b)*

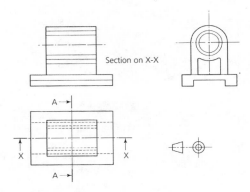

Figure 5.34 *Exercise 5.5*

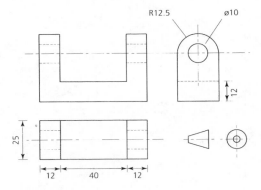

Figure 5.35 *Exercise 5.6(a)*

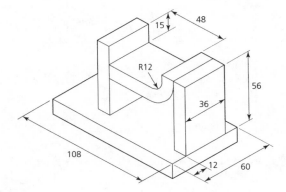

Figure 5.36 *Exercise 5.6(b)*

(ii) *third angle* orthographic projection with the necessary dimensions so that your sketch can be used as a detail drawing for the manufacture of the component.

6 Measuring

When you have read this chapter you should understand:

- What is meant by linear measurement.
- How to make linear measurements.
- What is meant by angular measurement.
- How to make angular measurements.
- The factors affecting accuracy of measurement.
- The terminology of measurement.
- The general rules for accurate measurement.
- How to measure workpieces having square, rectangular, circular and irregular-shaped sections.

6.1 Introduction

Measuring can be considered to be the most important process in engineering. Without the ability to measure accurately, we cannot:

- Mark out components as described in Chapter 7.
- Set up machines correctly to produce components to the required size and shape.
- Check components whilst we are making them to ensure that they finally end up the correct size and shape.
- Inspect finished components to make sure that they have been correctly manufactured.

6.2 Linear measurement

When you measure length, you measure the shortest distance in a straight line between two points, lines or faces. It doesn't matter what you call this distance (width, thickness, height, breadth, depth or diameter) it is still a measurement of length. There are two systems for the measurement of length, the *end system* of measurement and the *line system* of measurement. The end system of measurement refers to the measurement of distance between two faces of a component, whilst the line system of measurement refers to the measurement of the distance between two lines or marks on a surface. No matter what system is used, measurement of length is the comparison of the size of a component or a feature of a component and a known standard of length. In a workshop this may be a steel rule or a micrometer caliper, for example. These, in turn, are directly related to fundamental international standards of length.

In order for world trade to flourish it is necessary for national standards to be interchangeable or 'harmonized'. In the UK this is the responsibility of the British Standards Institution (BSI) which works in conjunction with the International Standards Organization (ISO) and European Community standards committees. Such international standardization is essential to ensure the *interchangeability* of components and equipment manufactured in different countries. The units of the *Système Internationale d'Unites* (SI) are now used throughout the world.

The fundamental unit of length is the *metre* and, currently, this is defined as:

> *the length of a path travelled by laser light in 1/299 792 458 seconds. The light being realized through the use of an iodine stabilized helium–neon laser.*

The international standard yard is defined as 0.9144 metre. Whilst units based on the metre are used worldwide, units based on the international standard yard are mainly used in the UK and the USA.

6.1.1 Steel rules (use of)

The steel rule is frequently used in workshops for measuring components of limited accuracy quickly. The quickness and ease with which it can be used, coupled with its low cost, makes it a popular and widely used measuring device. Metric rules may be obtained in various lengths from 150 mm to 1000 mm (1 metre). Imperial rules may be obtained in various lengths from 6 inch to 36 inch (1 yard). It is convenient to use a rule engraved in both systems, one system on the front and the other on the back.

Steel rules may be 'rigid' or 'flexible' depending upon their thickness and the 'temper' of the steel used in their manufacture. When choosing a steel rule the following points should be looked for. It should be:

- Made from hardened and tempered, corrosion resistant spring steel.

- Engine divided. That is, the graduations should be precision engraved into the surface of the metal.

- Ground on the edges so that it can be used as a straight edge when scribing lines or testing a surface for flatness.

- Ground on one end so that this end can be used as the zero datum when taking measurements from a shoulder.

- Satin chrome finished so as to reduce glare and make the rule easier to read, also to prevent corrosion.

No matter how accurately a rule is made, all measurements made with a rule are of limited accuracy. This is because of the difficulty of sighting the graduations in line with the feature being measured. Some ways of minimizing sighting errors are shown in Fig. 6.1.

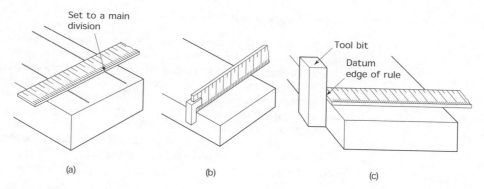

Figure 6.1 *Use of a rule – measuring the distance between: (a) two scribed lines; (b) two faces using a hook rule; (c) two faces using a steel rule and a tool bit as an abutment*

When using a rule to make direct measurements, as in Fig. 6.1(a), the accuracy of measurement depends upon the *visual alignment* of a mark or surface on the work with the corresponding graduation on the rule. This may appear relatively simple but, in practice, errors can very easily occur. These errors can be minimized by using a thin rule and keeping your eyes directly above and at 90° to the mark on the work. If you look at the work and the rule from an angle, you will get a false reading. This is known as *parallax* error. Figures 6.1(b) and 6.1(c) show two ways of aligning the datum (zero) end of the rule with the edge of the component to eliminate one source of sighting error.

6.1.2 Steel rule (care of)

A good rule should be looked after carefully to prevent wear and damage to its edges and to the datum end. It should never be used as a scraper or as a screwdriver, and it should never be used to clean the swarf out of the T-slots in the tables of machine tools. After use, plain steel rules should be lightly oiled to prevent rusting. Dulling of the surfaces will make the scales difficult to read. There is no need to oil satin-chrome plated rules, just wipe them clean.

6.1.3 Line and end measurement

Linear distances sometimes have to be measured between two lines, sometimes between two surfaces and sometimes between a combination of line and surface. Measurement between two lines is called *line measurement*. Measurement between two surfaces is called *end measurement*. It is difficult to convert between end systems of measurement and line systems of measurement and vice versa. For example, a rule (which is a line system measuring device) is not convenient for the direct measurement of distances between two edges. Similarly, a micrometer (which is an end system measuring device) would be equally inconvenient if used to measure the distance between two lines. The measuring device must always be chosen to suit the job in hand.

6.1.4 Calipers and their use

Calipers are used in conjunction with a rule so as to transfer the distance across or between the faces of a component in such a way as to reduce sighting errors. That is, to convert from end measurement to line measurement. Firm-joint calipers are usually used in the larger sizes and spring-joint calipers are used for fine work. Examples of internal and external calipers of both types are shown in Fig. 6.2 together with examples of their uses.

The accurate use of calipers depends upon practice, experience, and a highly developed sense of feel. When using calipers, the following rules should be observed:

- Hold the caliper gently and near the joint.

- Hold the caliper square (at right angles) to the work.

- No force should be used to 'spring' the caliper over the work. Contact should only just be felt.

- The caliper should be handled and laid down gently to avoid disturbing the setting.

- Lathe work should be *stationary* when taking measurements. This is essential for *safety* and *accuracy*.

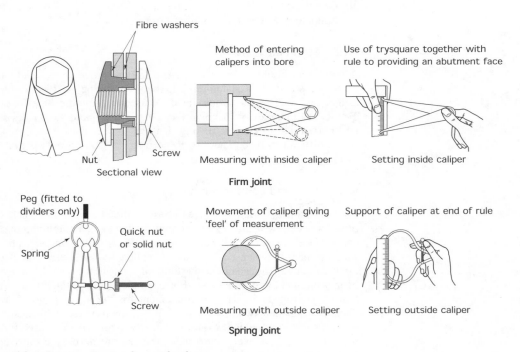

Figure 6.2 *Construction and use of calipers*

6.1.5 The micrometer caliper (use of)

Most engineering work has to be measured to much greater accuracy than it is possible to achieve with a rule, even when aided by the use of calipers. To achieve this greater precision, measuring equipment of greater accuracy and sensitivity has to be used. One of the most familiar measuring instruments used in engineering workshops is the *micrometer caliper*. This is frequently referred to as a 'micrometer' or simply a 'mike'. The constructional details of a typical micrometer caliper are shown in Fig. 6.3.

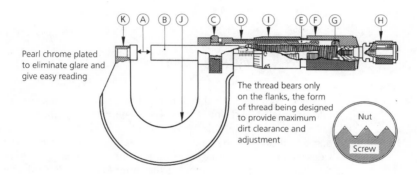

Pearl chrome plated to eliminate glare and give easy reading

The thread bears only on the flanks, the form of thread being designed to provide maximum dirt clearance and adjustment

Nut
Screw

A *Spindle and anvil faces* – Glass hard and optically flat, also available with tungsten carbide faces
B *Spindle* – Thread ground and made from alloy steel, hardened throughout, and stabilised
C *Locknut* – Effective at any position. Spindle retained in perfect alignment
D *Barrel* – Adjustable for zero setting. Accurately divided and clearly marked, pearl chrome plated
E *Main nut* – Length of thread ensures long working life
F *Screw adjusting nut* – For effective adjustment of main nut
G *Thimble adjusting nut* – Controls position of thimble
H *Ratchet* – Ensures a constant measuring pressure
I *Thimble* – Accurately divided and every graduation clearly numbered
J *Steel frame* – Drop forged
K *Anvil end*– Cutaway frame facilitates usage in narow slots

Figure 6.3   *The micrometer caliper (source: Moore and Wright)*

The operation of this instrument depends upon the principle that the distance a nut moves along a screw is proportional to the number of revolutions made by the nut and the lead of the screw thread. Therefore by controlling the number of complete revolutions made by the nut and the fractions of a revolution made by a nut, the distance it moves along the screw can be accurately controlled. It does not matter whether the nut rotates on the screw or the screw rotates in the nut, the principle of operation still holds good.

In a micrometer caliper, the screw thread is rotated by the thimble which has a scale that indicates the partial revolutions. The barrel of the instrument has a scale which indicates the 'whole' revolutions. In a standard metric micrometer caliper the screw has a lead of 0.5 millimetre and the thimble and barrel are graduated as in Fig. 6.4.

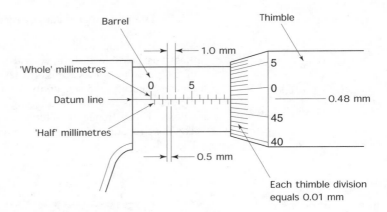

Figure 6.4 *Micrometer scales (metric)*

Since the lead of the screw of a standard metric micrometer is 0.5 millimetre and the barrel divisions are 0.5 millimetre apart, one revolution of the thimble moves the thimble along the barrel a distance of one barrel division (0.5 mm). The barrel divisions are placed on alternate sides of the datum line for clarity. Further, since the thimble has 50 divisions and one revolution of the thimble equals 0.5 millimetre, then a movement of *one thimble division* equals: 0.5 millimetre/50 divisions = 0.01 millimetre.

A metric micrometer caliper reading is given by:

- The largest visible 'whole' millimetre graduation visible on the barrel, *plus*

- The next 'half' millimetre graduation, if this is visible, *plus*

- The thimble division coincident with the datum line.

Therefore the micrometer scales shown in Fig. 6.5 read as follows:

$$9 \text{ 'whole' millimetres} = 9.00$$

$$1 \text{ 'half' millimetre} = 0.50$$

$$48 \text{ hundredths of a millimetre} = \underline{0.48}$$

$$= \underline{\underline{9.98}} \text{ mm}$$

Figure 6.5 shows the scales for a micrometer graduated in 'inch' units. The micrometer screw has 40 TPI (threads per inch), therefore the lead of the screw is 1/40 inch (0.025 inch). The barrel graduations are 1/10 inch subdivided into 4. Therefore each subdivision is 1/40 inch (0.025 inch) and represents one revolution of the thimble. The thimble carries 25 graduations. Therefore one thimble graduation equals a movement of 0.025 inch/25 = 0.001 inch. This is one-thousandth part of an inch and

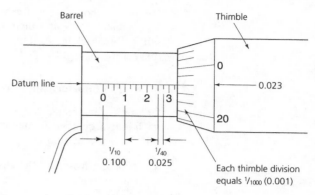

Figure 6.5 *Micrometer scales (English)*

is often referred to by engineers as a 'thou'. Thus 0.015 inch could be referred to as 15 'thou'.

An inch micrometer reading is given by:

• The largest visible 1/10 inch (0.1 inch) division, *plus*

• The largest visible 1/40 inch (0.025 inch) division, *plus*

• The thimble division coincident with the datum line.

Therefore the micrometer scales shown in Fig. 6.6 read as follows:

$$3 \text{ tenths of an inch} = 0.300$$
$$1 \text{ fortieth of an inch} = 0.025$$
$$23 \text{ thousandths of an inch} = \underline{0.023}$$
$$= \underline{0.348} \text{ inch}$$

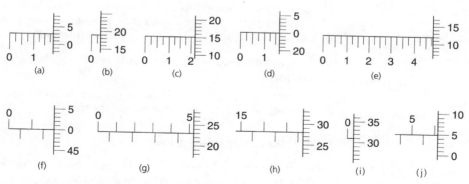

Figure 6.6 *Micrometer caliper reading exercises*

Figure 6.6 shows some further examples of English (inch) and metric micrometer scales and their readings. Try to work them out for yourself before looking up the correct readings at the end of this chapter (page 186).

6.1.6 Micrometer caliper (care of)

Unless a micrometer caliper is properly looked after it will soon lose its initial accuracy. To maintain this accuracy you should observe the following precautions:

- Wipe the work and the anvils of the micrometer clean before making a measurement.

- Do not use excessive measuring pressure, two 'clicks' of the ratchet are sufficient.

- Do not leave the anvil faces in contact when not in use.

- When machining, stop the machine before making a measurement. Attempting to make a measurement with the machine working can ruin the instrument and also lead to a serious accident. This rule applies to all measuring instruments and all machines.

Although easy to read and convenient to use, micrometer calipers have two disadvantages:

- A limited range of only 25 millimetres. Thus a range of micrometers is required, for example: 0–25 millimetres, 25–50 millimetres, 50–75 millimetres, and so on.

- Separate micrometers are required for internal and external measurements. The micrometer caliper so far described can be used only for external measurements.

6.1.7 Internal micrometer

An internal micrometer is shown in Fig. 6.7(a). It is used for measuring bore diameters and slot widths from 50 millimetres to 210 millimetres. For any one extension rod its measuring range is 20 millimetres. A range of extension rods in stepped lengths is provided in the case with the measuring head. It suffers from two important limitations.

- It cannot be used to measure small holes less than 50 millimetres diameter.

- It cannot be easily adjusted once it is in the hole and this affects the accuracy of contact 'feel' that can be obtained.

6.1.8 Micrometer cylinder gauge

Figure 6.7(b) shows the principle of the micrometer cylinder gauge. It is used for measuring the diameters of holes to a high degree of accuracy. It uses a micrometer-controlled wedge to expand three equi-spaced anvils

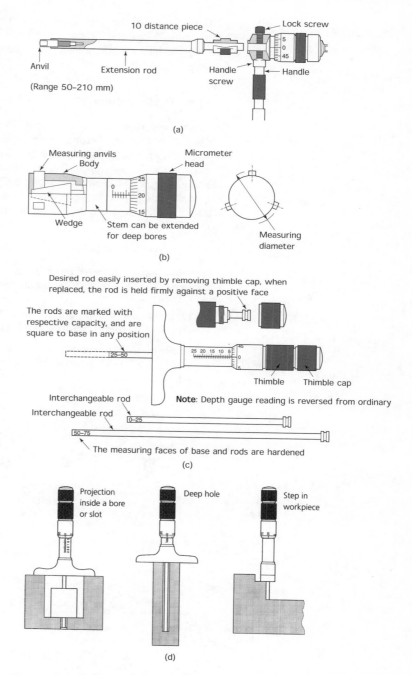

Figure 6.7 *Further applications of the micrometer principle: (a) the internal micrometer; (b) the micrometer cylinder gauge; (c) micrometer depth gauge; (d) application of the micrometer depth gauge*

until they touch the walls of the bore. Unfortunately it has only a limited measuring range and the range cannot be extended by the use of extension rods (see internal micrometer). A separate instrument has to be used for each range of hole sizes.

6.1.9 Depth micrometer

This is used for measuring the depth of holes and slots. You must take care when using a depth micrometer because its scales are reversed when compared with the familiar micrometer caliper. Also the measuring pressure tends to lift the micrometer off its seating. A depth micrometer is shown in Fig. 6.7(c). The measuring range is 25 millimetres for any given rods. Typical rods give a range of 0 to 25 mm, 25 to 50 mm, 50 to 75 mm. Some applications of a depth micrometer are shown in Fig. 6.7(d).

6.1.10 Vernier calipers

Although more cumbersome to use and rather more difficult to read, the vernier caliper has three main advantages over the micrometer caliper.

● One instrument can be used for measurements ranging over the full length of its main (beam) scale. Figure 6.8(a) shows a vernier caliper.

● It can be used for both internal and external measurements as shown in Fig. 6.8(b). Remember that for internal measurements you have to add the combined thickness of the jaws to the scale readings.

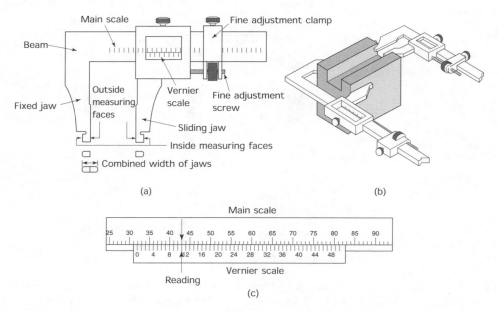

Figure 6.8 *The vernier caliper: (a) construction; (b) use; (c) vernier scale (50 divisions)*

- One instrument can be used for taking measurements in both inch units and in metric dimensional systems.

The measuring accuracy of a vernier caliper tends to be of a lower order than that obtainable with a micrometer caliper because:

- It is difficult to obtain a correct 'feel' with this instrument due to its size and weight.

- The scales can be difficult to read accurately even with a magnifying glass.

All vernier type instruments have two accurately engraved scales. A main scale marked in standard increments of measurement like a rule, and a vernier scale that slides along the main scale. This vernier scale is marked with divisions whose increments are slightly smaller than those of the main scale. Some vernier calipers are engraved with both inch and millimetre scales.

In the example shown in Fig. 6.8(c) the main scale is marked off in 1.00 mm increments, whilst the vernier scale has 50 divisions marked off in 0.98 mm increments. This enables you to read the instrument to an accuracy of $1.00 - 0.98 = 0.02$ mm. The reading is obtained as follows:

- Note how far the zero of the vernier scale has moved along the main scale (32 'whole' millimetres in this example).

- Note the vernier reading where the vernier and main scale divisions coincide (11 divisions in this example). You then multiply the 11 divisions by 0.02 mm which gives 0.22 mm.

- Add these two readings together:

$$32 \text{ 'whole' millimetres} = 32.00 \text{ mm } plus$$

$$11 \text{ vernier divisions} = 00.22 \text{ mm}$$

thus the reading shown in Fig. 6.9(c) = 32.22 mm

Always check the scales before use as there are other systems available and not all vernier scales have 50 increments. This is particularly the case in some cheap instruments. Also check that the instrument reads zero when the jaws are closed. If not, then the instrument has been strained and will not give a correct reading. There is no means of correcting this error and the instrument must be scrapped. Since they are expensive, it is essential to treat them with care. Figures 6.9 and 6.10 show some additional vernier-caliper scales in metric and inch units. Try to work them out for yourself before looking at the correct readings given at the end of this chapter (page 186).

As for all measuring instruments vernier calipers must be treated with care and cleaned before and after use. They should always be kept in the case provided. This not only protects the instrument from damage, it also supports the beam and prevents it from becoming distorted.

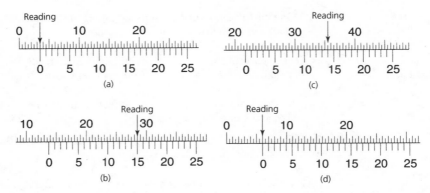

Figure 6.9 *Vernier scales (metric) reading exercises. (Note: The scales shown in all these exercises have a reading accuracy of 0.02 mm)*

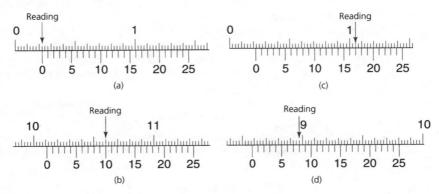

Figure 6.10 *Vernier scales (English) reading exercises. (Note: The scales shown in all these exercises have a reading accuracy of 0.001 inch)*

The vernier principle can also be applied to height gauges and to depth gauges. Some uses of the vernier height gauge are described later in this chapter and in Chapter 7.

6.1.11 Dial test indicators (DTI)

Dial test indicators are often referred to as 'clocks' because of the appearance of the dial and pointer. They measure the displacement of a plunger or stylus and indicate the magnitude of the displacement on a dial by means of a rotating pointer. There are two main types of dial test indicator.

Plunger type

This type of instrument relies upon a rack and pinion mechanism to change the linear (straight-line) movement of the plunger into rotary motion for the pointer. A gear train is used to magnify the movement of the pointer. This type of instrument has a long plunger movement and is, therefore, fitted with a secondary scale to count the number of revolutions made by the main pointer. A large range of dial diameters and markings is available. Figure 6.11(a) shows a typical example of this type of instrument and Fig. 6.11(b) shows how you can use one of these instruments to make comparative measurements. Dial test indicators are also widely used for setting up workpieces, and aligning work holding devices on machine tools will be described in the later chapters of this book.

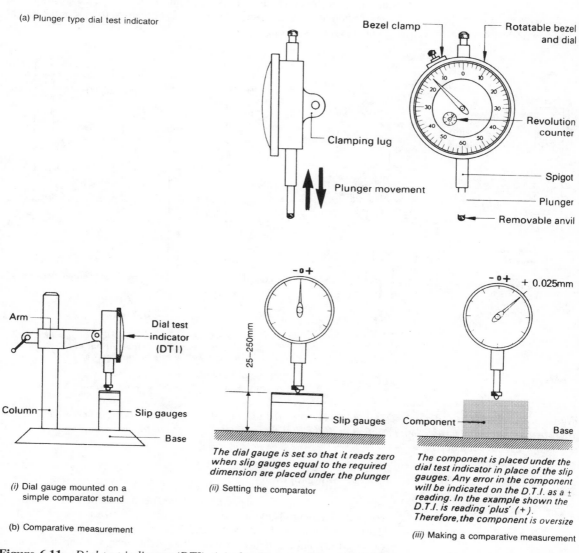

Figure 6.11 *Dial test indicator (DTI): (a) plunger type; (b) comparative measurement*

Lever type

This type of instrument uses a lever and scroll to magnify the displacement of the stylus. Compared with the plunger type, the lever type instrument has only a limited range of movement. However, it is extremely popular for inspection and machine setting because it is more compact and the scale is more conveniently positioned for these applications. Figure 6.12(a) shows a typical example of this type of instrument and Fig. 6.12(b) shows an application of its use. In this example the DTI is mounted on a vernier height gauge, and ensures that the measuring, contact, pressure over H_1 and H_2 is constant. That is, in each position, the vernier height gauge is adjusted until the DTI reads zero before the height gauge reading is taken.

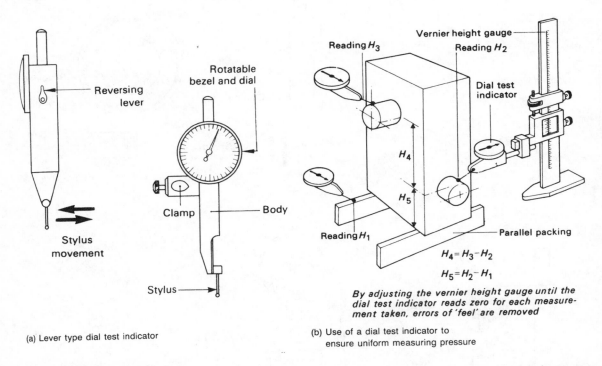

(a) Lever type dial test indicator

(b) Use of a dial test indicator to ensure uniform measuring pressure

Figure 6.12 *Dial test indicator (DTI): (a) lever type; (b) use of a DTI to ensure uniform measuring pressure – by adjusting the vernier height gauge until the dial test indicator reads zero for each measurement taken, errors of 'feel' are removed*

6.1.12 Slip gauges

Slip gauges are blocks of steel that have been hardened and stabilized by heat treatment. They are ground and lapped to size to very high standards of accuracy and surface finish. They are the most accurate standards of length available for use in workshops. The accuracy and finish is so high that two or more slip gauges may be *wrung* together. The method

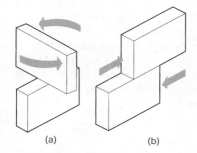

Figure 6.13 *Slip gauges: (a) 'wring' the gauges together with a rotary motion to assemble them; (b) slide the gauges to separate them. (Note: Pulling the slip gauges apart damages the gauging faces)*

of wringing slip gauges together is shown in Fig. 6.13(a). When correctly cleaned and wrung together, the individual slip gauges adhere to each other by molecular attraction and, if left like this for too long, a partial cold weld will take place. If this is allowed to occur, the gauging surfaces will be irreparably damaged when the blocks are separated. Therefore, immediately after use, the gauges should be separated carefully by sliding them apart as shown in Fig. 6.13(b). They should then be cleaned, smeared with petroleum jelly (vaseline) and returned to their case. A typical 78 piece metric set of slip gauges is listed in Table 6.1.

TABLE 6.1 *Metric slip gauges*

Range (mm)	Steps (mm)	Pieces
1.01 to 1.49	0.01	49
0.50 to 9.50	0.50	19
10.00 to 50.00	10.00	5
75.00 and 100.00	–	2
1.002 5	–	1
1.005	–	1
1.007 5	–	1

In addition, some sets also contain *protector slips* that are 2.50 mm thick and are made from a hard, wear resistant material such as tungsten carbide. These are added to the ends of the slip gauge stack to protect the other gauge blocks from wear. Allowance must be made for the thickness of the protector slips when they are used.

Slip gauges are wrung together to give a stack of the required dimension. In order to achieve the maximum accuracy the following precautions must be preserved:

- Use the minimum number of blocks.

- Wipe the measuring faces clean using a soft clean chamois leather.

- *Wring* the individual blocks together.

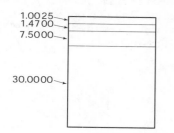

Figure 6.14 *Building up slip gauges*

Let's see how we can build up a stack of slip gauges to give a dimension of 39.9725 mm. This is shown in Fig. 6.14 and four slips are the minimum we can use in this example.

- The first slip selected always gives the right-hand digit(s). In this case 1.0025 mm.

- The second slip and the third slip have been chosen to give the remaining decimal places (1.470 + 7.500 = 8.970 mm).

- The fourth slip provides the balance of the whole number (39.000 − 1.0025 − 1.470 − 7.500 = 30 mm). Thus the fourth slip is 30 mm. All these sizes are available in the set listed in Table 6.1.

- If protector slips had been used (2×2.5 mm $= 5.0$ mm) then the 7.500 slip would have been replaced by a 2.50 mm slip.

Slip gauges come in various grades – workshop, inspection and standards room – and their accuracy and cost increases accordingly. They may be used directly for checking the width of slots. They may also be used in conjunction with a DTI for measuring heights and they may also be used for setting comparators as was shown in Fig. 6.11.

6.3 Measuring angles

Angles are measured in degrees and fractions of a degree. One degree of arc is 1/360 of a complete circle. One degree of arc can be subdivided into minutes and seconds (not to be confused with minutes and seconds of time):

60 seconds ($''$) of arc $= 1$ minute ($'$) of arc

60 minutes ($'$) of arc $= 1$ degree ($^\circ$) of arc

With the introduction of calculators and computers, decimal fractions of a degree are also used. However, 1 minute of arc equals 0.0166666° recurring so there is no correlation between the two systems of subdividing a degree.

6.3.1 Right angles

A right angle is the angle between two surfaces that are at 90° to each other. Such surfaces may also be described as being *mutually perpendicular*. The use of engineers' try-squares and their use for scribing lines at right angles to the edge of a component will be described in Chapter 7. Figure 6.15(a) shows a typical engineer's try-square.

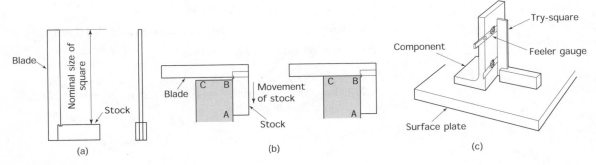

Figure 6.15 *The try-square (a), its use (b) and (c)*

Note that a try-square is not a measuring instrument. It does not measure the angle. It only indicates whether or not the angle being checked is a right angle. In Fig. 6.15(b), the stock is placed against the edge AB of

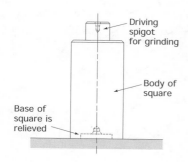

Figure 6.16 *Cylinder square*

the work and slid gently downwards until the blade comes into contact with the edge BC. Any lack of squareness will allow light to be seen between the edge BC and the try-square blade.

It is not always convenient to hold large work and a try-square up to the light. Figure 6.15(c) shows an alternative method using a surface plate as a datum surface. The squareness of the component face is checked with feeler gauges as shown. If the face is square to the base, the gap between it and the try-square blade will be constant.

Try-squares are precision instruments and they should be treated with care if they are to retain their initial accuracy. They should be kept clean and lightly oiled after use. They should not be dropped, nor should they be kept in a draw with other bench tools that may knock up burrs on the edges of the blade and stock. They should be checked for squareness at regular intervals. In addition to try-squares, prismatic squares and cylinder squares may be used for checking large work. Figure 6.16 shows a typical cylinder square.

6.3.2 Angles other than right angles (plain bevel protractor)

Figure 6.17 shows a simple bevel protractor for measuring angles of any magnitude between 0° and 180°. Such a protractor has only limited accuracy (±0.5°).

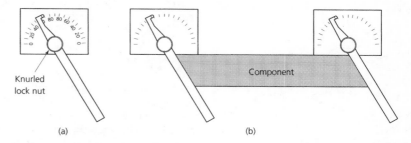

Figure 6.17 *The plain bevel protractor (a), and its use in checking angles (b)*

6.3.3 Angles other than right angles (vernier protractor)

Where greater accuracy is required the vernier protractor should be used. The scales of a vernier protractor are shown in Fig. 6.18. The main scale is divided into degrees of arc, and the vernier scale has 12 divisions each side of zero. These vernier scale divisions are marked 0 to 60 minutes of arc, so that each division is 1/12 of 60, that is 5 minutes of arc. The reading for a vernier protractor is given by the sum of:

- The largest 'whole' degree on the main scale as indicated by the vernier zero mark.

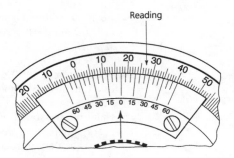

Figure 6.18 *Vernier protractor scales*

- The reading of the vernier scale division in line with a main scale division.

Thus the reading for the scales shown in Fig. 6.18 is:

$$17 \text{ 'whole' degrees} = 17° \ 00'$$

$$\text{vernier 25 mark in line with main scale} = \underline{00 \ \ 25'}$$

$$\text{Total angle} = \underline{17° \ 25'}$$

Vernier protractors are also available which can be read in degrees and decimal fractions of a degree.

6.3.4 Sine bar

Use of a sine bar is a simple but very accurate method of measuring and checking angles. Figure 6.19(a) shows a typical sine bar and Fig. 6.19(b) shows the principle of its use. The sine bar, slip gauges and the datum surface on which they stand form a right-angled triangle with the sine bar as the hypotenuse. Remember that the hypotenuse is the side opposite the right angle in a right-angled triangle.

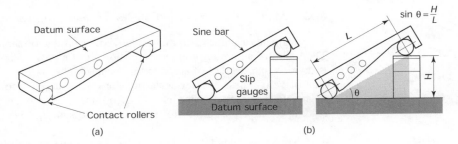

Figure 6.19 *The sine bar (a) and the principle of its use (b)*

Since: $\sin \theta = \dfrac{\text{opposite side}}{\text{hypotenuse}}$

Then: $\sin \theta = \dfrac{\text{height of slip gauges}}{\text{nominal length of sine bar}}$

$\qquad\quad = \dfrac{H}{L}$

Figure 6.20 shows a component being checked. The slip gauges are chosen to incline the sine bar at the required angle. The component is then placed on the sine bar. The height over the component is checked with a DTI mounted on a surface gauge or a vernier height gauge. If the component has been manufactured to the correct angle, then the DTI will read the same at each end of the component. Any difference in the readings indicates the magnitude of error in the angle of the component. Try working out the height of the slip gauges you would require to give an angle of $\theta = 25°$ if the nominal length (L) of the sine bar is 200 mm. Also state how you would build up the slip gauge stack. The answers are given at the end of this chapter (page 187).

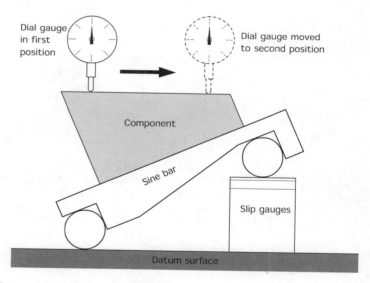

Figure 6.20 *Use of the sine bar*

6.3.5 Taper plug and ring gauges

Figure 6.21 shows typical taper plug and ring gauges. These cannot measure the angle of taper but they can indicate whether or not the taper is of the correct diameter. The gauges are 'stepped' as shown. If the component is within its 'limits of size' then the end of the taper will lie within the step.

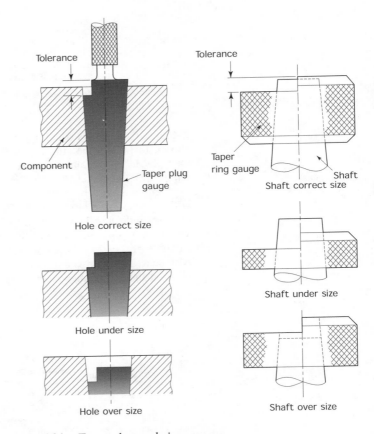

Figure 6.21 *Taper plug and ring gauges*

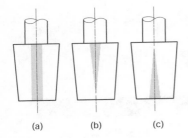

Figure 6.22 *Checking the angle of taper: (a) 'smear' indicates that the hole has the same taper as the plug gauge; (b) 'smear' indicates that the hole has a smaller angle of taper than the gauge; (c) 'smear' indicates that the hole has a larger angle of taper than the gauge*

As already stated, taper plug and ring gauges cannot measure the angle of taper, but they can be used to check the angle as shown in Fig. 6.22. Although a plug gauge is shown, a ring gauge can be used in a similar manner.

Plug gauge

- 'Blue' the gauge with a light smear of engineer's 'blue' and insert the gauge into the hole.

- Remove the gauge taking care not to rock or rotate the plug gauge.

- Wipe the gauge clean of any remaining 'blue'.

- Reinsert the gauge carefully into the hole.

- Upon withdrawing the gauge the smear left upon it will indicate the area of contact. This is interpreted as shown in Fig. 6.22.

Ring gauge

- Lightly 'blue' the shaft and insert it carefully into the ring gauge.
- Remove the shaft and wipe it clean.
- Reinsert the shaft into the gauge.
- Withdraw the shaft and the smear will indicate the area of contact.
- Interpretation of the smear is similar to that when a plug gauge was used.

6.4 Miscellaneous measurements

In addition to the linear and angular measurements described so far, other dimensional properties also have to be considered. Let's now look at some of these.

6.4.1 Flatness

A flat surface lies in a true plane. However, appearances can be deceptive. Figure 6.23 shows a surface that is definitely not flat. Yet, when checked with a rule or a straight edge parallel to its edges along the lines called *generators* it would appear to be flat. It is only when it is checked from corner to corner diagonally that the out-of-flatness shows up.

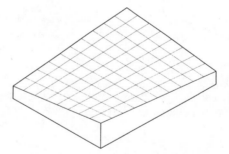

Figure 6.23 *Lack of flatness generated by straight lines and difficult to detect with a straight edge*

6.4.2 Parallelism

Parallelism is the constancy of distance between two lines or surfaces. Parallelism can be measured in a number of ways depending upon the job in hand. Some examples are shown in Fig. 6.24.

6.4.3 Concentricity

Concentricity implies a number of diameters having a common axis. Figure 6.25 shows various ways of testing for concentricity. Figure 6.25(a) shows that a bush with concentric diameters will have

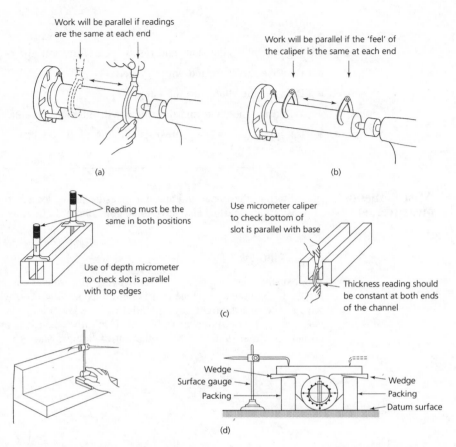

Figure 6.24 *Checking for parallelism: (a) with an indicating instrument (micrometer); (b) with a non-indicating instrument (caliper); (c) rectangular components; (d) with a scribing block (surface gauge)*

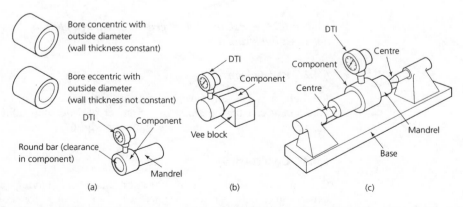

Figure 6.25 *Testing for concentricity: (a) constant wall thickness; (b) solid component; (c) bored component*

a constant wall thickness. If it does not have a constant wall thickness then the bore and the outer diameter will not be concentric. The bush does not have to be a close fit on the mandrel in this example. Figure 6.25(b) shows a solid component being checked with a DTI and a Vee block. The reading of the DTI must be constant if the diameters are concentric. Figure 6.25(c) shows a component being checked on a mandrel supported between bench centres.

6.4.4 Roundness

To test for roundness, a component has to be checked under a DTI whilst being supported in a Vee block. Any out-of-roundness will cause the component to ride up and down in the Vee block and this will show up as a variable reading on the DTI.

6.4.5 Profiles

The profile of a component is its outline shape. Simple radii can be checked with standard radius gauges as shown in Fig. 6.26(a). More complex profiles can be checked using a half template as shown in Fig. 6.26(b). This template has to be made specifically for the job in hand. For the more accurate checking of profiles an optical projector has to be used. However, optical projectors are beyond the scope of this book.

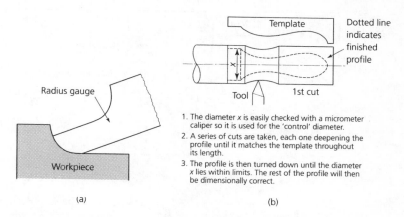

1. The diameter x is easily checked with a micrometer caliper so it is used for the 'control' diameter.
2. A series of cuts are taken, each one deepening the profile until it matches the template throughout its length.
3. The profile is then turned down until the diameter x lies within limits. The rest of the profile will then be dimensionally correct.

(a)　　　　　(b)

Figure 6.26 *Checking a profile: (a) checking a radius with a radius gauge; (b) use of template to turn profile*

6.5 Limits and fits

The upper and lower sizes of a dimension are called the *limits* and the difference in size between the limits is called the *tolerance*. The terms associated with limits and fits can be summarized as follows:

- *Nominal size*. This is the dimension by which a feature is identified for convenience. For example, a slot whose actual width is 25.15 millimetres would be known as the 25 millimetre wide slot.

- *Basic size*. This is the exact functional size from which the limits are derived by application of the necessary allowance and tolerances. The basic size and the nominal size are often the same.

- *Actual size*. The measured size corrected to what it would be at 20°C.

- *Limits*. These are the high and low values of size between which the size of a component feature may lie. For example, if the lower limit of a hole is 25.05 millimetres and the upper limit of the same hole is 25.15 millimetres, then a hole which is 25.1 millimetres diameter is *within limits* and is acceptable. Examples are shown in Fig. 6.27(a).

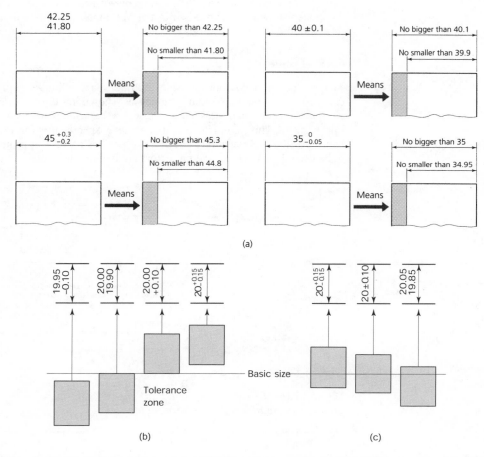

Figure 6.27 *Toleranced dimensions: (a) methods of tolerancing; (b) unilateral tolerance; (c) bilateral tolerance*

- *Tolerance*. This is the difference between the limits of size. That is, the upper limit minus the lower limit. Tolerances may be bilateral or unilateral as shown in Fig. 6.27(b).

- *Deviation.* This is the difference between the basic size and the limits. The deviation may be symmetrical, in which case the limits are equally spaced above and below the basic size. For example, 50.00 ± 0.15 mm. Alternatively, the deviation may be asymmetrical, in which case the deviation may be greater on one side of the basic size than on the other, e.g. 50.00 + 0.25 or −0.05.

- *Mean size.* This size lies halfway between the upper and lower limits of size and must not be confused with either the nominal size or the basic size. It is only the same as the basic size when the deviation is symmetrical.

- *Minimum clearance (allowance).* This is the clearance between a shaft and a hole under maximum metal conditions. That is, the largest shaft in the smallest hole that the limits will allow. It is the tightest fit between shaft and hole that will function correctly. With a *clearance fit* the allowance is positive. With an *interference fit* the allowance is negative. These types of fit are discussed in the next section.

6.6 Classes of fit

Figure 6.28(a) shows the classes of fit that may be obtained between mating components. In the *hole basis system* the hole size is kept constant

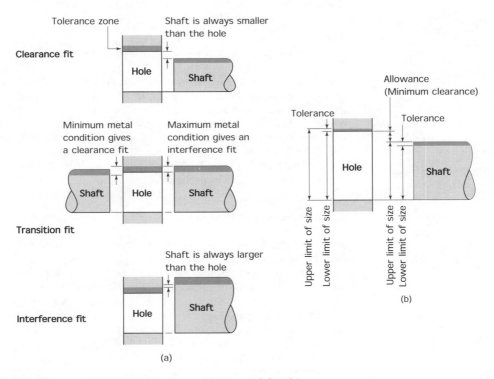

Figure 6.28 *Classes of fit (a), terminology of limits and fits (b)*

and the shaft size is varied to give the required class of fit. In an *interference fit* the shaft is always slightly larger than the hole. In a *clearance fit* the shaft is always slightly smaller than the hole. A *transition fit* occurs when the tolerances are so arranged that under maximum metal conditions (largest shaft: smallest hole) an interference fit is obtained, and that under minimum metal conditions (largest hole: smallest shaft) a clearance fit is obtained. The hole basis system is the most widely used since most holes are produced using standard tools such as drills and reamers. It is then easier to vary the size of the shaft by turning or grinding to give the required class of fit.

In a *shaft basis system* the shaft size is kept constant and the hole size is varied to give the required class of fit. Again, the classes of fit are: *interference fit*, *transition fit*, and *clearance fit*. Figure 6.28(b) shows the terminology relating to limits and fits.

6.7 Accuracy

The greater the accuracy demanded by a designer, the narrower will be the tolerance band and the more difficult and costly it will be to manufacture the component within the limits specified. Therefore, for ease of manufacture at minimum cost, a designer never specifies an accuracy greater than is necessary to ensure the correct functioning of the component. The more important factors affecting accuracy when measuring components are as follows.

6.7.1 Temperature

All metals and alloys expand when heated and contract when cooled. This is why measuring should take place in a constant temperature environment. You may have noticed that when you are machining materials in a workshop they often become hot. A component which has been heated by the cutting process will shrink whilst cooling to room temperature. This may result in a component that was within limits when measured on the machine but found to be undersize when it is checked in the temperature-controlled inspection room.

6.7.2 Accuracy of equipment

Since it is not possible to manufacture components to an exact size nor is it possible to measure them to an exact size, it follows that neither can measuring equipment be made to an exact size. Therefore measuring equipment also has to be manufactured to toleranced dimensions. In order that this has the minimum effect upon the measurement being made, *the accuracy of a measuring instrument should be about ten times greater than the accuracy of the component being measured.*

Measuring equipment should be checked regularly against even more accurate equipment. Where possible any errors should be corrected by adjustment. If this is not possible, and the error has reached significant proportions, the instrument has to be discarded.

6.7.3   Reading errors

There are two main reading errors:

- Misreading the instrument scales. Vernier scales are particularly difficult to read unless you have very good eyesight, so it is advisable to use a magnifying glass. Good lighting is also essential.
- Parallax (sighting errors) when using rules and similar scales. Care must be taken to ensure that your eye is over the point of measurement.

6.7.4   Type of equipment

It is possible to measure linear dimensions and angles with a variety of instruments. However, the accuracy of measurement is always lower than the reading accuracy and will depend, largely, upon the skill of the user. You must always match the instrument you use to the job in hand. It would be futile to try to measure an accurately machined dimension of 25.00 ± 0.02 millimetres with a rule and calipers. On the other hand, it would be a waste of time to use a vernier caliper when measuring a piece of bar in the stores to see if you could cut a 75 millimetre long blank from it. A rule would be quite adequate for this latter application.

6.7.5   Effect of force

The use of excessive force when closing the measuring instrument on the workpiece being measured can cause distortion of both the workpiece and of the measuring instrument resulting in an incorrect reading. In the worst case the distortion is permanent and either the workpiece or the measuring instrument or both will become worthless and have to be destroyed.

Some instruments are fitted with devices that ensure a correct and safe measuring pressure automatically. For example, three 'clicks' of the ratchet of a micrometer caliper applies the correct measuring force. The bench micrometer shown in Fig. 6.29 has a measuring force indicator (fiducial indicator) in place of the fixed anvil. When the pointers are in line, the correct measuring pressure is being applied.

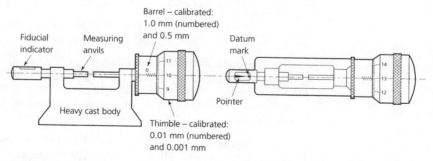

Figure 6.29   *The bench micrometer: the fiducial indicator removes errors of 'feel' – the micrometer is 'zeroed' with the pointer of the fiducial indicator in line with its datum mark and all subsequent measurements are made with the pointer in this position; this ensures constant measuring pressure*

The contact area of the jaws or anvils of the measuring instrument can also influence the measuring pressure. This is because pressure is defined as force per unit area and, for any given measuring force, the contact pressure varies inversely as the contact area. Reduce the area and the measuring pressure is increased. Increase the contact area and the pressure is reduced. A spherically ended stylus will, in theory, result in point contact and this will give rise to an infinitely high measuring pressure. In practice the spherical end on the stylus tends to sink into the surface being measured, thus increasing the contact area. At the same time the spherical end of the stylus tends to flatten and this, again, increases the contact area. Any increase in the contact area results in a decrease in measuring pressure and a balance is automatically achieved between the measuring pressure and the resistance to deformation of the material of the component being measured. Such deformation introduces measuring errors and damage to the finished surfaces of the component being measured. Such effects are marginal where components are made from relatively hard metals but they must be taken into account when measuring components made from softer materials such as some plastics.

6.7.6 Correct use of measuring equipment

No matter how accurately measuring equipment is made, and no matter how sensitive it is, one of the most important factors affecting the accuracy of measurement is the skill of the user. The more important procedures for the correct use of measuring equipment can be summarized as follows.

- The measurement must be made at right angles to the surface of the component.

- The use of a constant measuring pressure is essential. This is provided automatically with micrometer calipers by means of their ratchet. With other instruments such as plain calipers and vernier calipers the measuring pressure depends upon the skill and 'feel' of the user. Such skill comes only with practice and experience.

- The component must be supported so that it does not distort under the measuring pressure or under its own weight.

- The workpiece must be thoroughly cleaned before being measured, and coated with oil or a corrosion inhibiting substance immediately after inspection. Ideally, gloves should be worn so that the acid in your perspiration does not corrode the cleaned surfaces of the instruments and the workpiece.

- Measuring instruments must be handled with care so that they are not damaged or strained. They must be cleaned and kept in their cases when not in use. Their bright surfaces should be lightly smeared with petroleum jelly (vaseline). Measuring instruments must be regularly checked to ensure that they have not lost their initial accuracy. If an error is detected the instrument must be taken out of service immediately so that the error can be corrected. If correction is not possible the instrument must be immediately discarded.

6.8 Terminology of measurement

Indicated size

This is the size indicated by the scales of a measuring instrument when it is being used to measure a workpiece. The indicated size makes no allowance for any incorrect use of the instrument, such as the application of excessive contact pressure.

Reading

This is the size as read off the instrument scales by the operator. Errors can occur if the scales are misread, for example sighting (parallax) errors can occur when measuring with a rule. Vernier scales are particularly easy to misread in poor light. A magnifying lens is helpful even in good light and even if you have good eyesight. Electronic measuring instruments with digital readouts overcome many of these reading difficulties.

Reading value

This is also called the 'reading accuracy'. This is the smallest increment of size that can be read directly from the scales of the instrument. It will depend upon the layout of the scales. A micrometer caliper normally has a reading value of 0.01 millimetre. A bench micrometer fitted with a fiducial indicator normally has a reading value of 0.001 millimetre. A vernier caliper with a 50 division vernier scale normally has a reading value of either 0.01 millimetre or 0.02 millimetre depending upon how the scales are arranged.

Measuring range

This is the range of sizes that can be measured by any given instrument. It is the arithmetical difference between the largest size which can be measured and the smallest size which can be measured. For example, a 50 mm to 75 mm micrometer has a measuring range of 75 mm − 50 mm = 25 mm.

Measuring accuracy

This is the actual accuracy expected from a measuring instrument after taking into account all the normal errors of usage. It can never be better than the indicated size.

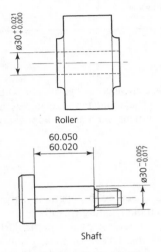

Roller

60.050
60.020

Shaft

Figure 6.30 *Exercise 6.1(a)*

Exercises

6.1 *Limits of size*
  (a) Figure 6.30 shows a roller and its shaft. Complete the associated table from the dimensions given.
  (b) The limits of size for the width of a component lie between 11.5 mm and 12.5 mm. With the aid of sketches show THREE ways in which these limits of size may be applied to the dimension.
  (c) With the aid of sketches, show what is meant by:
    (i) a clearance fit;
    (ii) a transition fit;
    (iii) an interference fit.
  (d) Which of the classes of fit listed in exercise (c) would be required for:
    (i) a pulley that is free to run on its shaft;
    (ii) a drill bush that has to be pressed into the bushplate of a drilling jig.

6.2 *Measuring equipment*
  (a) List the most important features of an engineer's rule. State briefly how it should be cared for to maintain its accuracy.
  (b) Explain briefly what are the main causes of reading error when using a steel rule and how these errors can be minimized.
  (c) Sketch the following measuring tools showing how they are used:
    (i) firm-joint calipers;
    (ii) odd-leg (jenny) calipers.
  (d) With the aid of sketches show how an engineer's try-square is used to check the squareness of a rectangular metal blank.

6.3 *Measuring instruments*
  (a) Sketch a micrometer caliper and:
    (i) name its more important features;
    (ii) show how the scales are arranged for metric readings;
    (iii) show how the scales are arranged for 'inch' readings.
  (b) With the aid of sketches, explain how the scales of a depth micrometer differ from a micrometer caliper.
  (c) Write down the micrometer readings shown in Fig. 6.31(a).
  (d) Sketch a vernier caliper that can be used for internal and external measurements, and also depth measurements. Name its more important features.
  (e) Write down the vernier readings shown in Fig. 6.31(b).
  (f) With the aid of sketches show how a plain bevel protractor is used to measure angles.

6.4 *Gauge blocks*
  (a) Using the slip gauges (gauge blocks) listed in Table 6.1 of the text, select a suitable set of gauge blocks to make up the dimension of 34.147 mm:
    (i) without using protector slips;
    (ii) using protector slips.

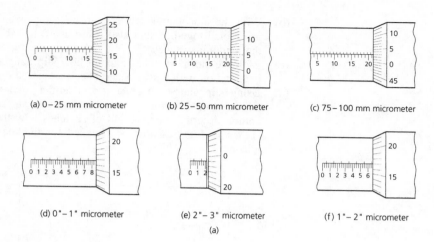

(a) 0 – 25 mm micrometer

(b) 25 – 50 mm micrometer

(c) 75 – 100 mm micrometer

(d) 0" – 1" micrometer

(e) 2" – 3" micrometer

(f) 1" – 2" micrometer

(a)

Figure 6.31(a)   *Exercise 6.3(c)*

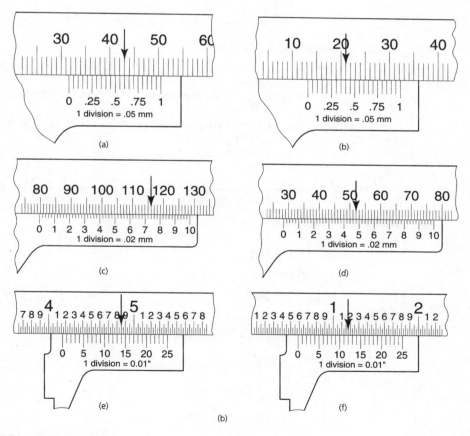

(a)

(b)

(c)

(d)

(e)

(f)

(b)

Figure 6.31(b)   *Exercise 6.3(e)*

(b) With the aid of a sketch explain how slip gauges should be assembled together, and also taken apart, to avoid damage to the gauging surfaces.

(c) With the aid of sketches explain how slip gauges are used in conjunction with a sine bar to check a tapered component.

(d) Using slip gauges, a lever type (Verdict) dial test indicator (DTI) mounted on a scribing block, and a surface plate as a datum, describe with the aid of sketches how the component shown in Fig. 6.32 can be checked for thickness and parallelism.

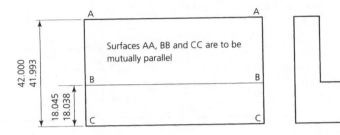

Figure 6.32 *Exercise 6.4(d)*

6.5 *Miscellaneous measuring devices*
With the aid of sketches show/explain how the following measuring devices are used.

(a) A taper plug gauge (stepped) to check the size and angle of taper of a tapered bore.

(b) Feeler gauges.

(c) Radius gauges.

Answers   **Figure 6.6**

(a) 0.178 inch

(b) 0.044 inch

(c) 0.215 inch

(d) 0.175 inch

(e) 0.487 inch

(f) 2.00 mm

(g) 5.23 mm

(h) 17.78 mm

(i) 0.31 mm

(j) 6.05 mm

Figure 6.9

(a)   3.50 mm

(b)   13.80 mm

(c)   21.78 mm

(d)   6.00 mm

Figure 6.10

(a)   0.225 inch

(b)   10.110 inch

(c)   0.217 inch

(d)   8.583 inch

Figure 6.20

H = 84.52 mm

Use the following slip gauges

  1.02 mm
  0.50 mm
  8.00 mm
 75.00 mm
─────────────
 84.52 mm
═════════════

7 Marking out

When you have read this chapter you should be able to understand how to:

- Identify and select marking-out tools for making lines.
- Identify and select marking-out equipment for providing guidance.
- Identify and select marking-out equipment for providing support.
- Identify and select different types of datum.
- Identify and use different co-ordinate systems.
- Mark out workpieces having square, rectangular, circular and irregular-shaped sections.

7.1 Marking-out equipment (tools for making lines)

Marking out is, essentially, drawing on metal so as to provide guide lines for a fitter or a machinist to work to. A pencil line would not be suitable. The hard metal surface would soon make a pencil blunt and the line would become thick and inaccurate; also a pencil line is too easily wiped off a metal surface. Usually the line is scribed using a sharp pointed metal tool, such as a scriber, that cuts into the surface of the metal and leaves a fine, permanent line.

7.1.1 Scriber

This is the basic marking-out tool. It consists of a handle with a sharp point. The pointed end is made from hardened steel so that it will stay sharp in use. Engineers' scribers usually have one straight end and one hooked end, as shown in Fig. 7.1. It is essential that the scribing point is kept sharp. Scribing points should not be sharpened on a grinding machine. The heat generated by this process tends to soften the point of the scriber so that it soon becomes blunt. The scribing point should be kept needle sharp by the use of an oil stone (see Fig. 7.27).

7.1.2 Centre and dot punches

Typical centre and dot punches are shown in Fig. 7.2. They are used for making indentations in the surface of the metal. There are two types of punch. Figure 7.2(a) shows a dot punch. This has a relatively fine point of about 60° or less and is used for locating the legs of such instruments as dividers and trammels. Figure 7.2(b) shows a centre punch. This is heavier than a dot punch and has a less acute point (usually 90° or greater). It is used to make a heavy indentation suitable for locating the point of

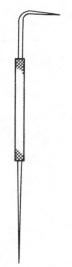

Figure 7.1 *Scriber*

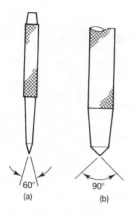

Figure 7.2 *Punches: (a) dot punch; (b) centre punch*

a twist drill. Another use for a dot punch is for 'preserving' a scribed 8 (page 212) line as shown in Fig. 7.28 (page 212). This use will be considered in greater detail towards the end of this chapter.

The correct way to use a dot punch is shown in Fig. 7.3. Usually the position for making a dot mark is at the junction of a pair of scribed lines at right angles to each other.

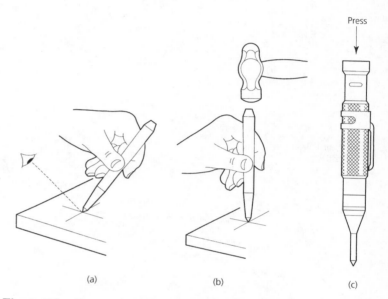

Figure 7.3 *Correct way to use dot and centre punches*

- You hold the punch so that it is inclined away from you. This enables you to see when the point of the punch is at the junction of the scribed lines as shown in Fig. 7.3(a).

- You then carefully bring the punch up to the vertical taking care not to move the position of the point.

- You then strike the punch lightly and squarely with a hammer as shown in Fig. 7.3(b).

- Check the position of the dot with the aid of a magnifying glass. Draw the dot over if it is slightly out of position.

For rough work you can use a centre punch in the same way but you need to hit it harder with a heavier hammer if you are to make a big enough indentation to guide the point of a drill. Because of the difficulty in seeing the point of a centre punch it is preferable to make a dot punch mark and, when you are satisfied that it is correctly positioned, you can enlarge the dot mark with a centre punch. The centre punch is correctly positioned when you feel its point 'click' into the mark left by the dot punch.

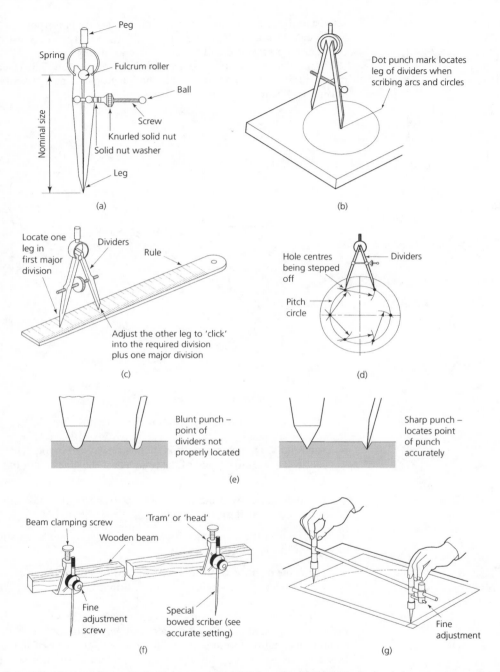

Figure 7.4 *Dividers and trammels: (a) parts of a divider; (b) scribing a circle; (c) setting a required radius; (d) stepping off hole centres; (e) location of divider point; (f) trammel or beam compass; (g) adjustment of trammel*

Figure 7.3(c) shows an automatic dot punch. This has the advantage that it can be used single handed and it is less likely to skid across the surface of the work. The punch is operated by downward pressure that releases a spring loaded hammer in its body. No separate hammer is required.

7.1.3 Dividers and trammels

These instruments are used for marking out circles and arcs of circles. A typical pair of dividers and the names of its component parts are shown in Fig. 7.4(a). Dividers are used to scribe circular lines as shown in Fig. 7.4(b). They are set to the required radius as shown in Fig. 7.4(c). They are also used for stepping off equal distances (such as hole centres along a line or round a pitch circle) as shown in Fig. 7.4(d). The leg about which the dividers pivot is usually located in a fine centre dot mark. To locate the point of this leg accurately it is essential to use a sharp dot punch as shown in Fig. 7.4(e).

Trammels are used for scribing large diameter circles and arcs that are beyond the range of ordinary dividers. They are also called beam compasses when the scribing points are located on a wooden beam as shown in Fig. 7.4(f). Trammels have a metal beam usually in the form of a solid rod or a tube. This often carries a scale and one of the scribing points is fitted with a vernier scale and a fine adjustment screw for accurate setting as shown in Fig. 7.4(g).

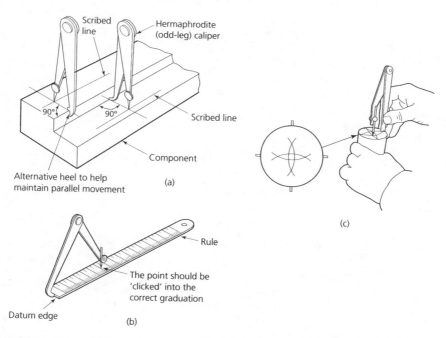

Figure 7.5 *Hermaphrodite (odd-leg) calipers: (a) scribing lines parallel to an edge; (b) setting odd-leg calipers; (c) finding the centre of a bar*

7.1.4 Hermaphrodite calipers

These are usually called odd-leg calipers or jenny calipers. They consist of one caliper leg and one divider leg and are used for scribing lines parallel to an edge as shown in Fig. 7.5(a). They are set to the required size as shown in Fig. 7.5(b).

7.1.5 Scribing block

A scribing block or surface gauge is used for marking out lines parallel to a datum surface or a datum edge. The parts of a typical scribing block are shown in Fig. 7.6(a) and some typical applications are shown in Fig. 7.6(b). Normally the scribing point is set to mark a line at a given height above the base of the instrument. This line will be marked parallel to the surface along which the base of the instrument is moved. When a line parallel to a datum edge is required, the edge pins are lowered. These pins are then kept in contact with the datum edge as the scribing block is moved along the work.

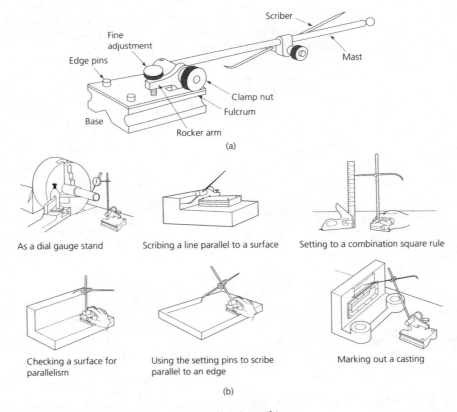

Figure 7.6 *The surface gauge (a) and typical applications (b)*

7.1.6 Vernier height gauge

The vernier height gauge was introduced in Chapter 6 as a measuring instrument. It is also used for scribing lines parallel to a datum surface in a similar manner to a scribing block. However, unlike a scribing block that has to be set to a separate steel rule, a vernier height gauge has a built-in main scale and vernier scale so that it can be set to a high degree of accuracy. The setting and reading of vernier scales was described in Chapter 6. The height gauge is fitted with a removable, sharpened nib. This is set to the required height by the scales provided. To scribe a line parallel to the datum surface, as shown in Fig. 7.7, the following procedure is used.

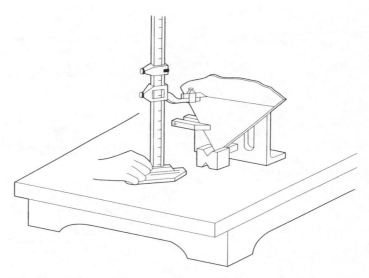

Figure 7.7 *Use of a vernier height gauge to scribe a line parallel to a datum surface*

- Set the nib of the height gauge to the correct distance from the base of the instrument.

- Keep the base of the height gauge firmly on the datum surface on which it and the work are standing.

- Keep the scribing nib firmly in contact with the work surface.

- Move the height gauge across the datum surface so that the scribing nib slides across the work. Keep the nib at an angle to the work surface so that the nib trails the direction of movement.

- To sharpen the nib without losing the zero setting of the instrument, see Section 7.7, Fig. 7.27(b).

7.2 Marking-out equipment (tools for providing guidance)

You cannot draw a straight line with a scriber without the help of some form of straight edge to guide the scriber. Let's now consider the tools that provide guidance for the scribing point.

7.2.1 Rule and straight edge

Where a straight line is required between two points, a rule can be used or, for longer distances, a straight edge. The correct way to use a scriber is shown in Fig. 7.8(a). The scriber is always inclined away from any guidance edge. Its point should always trail the direction of movement to prevent it 'digging in' to the metal surface so that it produces a poor line and damages the scribing point.

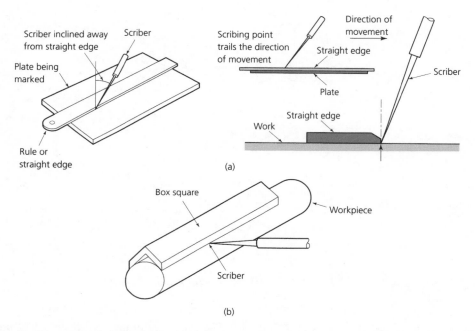

Figure 7.8 *Scribing straight lines: (a) scribing a straight line using a rule as a straight edge; (b) scribing a straight line using a box square*

7.2.2 Box square

This is also known as a key seat rule. It is used for marking and measuring lines scribed parallel to the axis of a cylindrical component such as a shaft. A typical box square and its method of use is shown in Fig. 7.8(b).

7.2.3 Try-square

When you need to scribe a line at 90° to a datum edge a try-square is used as shown in Fig. 7.9. A line scribed at 90° to an edge or another

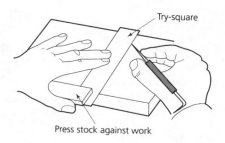

Press stock against work

Figure 7.9 *Scribing a line perpendicular to an edge*

line is said to be at *right angles* to that edge or line or it is said to be *perpendicular* to that edge or line. They both mean the same thing.

7.2.4 Combination set

This is shown in Fig. 7.10(a). It consists of a strong, relatively thick and rigid rule together with three 'heads' that are used individually but in conjunction with the rule.

- The square head can be clamped to the rule at any point along its length. It can either be used as a try-square (90°) or as a mitre square (45°) as shown in Fig. 7.10(b).

- The centre head or centre finder can also be clamped to the rule at any point along its length. The edge of the blade that passes through the centre of the centre finder also passes through the centre

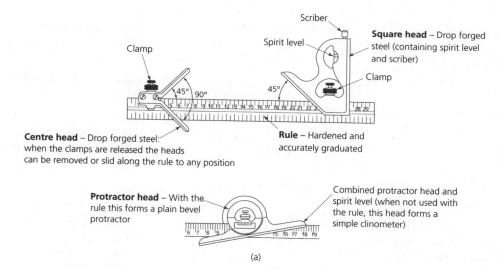

(a)

Figure 7.10 *The combination set: (a) construction; (b) uses; (c) finding the centre of a circular component*

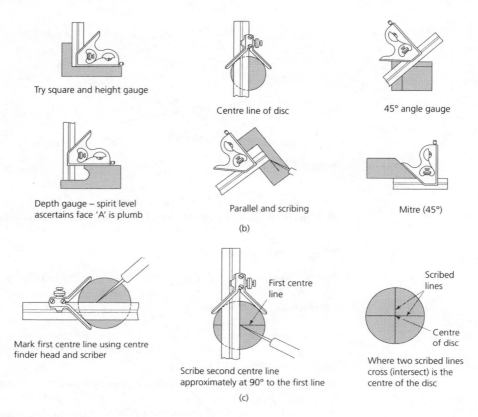

Try square and height gauge

Centre line of disc

45° angle gauge

Depth gauge – spirit level
ascertains face 'A' is plumb

Parallel and scribing

(b)

Mitre (45°)

Mark first centre line using centre
finder head and scriber

First centre
line

Scribe second centre line
approximately at 90° to the first line

(c)

Scribed
lines

Centre
of disc

Where two scribed lines
cross (intersect) is the
centre of the disc

Figure 7.10   *(continued)*

of the cylindrical workpiece. The centre of the cylindrical workpiece is found by scribing two lines at right angles to each other as shown in Fig. 7.10(c). The lines intersect at the centre of the workpiece.

- A protractor head is also supplied and this is used for marking out lines that are at any angle other than at 90° or 45° to the datum surface or edge.

- The square head and the protractor head are supplied with spirit (bubble) levels for setting purposes. However, they are only of limited accuracy.

7.3 Marking-out equipment (tools for providing support)

When marking out a component, it is essential that the blank is properly supported. As well as keeping the workpiece rigid and in the correct position, the supporting surface may also provide a datum from which to work. A datum is a line, surface or edge from which measurements are taken, but more about that in Section 7.4.

7.3.1 Surface plate and tables

Surface plates are cast from a stable cast iron alloy and are heavily ribbed to make them rigid. An example is shown in Fig. 7.11(a). They are used on the bench to provide a flat surface for marking out small workpieces. They are very heavy and should only be moved with care, preferably by two or more persons in the larger sizes.

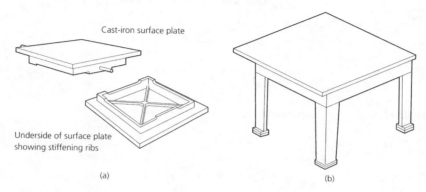

Cast-iron surface plate

Underside of surface plate
showing stiffening ribs

(a)

(b)

Figure 7.11 *Surface plate (a) and marking out table (b)*

Surface tables (marking-out tables), such as the one shown in Fig. 7.11(b), are used for providing a support and datum surface when marking out larger workpieces. A marking-out table is of heavy and rigid construction. The working surface may be of cast iron machined or ground flat. Plate glass and granite are also used because of their smoothness and stability. They do not give such a nice 'feel' as cast iron when moving the instruments upon them. This is because cast iron is self-lubricating.

The working surface must be kept clean and in good condition. Nothing must be allowed to scratch or damage the table and heavy objects must be slid gently onto the table from the side. Clean the table before and after use and make sure all sharp corners and rough edges are removed from the workpiece before it is placed on the table. Keep the table covered when it is not in use. Oil the working surface of the table if it is not to be used for some time.

7.3.2 Angle plates

These are also made from good quality cast iron and the working faces are machined at right angles to each other. The ends are also machined so that the angle plate can be stood on end when it is necessary to turn the work clamped to it through 90°. Figure 7.12(a) shows a typical angle plate being used to support work perpendicular to the datum surface of a marking-out table.

Figure 7.12(b) shows an adjustable angle plate. It is used for supporting work at any angle other than at 90° to the datum surface of a marking-out table. There is usually a scale that can be used for initial setting. It is only of limited accuracy and a vernier protractor should be used as shown for more accurate setting.

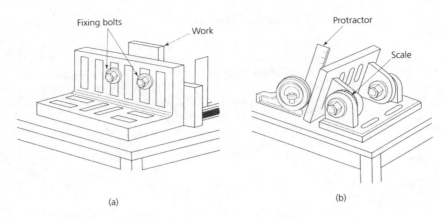

Figure 7.12 *Angle plate (a), adjustable angle plate (b)*

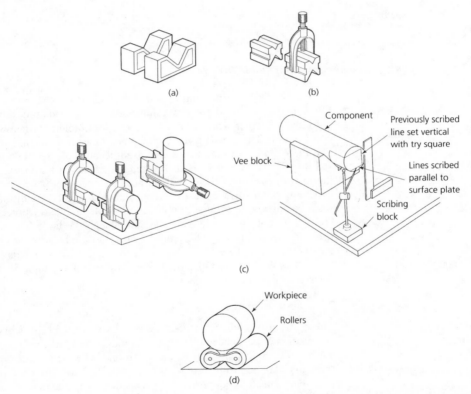

Figure 7.13 *Vee blocks and linked rollers: (a) plain vee blocks; (b) slotted vee blocks with 'horseshoe' clamp; (c) uses of vee blocks; (d) use of linked rollers*

7.3.3 Vee blocks

Vee blocks are used for supporting cylindrical workpieces so that their axes (plural of axis) are parallel to the datum surface. They also prevent the work from rolling about. Figure 7.13(a) shows a pair of plain vee blocks and Fig. 7.13(b) shows a pair of slotted vee blocks with 'horseshoe' clamps. Vee blocks are always manufactured as a matched pair and they should be kept as a matched pair. This ensures the axis of the work is parallel to the datum surface of the marking-out table. Figure 7.13(b) shows some applications of vee blocks. As well as vee blocks, linked rollers are also used for supporting cylindrical work as shown in Fig. 7.13(d).

7.3.4 Parallels

These are parallel strips of hardened and ground steel of square or rectangular section. They are used for supporting and raising work. They are manufactured in various sizes and, like vee blocks, are always manufactured in pairs. This ensures the supported work is always parallel to the datum surface of the marking-out table.

7.3.5 Jacks, wedges and shims

Adjustable screw jacks are used to provide additional support for heavy castings, as shown in Fig. 7.14. Without the jack, the overhanging weight of the casting would make it unstable so that it would tend to fall over.

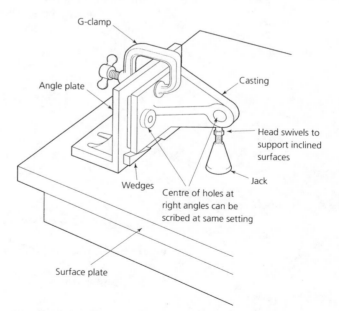

Figure 7.14 *Supporting larger work*

Wedges are also useful in levelling heavy components, as shown in Fig. 7.14. Where wedges are too thick, shims can be used. Shims are cut from thin hard-rolled brass or steel strip. The strip is supplied in graded thicknesses. They are used for packing the work level. It is always better to use one thick shim than two or more thin shims.

7.4 The purposes, advantages and disadvantages of manual marking out

For most jobbing work, prototype work, toolroom work and small quantity production, components are usually marked out as a guide to manufacture. The purposes, advantages and disadvantages of manual marking out can be summarized as follows.

7.4.1 Purposes and advantages

- To provide guide lines that can be worked to, and which provide the only control for the size and shape of the finished component. This is suitable only for work of relatively low accuracy.

- To indicate the outline of the component to a machinist as an aid for setting up and roughing out. The final dimensional control would come, in this instance, from precision instruments used in conjunction with the micrometer dials of the machine itself.

- To ensure that adequate machining allowances have been left on castings and forgings before expensive machining operations commence. The features checked are surfaces, webs, flanges, cored holes and bosses. In the example shown in Fig. 7.15, it is obvious that the base will not clean up. Neither is the web central nor will the bored hole be central in the boss. There would be no point in machining this casting.

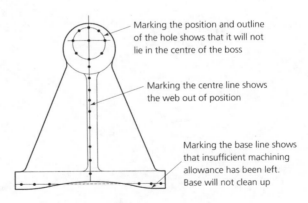

Marking the position and outline of the hole shows that it will not lie in the centre of the boss

Marking the centre line shows the web out of position

Marking the base line shows that insufficient machining allowance has been left. Base will not clean up

Figure 7.15 *Checking a clamp*

7.4.2 Disadvantages

- Scribed lines cut into the surface of the workpiece and deface the surface of the metal. Where the surface finish is important, allowance must be left for surface grinding to remove the scribed marks on completion of the component. Any marks cut into the surface of the metal are a potential source of fatigue failure and cracking during heat treatment and bending.

- The above disadvantages cannot be overcome by drawing with a pencil as this would not be sufficiently permanent nor sufficiently accurate. The only exception is in sheet metal work where fold lines are drawn with a soft pencil to avoid cutting through the protective coating of tin (tin-plate) or of zinc (galvanized sheet). Damage to such coatings leads to failure through corrosion.

- Centre punch marks may not control the drill point with sufficient accuracy unless the metal is heavily indented and, even then, total control cannot be guaranteed.

- Centre punching can cause distortion of the work. If the work is thick and the mark is not near the edges, a burr will still be thrown up round the punch mark. When the mark is near the edge of the metal – especially thin metal – the edge of the metal will swell out adjacent to the mark. This can cause inaccuracies if the distorted metal is a datum surface. Thin material, such as sheet metal, may buckle and distort when centre punched. Only the lightest marks should be made in such material.

- The accuracy of a scribed line to rule accuracy is limited to about ± 0.5 mm. When using a vernier height gauge this improves to about ± 0.1 mm. In practice the accuracy depends upon the condition of the scribing point and the skill of the person using the equipment.

7.5 Types of datum

The term datum has already been used several times in this chapter. It has also been described as a point, line or edge from which measurements are taken. Let's now examine the different types of datum in more detail.

- *Point datum*. This is a single point from which dimensions can be taken when measuring and marking out. For example, the centre point of a pitch circle.

- *Line datum*. This is a single line from which or along which dimensions are taken when measuring and marking out. It is frequently the centre line of a symmetrical component.

- *Edge datum*. This is also known as a *service edge*. It is a physical surface from which dimensions can be taken. This is the most widely used datum for marking out. Usually two edges are prepared at right angles to each other. They are also referred to as *mutually perpendicular* datum edges. These two edges ensure that the distances marked out from them are also at right angles to each other.

- *Surface datum*. For example, this can be the working surface of a surface plate or a marking-out table. It provides a common datum to support the work and the measuring and marking-out equipment in the same plane. For example, if you set your work with its datum edge on the surface datum of the marking-out table, and you set your surface gauge or scribing block to 25 mm, then the line you scribe on your work will be 25 mm from its datum edge. This is because the datum surface of the foot of the surface gauge and the datum surface of your work are both being supported in the same plane by the surface plate or marking-out table, as shown in Fig. 7.16.

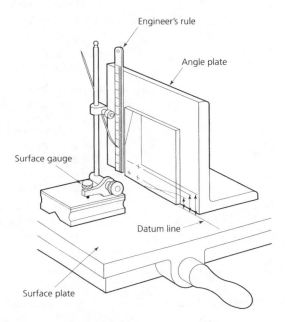

Figure 7.16 *Marking out from a datum surface*

7.5.1 Co-ordinates

The distance from a datum to some feature such as the centre of a hole is called an *ordinate*. In practice, two such dimensions are required to fix the position of a feature on a flat surface. These two ordinates are called *co-ordinates*. There are two systems of co-ordinates in common use.

7.5.2 Rectangular co-ordinates

The feature is positioned by a pair of ordinates (co-ordinates) lying at right angles to each other and at right angles to the two axes or datum edges from which they are measured. This system requires the preparation of two mutually perpendicular datum edges before marking out can commence. Figure 7.17(a) shows an example of the centre of a hole dimensioned by means of rectangular co-ordinates. Sometimes rectangular co-ordinates are called *Cartesian* co-ordinates.

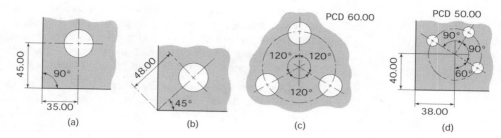

Figure 7.17 *Co-ordinates: (a) rectangular co-ordinates; (b) polar co-ordinates; (c) polar co-ordinates applied to holes; (d) combined co-ordinates (Note: PCD = pitch circle diameter: dimensions in millimetres)*

7.5.3 Polar co-ordinates

In this instance the co-ordinates consist of a linear (straight line) distance and an angular displacement. Figure 7.17(b) shows how the centre of a hole can be dimensioned using polar co-ordinates. Dimensioning by this technique is often employed when holes are located around a pitch circle or when machining is taking place on a rotary table. Figure 7.17(c) shows how polar co-ordinates are used to position holes around a pitch circle. In this example, the linear dimension is the radius of the pitch circle measured from a point datum at its centre. In practice, polar co-ordinates are rarely used in isolation. They are usually combined with rectangular co-ordinates as shown in Fig. 7.17(d).

7.6 Techniques for marking out

Having familiarized ourselves with the equipment used for marking out, the types of datum and the systems of co-ordinates, it is time to apply this knowledge to some practical examples.

7.6.1 Surface preparation

- Before commencing to mark out a metal surface, the surface must be cleaned and all oil, grease, dirt and loose material removed.

- A dark pencil line shows up clearly on white paper because of the colour contrast. Since scribed lines cut into the metal surface there is very little colour contrast and they do not always show up clearly.

- To make the line more visible, the metal surface is usually coated in a contrasting colour. Large castings are usually whitewashed, but smaller steel and non-ferrous precision components are usually coated with a quick drying layout 'ink'.

- Avoid using the old-fashioned technique of copper plating the surface of a steel component with a solution of copper sulphate containing a trace of sulphuric acid. Although it leaves a very permanent coating, it can be used only on steels and it is corrosive if it gets on marking-out instruments. The coating can be removed only by using emery cloth or by grinding.

- Layout ink is available in a variety of colours and can be readily applied to a smooth surface using an aerosol can. The ink should be applied thinly and evenly. Two thin coats are better than one thick coat. Wait for the ink to dry before marking out. The ink can be removed with a suitable solvent when the component is finished.

- *Safety*. Direct the spray only at the workpiece, never at your work-mates. Obey the maker's instructions at all times. Use only if there is adequate ventilation. Avoid breathing in the solvent and the propellant gas.

7.6.2 Use of a line datum

Figure 7.18 shows a simple link involving straight lines, arcs, and circles. It is symmetrical about its centre line. There are several ways of marking out this component. For the moment a centre line datum will be used.

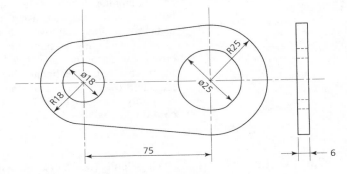

Figure 7.18 *Link: dimensions in millimetres*

Let's assume that we have a flat metal plate of the correct thickness and big enough from which to cut the link. The following operations refer to Fig. 7.19.

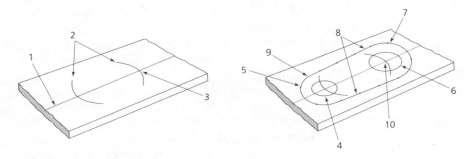

Figure 7.19 *Marking out from a centre line datum*

1. Clean the blank (plate) so as to remove all oil, grease and dirt. Remove all sharp corners for safety. Apply a light coating of layout

ink to the surface of the blank that is to be marked out. Using a steel rule as a straight edge scribe a centre line along the middle of the plate.

2. Set your dividers to the hole centre distance of 75 mm and step off this distance on the centre line. Leave sufficient room to strike the arcs that form the ends of the links.

3. Lightly dot punch the intersections of the centre line and the arcs you have struck with your dividers. These centre dots are used to locate the leg of the dividers in the following operations.

4. Set your dividers to 9 mm and scribe in the 18 mm diameter hole.

5. Set your dividers to 18 mm and, using the same centre dot as in (4), strike the smaller end radius.

6. Set your dividers to 12.5 mm and, using the other centre dot, scribe in the 25 mm diameter hole.

7. Set your dividers to 25 mm and, using the same centre dot as in (6), strike the larger end radius.

8. Scribe tangential lines to join the 18 mm and 25 mm end radii using your steel rule as a straight edge to guide the scriber.

9. Preserve the outline by dot punching as described in Section 7.1.2. The use of witness lines and marks is discussed further in Sections 7.6.7, 7.6.8, 7.6.9 and 7.6.10.

10. Enlarge the hole centre dot punch marks with a centre punch ready for drilling. This completes the marking out.

7.6.3 Use of a single edge datum

The following sequence of operations refers to Fig. 7.20. It assumes that the metal blank from which we are going to make the link has at least one straight edge. This would be the case if the blank was sawn from a piece of 75 mm by 6 mm bright-drawn, low carbon steel.

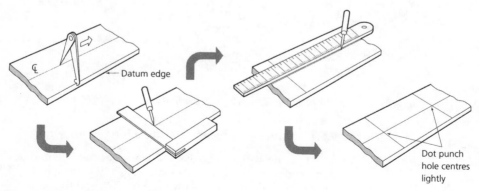

Figure 7.20 *Marking out from a datum edge*

1. Clean the sawn blank so as to remove all oil, grease and dirt. Remove all sharp corners for safety. Apply a light coat of layout ink. Use a steel rule as a straight edge to check the selected datum edge for flatness and straightness. Carefully remove any bruises with a fine file.

2. Scribe the centre line parallel to the datum edge using odd-leg calipers as shown.

3. Scribe the first centre line at right angles to the datum edge using a try-square to guide the scriber point and leaving room for striking the arc that forms the end of the link.

4. Measure and mark off the centre distance to the second hole either by using your rule and scriber as shown or by stepping off the distance with dividers set to 75 mm as in the previous example.

5. Scribe the second hole centre line at right angles to the datum edge using a try-square. Dot punch the centre points.

6. The remaining operations are the same as (4) to (10) inclusive in the previous example.

An alternative method is shown in Fig. 7.21. Clamping the blank to an angle plate provides the same effect as having a pair of mutually perpendicular datum edges. This enables us to scribe the centre lines at right angles to each other without the use of a try-square. By using a vernier height gauge the centre distance can be marked out much more accurately than by using a scribing block as shown below. The plate can be clamped by using small G-clamps as shown or by using toolmaker's clamps.

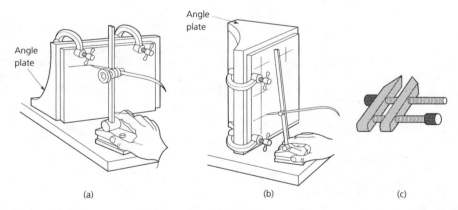

Figure 7.21   *Use of angle plate: (a) to provide mutually perpendicular surfaces; (b) toolmaker's clamp*

7.6.4   Mutually perpendicular datum edges

This time we will assume that our blank has two datum edges that are at right angles to each other; they are mutually perpendicular. The general set-up for marking out is shown in Fig. 7.22 and the following sequence of operations refers to Fig. 7.23.

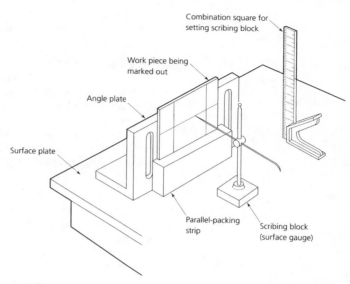

Combination square for setting scribing block

Work piece being marked out

Angle plate

Surface plate

Parallel-packing strip

Scribing block (surface gauge)

Figure 7.22 *Marking out from a datum surface – the surface plate provides the datum surface; all measurements are made from this surface; all lines scribed by the scribing block will be parallel to this surface*

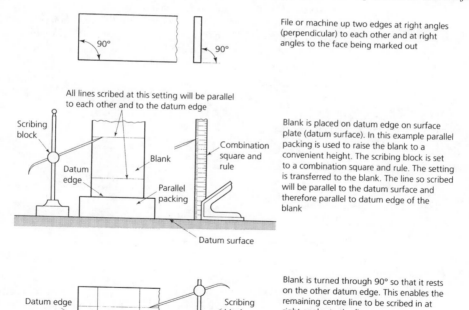

90°

90°

File or machine up two edges at right angles (perpendicular) to each other and at right angles to the face being marked out

All lines scribed at this setting will be parallel to each other and to the datum edge

Scribing block

Datum edge

Blank

Parallel packing

Combination square and rule

Datum surface

Blank is placed on datum edge on surface plate (datum surface). In this example parallel packing is used to raise the blank to a convenient height. The scribing block is set to a combination square and rule. The setting is transferred to the blank. The line so scribed will be parallel to the datum surface and therefore parallel to datum edge of the blank

Datum edge

Parallel packing

Scribing block

Datum surface

Blank is turned through 90° so that it rests on the other datum edge. This enables the remaining centre line to be scribed in at right angles to the first two

Figure 7.23 *Marking-out procedure when using a datum surface*

1. File or machine two edges at right angles to each other and to the surface being marked out. Remove all sharp edges, oil, grease and dirt from the blank and apply a light coat of layout ink.

2. The blank is placed on its end datum edge on a marking-out table as shown. A precision ground, parallel packing block is used to raise the work to a convenient height. The thickness of the packing must be measured and allowed for when setting the scribing point. The point of the scriber is set to the combination rule. Make sure the datum end of the rule is in contact with the surface of the marking-out table. A line is now scribed on the blank at this setting. The scribing point is raised by 75 mm and a second line is scribed as shown.

3. The blank is then turned through 90° so that it rests on the other datum edge. This enables the remaining centre line to be scribed at right angles to the first two. Where the lines intersect are the hole centres. Dot punch these centres lightly. The marking out of the link is completed as described in operations (4) to (10) inclusive in the first example. If greater accuracy is required a vernier height gauge is used in place of the scribing block.

7.6.5 Use of a point datum and tabulated data

Figure 7.24 shows a component that has been drawn using rectangular co-ordinates and absolute dimensioning for the hole centres. Each hole centre then becomes a *point datum* for the clusters of small holes. To avoid confusion on the drawing, the large number of repeated dimensions for the holes has been tabulated. This is referred to as tabulated data.

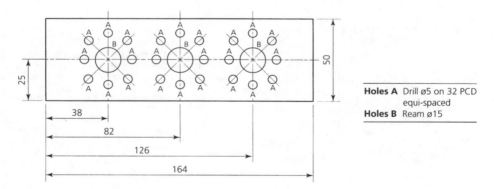

Holes A Drill ø5 on 32 PCD
equi-spaced
Holes B Ream ø15

Figure 7.24   *Tabulated data*

Because the major hole centres have been dimensioned using rectangular co-ordinates, they can be marked out as described previously. The dot punch marks at the intersection of the centre lines are used to locate the dividers. These are used to mark out the outline of the 15 mm diameter holes and also the 32 mm diameter pitch circles for the smaller holes. Since there are eight equi-spaced holes in each cluster, they will be at

45° to each other. We can mark out their centre positions using the square and mitre head from the combination set as shown in Fig. 7.25(a). Had there been six holes, their chordal distance would have been the same as the pitch circle radius. Therefore, after marking out the pitch circles, the hole centres could have been stepped off with the dividers at the same setting, as shown in Fig. 7.25(b).

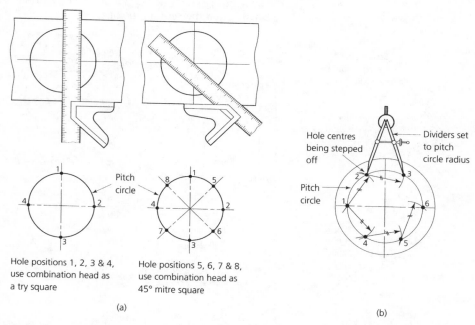

(a)

(b)

Figure 7.25 *Marking-out holes on a pitch circle: (a) use of combination square; (b) use of dividers*

Sometimes a drawing has to satisfy a family of similar components that only vary in size but not in shape. Such an example is shown in Fig. 7.26. This drawing has tabulated dimensions for the overall length and the hole centres. The width and thickness of the component remains constant and the holes are located on the centre line that is also constant.

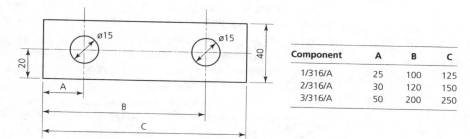

Component	A	B	C
1/316/A	25	100	125
2/316/A	30	120	150
3/316/A	50	200	250

Figure 7.26 *Tabulated dimensions*

7.6.6   Condition and care of equipment

Marking-out equipment should be kept in good condition if inaccuracies are to be avoided.

- As has been mentioned previously, the points of scribers and dividers should be kept needle sharp by regular dressing with a fine oil slip. This is shown in Fig. 7.27(a). Do not sharpen by grinding, the heat generated will soften the scribing point.

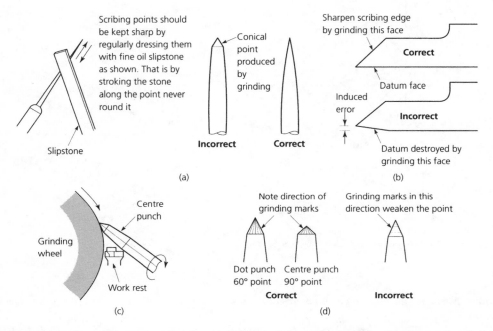

Figure 7.27   *Care of marking-out equipment: (a) sharpening scriber points; (b) sharpening height gauge scribing blades; (c) sharpening centre and dot punches; (d) correct dot and centre punch point configurations*

- The nib of the vernier height gauge should be sharpened by carefully grinding as shown in Fig. 7.27(b). Use a free cutting wheel to avoid overheating and softening the scribing edge. Use an appropriate silicon carbide (green grit) wheel if the nib is tungsten carbide tipped.

- When sharpening the point of a dot punch or a centre punch, the punch is presented to the abrasive wheel as shown in Fig. 7.27(c). This ensures that the grinding marks run down the point as shown in Fig. 7.27(d) and not round it.

- Rules should be kept clean. The datum end should be protected and *never* used as a makeshift screwdriver or for shovelling swarf out of the T-slot of a machine tool bed. The edges of a rule must also be kept in a good condition if it is to enable straight lines to be scribed or it is to be used as a straight edge.

- Try-squares must also be treated carefully and cleaned and boxed when not in use. They should never be dropped, mixed with other tools or used for any purpose other than for which they are designed.

- Angle plates must be kept clean and free from bruises. Bruises not only prevent proper contact between the angle plate and the work it is supporting, they also cause damage to the surface of the marking-out table on which they are supported.

- Surface plates and marking-out tables must also be treated with care as they provide the datum from which other dimensions are taken.

- Vee blocks must be kept boxed in pairs as originally supplied. They are made in matched pairs and must be kept together for the whole of their working lives. Vee blocks from two different sets will not necessarily support a shaft parallel to the datum surface on which the blocks are supported.

- Table 7.1 summarizes the more usual causes of faults and inaccuracies when marking out.

TABLE 7.1   *Faults and inaccuracies when marking out*

Fault	Possible cause	To correct
Inaccurate measurement	Wrong instrument for tolerance required	Check instrument is suitable for tolerance required
Scribed lines out of position	Incorrect use of instrument	Improve your technique
	Parallax (sighting) error	Use the scriber correctly
Lines not clear	Rule not square with datum edge	Use a datum block (abutment)
	Scribing point blunt	Sharpen the point of the scriber
	Work surface too hard	Use a surface coating (spray-on lacquer)
	Scribing tool lacks rigidity	Use only good-quality tools in good condition
Corrosion along scribed lines	Protective coating (tin plate) cut by using too sharp a scribing point	Use a pencil when marking coated materials
Component tears or cracks along scribed line when bent	Scribed line and direction of bend parallel to grain of material	Bend at right angles to grain of the material
	Scribed line cut too deeply	Mark bend lines with a pencil
Circles and arcs irregular and not clear	Scribing points blunt	Resharpen
	Instruments not rigid	Use only good quality dividers or trammels of correct size for job
	Centre point slipping	Use a dot punch to make a centre location
Centre punch marks out of position	Incorrect use of punch	Position punch so that point is visible and then move upright when point is correctly positioned
	Scribed lines not sufficiently deep to provide a positive point location	Ensure point can click into the junction of the scribed lines

7.6.7 Cutting and limit lines

The concept of dot punching scribed lines to preserve them has already been introduced. Let's now examine this technique more closely. Scribed lines are often marked with a dot punch as shown in Fig. 7.28. Small dot punch or 'pop' marks are made along a straight line at about 20 mm to 25 mm intervals and at corners as shown in Fig. 7.28(a). They should be closer together around curves and complex profiles. Be careful to locate the point of the dot punch accurately on the scribed line when dot punching. If the scribed line should become defaced or erased, it can be restored using a scriber to connect the dot marks again.

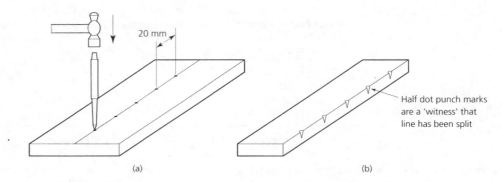

Figure 7.28 *Preserving a scribed line: (a) dot punching; (b) witness marks*

Another use for these 'pop' marks is as an aid to machining. If you machine down to a scribed line so as to 'split the line', there will be no line left to prove that you have worked accurately to the line. However, if the line has dot marks along it, and you have accurately split the line then half the marks are still visible to prove the accuracy of your work as shown in Fig. 7.28(b). For this reason such marks are often called *witness marks*.

7.6.8 Round holes – size and position

In theory all you need when marking out hole centres ready for drilling is a centre punch mark at the intersection of the centre lines as a guide for the drill point. Unfortunately drills have a habit of 'wandering' especially when starting a large drill with a centre punch mark. Therefore it is usual also to mark out the circle representing the hole, as shown in Fig. 7.29(a), using dividers. The hole is then dot punched. If the hole is drilled accurately, the dot punch marks should be split. However, this assumes that the:

- Centre lines are accurately marked out.

- Centre punch mark is exactly at the intersection of the centre lines.

- Dividers are exactly set to the hole radius.

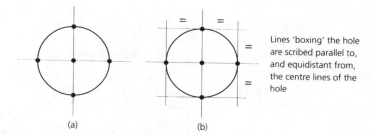

Lines 'boxing' the hole are scribed parallel to, and equidistant from, the centre lines of the hole

Figure 7.29 *Marking out round holes*

- Dividers do not 'wander' in the centre punch mark.
- 'Pop' marks around the circle are accurately positioned.

This is an awful lot of assumptions. For this reason it is better to 'box' the hole as shown in Fig. 7.29(b). Whilst the hole centres are being accurately marked out using rectangular co-ordinates, the vernier height gauge can also be used to accurately scribe lines either side of the centre lines at a distance equal to the radius of the hole. This produces an accurate box within which the drilled hole should lie.

7.6.9 Guide lines

Guide lines and witness lines are also used in conjunction with straight cutting lines as shown in Fig. 7.30. The guide line is scribed parallel to the cutting line or the limit line and it is positioned on the waste material side as shown in Fig. 7.30(a), therefore the guide line will be removed during machining. In the case of a drilled hole or a bore, the guide line is a circle slightly smaller than the finished size of the hole or bore. This is shown in Fig. 7.30(b).

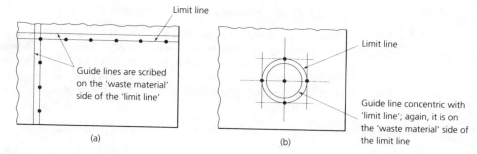

Limit line

Guide lines are scribed on the 'waste material' side of the 'limit line'

Limit line

Guide line concentric with 'limit line'; again, it is on the 'waste material' side of the limit line

Figure 7.30 *Guide lines*

The reason for providing a guide line is to provide a visual check that the work is correctly set and that machining is being carried out parallel to the cutting line or the limit line. This enables adjustments and corrections to be made before cutting to the final size. For this reason more than one guide line may be provided.

7.6.10   Witness lines

Witness lines are scribed parallel to the cutting or the limit line on the opposite side to the guide line as shown in Fig. 7.31. Therefore, when cutting is complete, they should still be present. They are used in conjunction with or in place of the dot punch witness marks described earlier. If cutting or machining has been successfully and correctly performed, the witness line should be parallel to the edge of the component and the correct distance from it. It remains as a witness to the accuracy of the fitting or machining processes used.

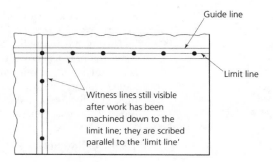

Figure 7.31   *Witness lines*

Witness lines are applied to a round hole on the opposite side of the limit line (outline) of the hole. That is, it will lie just outside the limit line, whilst the guide line (as previously described) will lie just inside the limit line. The circular or boxed lines can then act as a *witness* to the size and position of the drilled hole.

7.6.11   Line enhancement

The use of layout inks has already been discussed. However, their use can be messy and they tend to dissolve away with some coolants during cutting or be scratched away by the swarf during machining operations. For this reason it is sometimes better to enhance the line itself to give a colour contrast by rubbing one of the following substances into the scribed line.

- Engineer's blue will enhance the clarity of scribed lines on bright shiny metals.

- Chalk powder will enhance the clarity of scribed lines on dull dark metals such as grey cast iron.

- Graphite from crushed pencil leads can be used with good effect to enhance lines scribed on non-metallic materials.

Exercises **7.1** *Marking out and marking-out equipment*
(a) (i) List the reasons for marking out components ready for manufacture.
(ii) Explain why mass produced components are not marked out prior to manufacture.
(b) List the advantages and limitations of manual marking out in terms of accuracy and possible damage to the surfaces of the workpiece.
(c) Complete Table 7.2. It has been started to give you a guide.

TABLE 7.2 *Exercise 7.1(c)*

Technique	Equipment required
Straight lines	Rule and scriber
Circles and arcs	–
Lines parallel to an edge (not using a surface plate)	
Lines parallel to a surface plate	–
Lines parallel to angle sections	–
Lines along shafts parallel to each other and to the axis of the shaft	
Lines perpendicular to an edge	–

7.2 *Techniques for marking out*
(a) Draw up an operation schedule for marking out the component shown in Fig. 7.32, using its centre line as a datum. List the marking-out operations in the correct order and the equipment used.

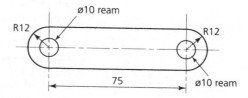

Figure 7.32 *Exercise 7.2(a)*

(b) With the aid of sketches explain how lines can be scribed parallel and perpendicular to a surface plate datum.
(c) State the purpose of a box square and, with the aid of sketches, show how it can be used.
(d) Describe the difference between a dot punch and a centre punch and explain their uses.

7.3 *Types of datum*
   (a) Copy and complete Table 7.3.

TABLE 7.3 *Exercise 7.3(a)*

Type of datum	Sketch of example
Edge of datum	
Line of datum	
	6 holes ø12 on 125 PCD

   (b) With the aid of sketches, describe how the component shown in Fig. 7.33 can be marked out on a surface table using the edge marked AA as a datum.
   (c) With the aid of sketches describe how a scribed line can be 'protected' using dot punch marks. Also describe how these dot punch marks can act as a 'witness' to show that a fitter or a machinist has worked correctly to a scribed line.

7.4 *Minimizing inaccuracies when marking out*
   (a) Explain what is meant by the term *parallax errors* when marking out using a steel rule. How can such errors be minimized?
   (b) Describe two ways in which a scribed line can be made to show up more clearly.
   (c) Describe TWO ways (other than those in (a) and (b)) by which marking-out inaccuracies can be minimized.

7.5 *Care of marking-out tools and equipment*
   (a) With the aid of sketches describe how the scribing points/edges of the following marking-out tools should be sharpened:
      (i) divider points;
     (ii) vernier height gauge nib;
    (iii) dot punch point.

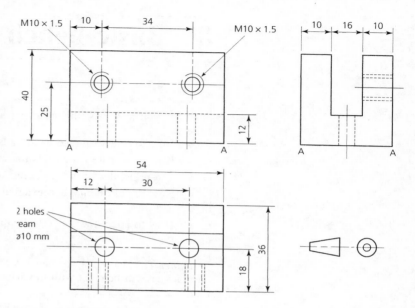

Figure 7.33 *Exercise 7.3(b)*

(b) Describe how marking-out tools and measuring instruments should be cared for and stored in order to maintain their accuracy and to maintain them in good condition.

8 Basic bench fitting

When you have read this chapter you should understand:

- How to select suitable hand tools for particular jobs.
- How to prepare hand tools for safe and effective use.
- The principles of metal cutting.
- How to cut internal and external screw threads using taps and dies.
- How to apply the above techniques in the production of typical workpieces.

(*Note:* The sharpening of bench tools on the off-hand grinding machine will be dealt with in Chapter 12.)

8.1 Relative merits and disadvantages of using hand tools

Despite the wide range of machine tools available, and despite the high rates of material removal that are possible with modern machine tools and cutters, bench fitting using hand tools still has a place in modern industry. Bench fitting is too slow and costly for batch and flowline production, but it has a place in the making of 'one-off' prototypes for research and development projects, and in jig and toolmaking.

8.1.1 Merits

- Hand tools are relatively cheap and versatile for making small components of complex shapes that would be difficult to hold on machines.

- Small and delicate components may not be strong enough to withstand the clamping and machining forces, hand processes will then be the only choice.

- Skilled craftspersons can work to relatively high levels of accuracy and finish using hand tools.

- No capital investment in costly plant is required.

- Hand tools are more easily maintained compared with machine tool cutters.

8.1.2 Disadvantages

- Compared with machining, the rate of material removal by hand tools is limited and production using hand tools is relatively slow.

- Compared with machining processes such as surface and cylindrical grinding, the accuracy and finish achieved even by a skilled craftsperson are limited.

- The unit cost of production by using hand tools is high because of the limited rate of material removal and the relatively high wages that can be commanded by skilled fitters and toolmakers.

8.2 The fitter's bench

The term *fitting* covers those operations that the engineering craftsperson performs by hand at the bench. The production of accurate components by hand demands levels of skill that takes many years of constant practice to acquire. The basic requirement of successful fitting is a properly designed work bench. There is no single design for an ideal bench. However, for accurate work it is generally accepted that:

- The bench must be made from heavy timbers on a strongly braced metal frame so that it is as solid and rigid as possible.

- It must be positioned so that there is adequate natural lighting supplemented as required by adequate, shadowless, artificial lighting.

- The height of the bench should allow the top of the vice jaws to be in line with the underside of the fitter's forearm when held parallel to the ground.

- There should be adequate storage facilities for small tools and instruments.

8.2.1 The fitter's vice

A fitter uses a parallel jaw vice of the type shown in Fig. 8.1(a). It is often fitted with a quick-release device that frees the screw from the nut so that the vice can be opened or closed quickly. This saves time when changing

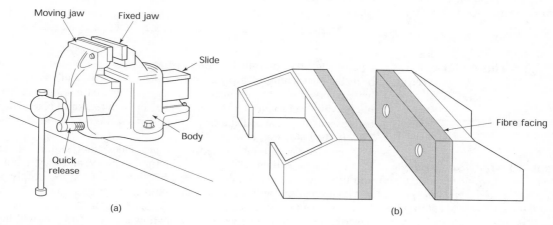

Figure 8.1 *Fitter's vice (a), vice shoes (b)*

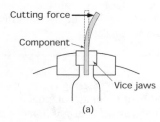

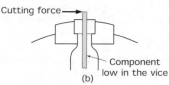

Figure 8.2 *Positioning work in the vice: (a) incorrect – if the cutting force is applied too far from the vice jaws, it will have insufficient 'leverage' to bend the component; even when the force is too small to bend the component, it will make it vibrate and give off an irritating squealing noise; (b) correct – when the component is held with the least possible overhang, the cutting force does not have sufficient 'leverage' to bend the component or to make it vibrate*

between wide and narrow work. For accurate work the vice must be kept in good condition as follows:

- Oil the screw and nut regularly.
- Oil the slideways regularly.
- Ensure that the vice is substantial enough for the work in hand.
- Heavy hammering and bending should be confined to the anvil and not performed on the vice.
- When chipping, the thrust of the chisel should be against the fixed jaw.
- Never hammer on the top surface of the slide.

8.2.2   Vice shoes

The jaws of a vice are serrated to prevent the work from slipping. However, these serrations can mark and spoil a finished surface. If the vice is to be used only for fine work and light cuts, the jaws can be surface ground flat and smooth. Alternatively, if the vice is going to be used for both rough and fine work, then vice shoes can be used. These can either be cast from a soft metal such as lead or they can be faced with fibre as shown in Fig. 8.1(b).

8.2.3   Using a vice

The vice should be securely bolted to the bench and should be positioned so that the fixed jaw is just clear of the edge of the bench. This allows long work to hang down clear of the bench. Work should be positioned in the vice so that the major cutting forces acting on the work are directed towards the fixed jaw. The work should always be held in a vice with a minimum of overhang as shown in Fig. 8.2. There is always a possibility that work protruding too far out of a vice will bend under the force of the cut. Also that the work will vibrate and produce an irritating squealing sound.

8.3   The metal cutting wedge

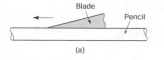

Figure 8.3 *The clearance angle (β): (a) no clearance (β = 0) – the blade skids along the pencil without cutting; (b) clearance (β > 0) – the blade bites into the pencil and cuts*

One of the first controlled cutting operations you performed must have been the sharpening of a pencil with a penknife. It is unlikely you will have received any formal instruction before your first attempt but, most likely, you soon found out (by trial and error) that the knife blade had to be presented to the wood at a definite angle if success was to be achieved. This is shown in Fig. 8.3.

If the blade is laid flat on the wood it just slides along without cutting. If you tilt it at a slight angle, it will bite into the wood and start to cut. If you tilt it at too steep an angle, it will bite into the wood too deeply and it will not cut properly. You will also find that the best angle will vary between a knife that is sharp and a knife that is blunt. A sharp knife will penetrate the wood more easily, at a shallower angle, and you will have more control. But look at that knife blade. It is the shape of a wedge. In

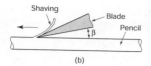

(b)

Figure 8.3 *(continued)*

8.4 The angles of a wedge-shaped cutting tool and their terminology

fact all cutting tools are wedge shaped (more or less), so let's now look at the angles of a typical metal cutting tool.

Having seen that a cutting tool is essentially wedge shaped, let's now see how this wedge shape affects the other cutting angles of a metal cutting tool.

8.4.1 Clearance angle

We have seen that for our knife to cut, we need to incline it to the surface being cut, and that we have to control this angle carefully for effective cutting. This angle is called the *clearance angle* and we give it the Greek letter 'beta' (β). All cutting tools have to have this angle. It has to be kept as small as possible to prevent the tool 'digging in'. At the same time it has to be large enough to allow the tool to penetrate the workpiece material. The clearance will vary slightly depending upon the cutting operation and the material being cut. It is usually about 5° to 7°.

8.4.2 Wedge angle

If, in place of our pencil, we tried to sharpen a point on a piece of soft metal (such as copper) with our knife we would find that the knife very quickly becomes blunt. If you examine this blunt edge under a magnifying glass, you will see that the cutting edge has crumbled away. To cut metal successfully, the cutting edge must be ground to a less acute angle to give it greater strength when cutting metal. This is shown in Fig. 8.4.

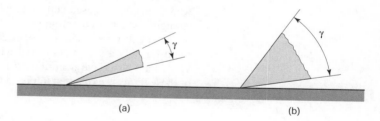

(a)   (b)

Figure 8.4 *Wedge (tool) angle (γ): (a) blade sharpened for cutting wood; (b) blade sharpened for cutting metal*

The angle to which the tool is ground is called the wedge angle or the tool angle and it is given the Greek letter 'gamma' (γ). The greater the wedge angle, the stronger will be the tool. Also, the greater the wedge angle the quicker the heat of cutting will be conducted away from the cutting edge. This will prevent the tool overheating and softening, and help to prolong the tool life. Unfortunately, the greater the wedge angle is made, the greater will be the force required to make the tool penetrate the workpiece material. The choice of the wedge angle becomes a compromise between all these factors.

8.4.3 Rake angle

To complete the angles associated with cutting tools, reference must be made to the rake angle. This is given the Greek letter alpha (α). The rake angle is very important, for it alone controls the geometry of the chip formation for any given material and, therefore, it controls the mechanics of the cutting action of the tool. The relationship of the rake angle to the angles previously discussed is shown in Fig. 8.5.

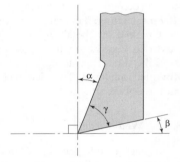

Material being cut	α
Cast iron	0°
Free-cutting brass	0°
Ductile brass	14°
Tin bronze	8°
Aluminium alloy	30°
Mild steel	25°
Medium-carbon steel	20°
High-carbon steel	12°
Tufnol plastic	0°

Figure 8.5 *Cutting tool angles: α = rake angle; β = clearance angle; γ = wedge or tool angle*

Increasing the rake angle increases the cutting efficiency of the tool and makes cutting easier. Since increasing the rake angle reduces the wedge angle, increased cutting efficiency is gained at the expense of tool strength. Again a compromise has to be reached in achieving a balance between cutting efficiency, tool strength and tool life.

So far only a single point tool with positive rake has been considered. Tools may also have neutral (zero) rake and negative rake. The meaning of these terms is explained in Fig. 8.6. It can be seen that the wedge angles

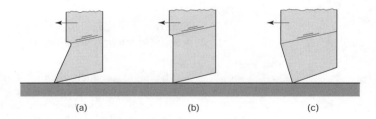

(a)   (b)   (c)

Figure 8.6 *Rake angles: (a) positive rake; (b) neutral (zero) rake; (c) negative rake*

for such tools is much more robust and it should come as no surprise that they are used for heavy cutting conditions. However, the cutting action of tools with neutral and negative rake angles is somewhat different to the positive rake geometry considered so far and is beyond the scope of this book.

8.5 The application of the basic cutting angles to hand tools

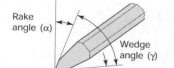

(a)

(b)

(c)

Figure 8.7 *The cold chisel*

Let's now consider how the basic principles of the metal cutting wedge can be applied to a range of standard bench tools.

8.5.1 Cold chisels

The basic wedge angle described above applies to all metal-cutting tools. Figure 8.7(a) shows how the point of a cold chisel forms a metal-cutting wedge with rake and clearance angles, and how the angle at which you present the chisel to the work (angle of inclination) affects the cutting action of the chisel.

In Fig. 8.7(b) the chisel is presented to the work so that the angle of inclination is too small. As a result, the rake angle becomes larger and the clearance angle disappears. This prevents the cutting edge of the chisel from biting into the work and the cut becomes progressively shallower until the chisel ceases to cut.

In Fig. 8.7(c) the chisel is presented to the work so that the angle of inclination is too large. As a result the effective rake angle becomes smaller and the effective clearance angle becomes larger. This results in the cutting edge of the chisel 'digging in' so that the cut becomes progressively deeper.

8.5.2 Files

Like any other cutting tool a file tooth must have correctly applied cutting angles. File teeth are formed by a chisel edge cutter so that the first or 'overcut' produces a single cut file or 'float' with the teeth at 70° to the edge of the file blank. Such files are not widely used except on soft materials such as copper and aluminium. The tooth form is less likely to become clogged up than the tooth form of the more commonly used double-cut file.

Most files have a second or 'up-cut' at 45° to the opposite side of the file blank so that the 'cuts' cross each other. Files manufactured in this manner are referred to as 'double-cut' files. Up-cutting gives the teeth a positive rake angle and a smoother cutting action. Double-cut files are suitable for use on tougher materials such as plain carbon steels and alloy steels. They are also suitable for use on cast iron and most non-ferrous metals.

8.5.3 Hacksaw blades

The teeth of a heavy duty hacksaw blade suitable for use on a power driven sawing machine is shown in Fig. 8.8(a). You will see that the

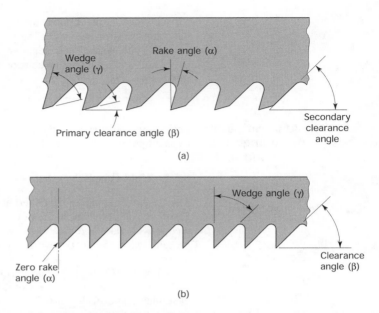

Figure 8.8 *Hacksaw blade teeth: (a) heavy duty power saw blade – tooth form gives high strength coupled with adequate chip clearance; (b) light duty hand saw blade showing simplified tooth form used for fine tooth blades*

teeth form a series of metal-cutting wedges. Since there are a series of metal-cutting edges this is called a *multi-tooth* cutting tool, compared with a chisel or a lathe tool which are called single-point cutting tools. Like all multi-tooth cutting tools designed to work in a slot, the power hacksaw blade has to be provided with chip (secondary) clearance as well as cutting (primary) clearance. The secondary clearance provides room for the chips to be carried out of the slot without clogging the teeth whilst, at the same time, maintaining a strong cutting edge.

The finer teeth of a hand saw blade have only a simple wedge shape as shown in Fig. 8.8(b). Chip clearance is provided by exaggerating the primary clearance. Although this weakens the teeth, their strength is adequate for a hand saw. In addition side clearance has to be provided to prevent the blade binding in the slot being cut. This is done by providing the teeth with a 'set', as described in Section 8.9.

8.6 Chipping

Chipping is the removal of metal by the use of cold chisels. The cutting action of a cold chisel has already been discussed. Now let's look at the chipping process. This process is used for rapidly breaking down a surface. It is the quickest way of removing metal by hand but the accuracy is low and the finish is poor. However, in some instances there are no alternatives. Figure 8.9 shows a selection of cold chisels and some typical chipping operations.

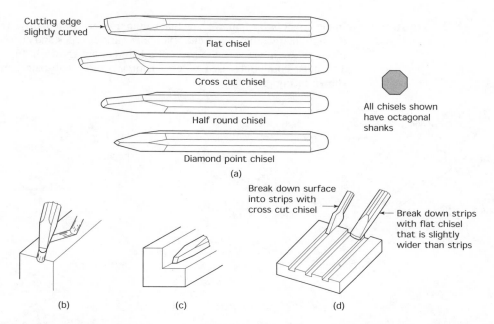

Figure 8.9 *Cold chisel types (a) and uses: (b) cutting an oil groove with a half-round chisel; (c) squaring out a corner with a diamond point chisel; (d) chipping a flat surface*

Safety – *When using a cold chisel:*

- *Do NOT chip towards your workmates.*

- *Always use a chipping screen (Fig. 8.10).*

- *Always wear goggles to protect your eyes from the flying splinters of metal (Fig. 8.10).*

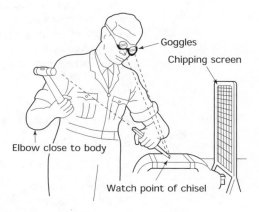

Figure 8.10 *Safety when using a cold chisel*

8.7 Hammers

In the previous section, we saw that hammers were used to drive the chisel through the material being cut. There are various types and sizes of hammer used by fitters, and the parts of a hammer are shown in Fig. 8.11(a). The most commonly used type of hammer is the ball-pein hammer as shown in Fig. 8.11(b).

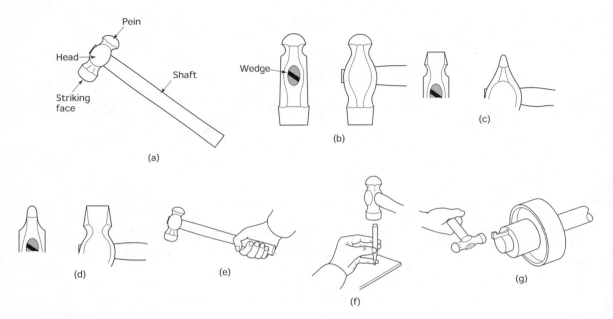

Figure 8.11 *Hammer construction (a), ball pein type (b), cross pein type (c), straight pein type (d), correct grip (e), used with another tool (f), used directly (g)*

If a hammer is too big, it will be clumsy to use and proper control cannot be exercised. If a hammer is too small it has to be wielded with so much effort that, again, proper control cannot be exercised. In both these instances the use of the incorrect size of hammer will result in an unsatisfactory job, possible damage to the work and possible injury to the user. Before using a hammer you must check it to make sure of the following:

- The handle (shaft) is not split.

- The head is not loose.

- The head is not cracked or chipped.

- Never 'strangle' a hammer by holding it too near the head. It should be held as shown in Fig. 8.11(e).

- A hammer is usually used to strike other tools such as chisels, drifts and centre punches as shown in Fig. 8.11(f).

You must be careful when a hammer is used to strike a component, such as a key or a dowel, directly (Fig. 8.11(g)) so that the component being struck is not bruised. Soft-faced hammers should be used when machined surfaces have to be struck. Soft-faced hammers are faced with various materials such as soft metals like brass and aluminium and non-metals such as plastic and rawhide. Some are made from solid rubber moulded onto the handle. However, these tend to bounce and it is difficult to deliver a dead blow. An improved design is hollow and loosely filled with lead shot. This type of rubber mallet will deliver a dead blow and also provide the protection against bruising of the solid rubber type. Alternatively a soft metal (brass, copper or aluminium) drift should be placed between the hammer head and the component being struck.

8.8 Filing

Filing operations can range from roughing down to fine and accurate finishing operations. There is a wide variety of files, and to specify any given file you must state the length, shape and grade of cut. The main features of a typical file are shown in Fig. 8.12.

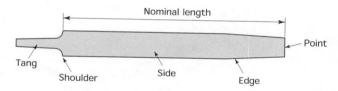

Figure 8.12 *Engineer's file*

8.8.1 Grade or cut

The *grade* or cut of a file depends upon its length. A long second-cut file can have a coarser cut than a short bastard-cut file. The most common cuts are:

- *Bastard cut* – general roughing out.

- *Second cut* – roughing out tough materials such as die steels and for finishing on less tough materials.

- *Smooth cut* – general finishing of precision components and for draw filing.

8.8.2 Types of file

The *shape* of the file selected is governed by its application. Figure 8.13 shows some of the more commonly used files and typical applications.

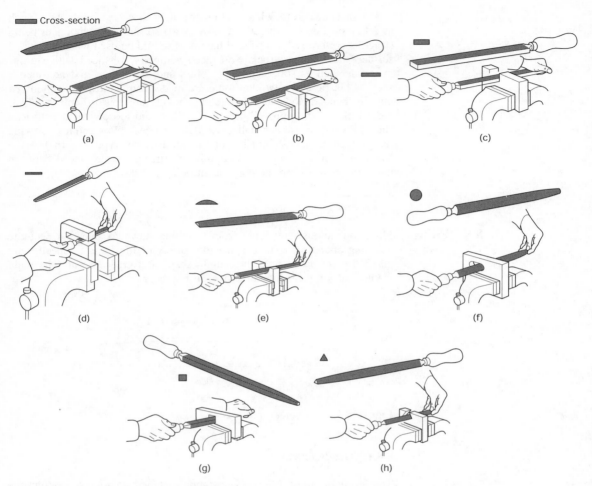

Figure 8.13 *Types of file and their applications: (a) flat file; (b) hand file; (c) pillar file; (d) ward file; (e) half-round file; (f) round file; (g) square file; (h) three-square file*

Flat file

A flat file is shown in Fig. 8.13(a). It tapers for the last third of its length and the last third of its thickness. It is double cut on both faces and single cut on both edges. It is used for the general filing of flat surfaces.

Hand file

A hand file is shown in Fig. 8.13(b). It is parallel in width but tapers slightly in thickness. It is double cut on both faces and is single cut on one edge only. The other edge is left smooth and is called a *safe edge*.

Pillar file

A pillar file is shown in Fig. 8.13(c). It is similar to a hand file but is narrower, thicker and does not taper. It is useful for work in narrow slots. Because of its thickness it is able to withstand a greater downward pressure and because it is narrower than a hand file it can 'bite' more readily into the metal.

Warding file

A warding file is shown in Fig. 8.13(d). It is similar in shape to a flat file but smaller and thinner, and it does not taper in thickness. It gets its name from the fact that it was originally used to file the slots between the 'teeth' or *wards* of keys for locks. It is used for filing flat surfaces in narrow slots.

Half-round file

A half-round file is shown in Fig. 8.13(e). Despite its name, it is not semi-circular in section. It is a segment of a circle. Half-round files are double cut on their flat side for general filing, but are single cut on the curved side. They taper in width and thickness for the last third of their length. Half-round files are used for filing concave surfaces and for working into corners.

Round file

A round file is shown in Fig. 8.13(f). This type of file is circular in cross-section and tapers for the last third of its length. Round files are used for opening out circular holes and for rounding internal corners. They are all single cut in the smaller sizes.

Square file

A square file is shown in Fig. 8.13(g). It is square in cross-section and tapers on all sides for the last third of its length. It is usually double cut on all four sides. It is used for filing square and rectangular holes, slots and grooves.

Three-square file

A three-square file is shown in Fig. 8.13(h). It is triangular in cross-section with all its angles at 60°. It is double cut on all three sides and tapers for the last third of its length. It is used for filing corners between 60° and 90°. For angles less than these either a half-round file or a knife-edge file has to be used.

8.8.3 Use of a file

A file can be controlled only if the fitter's body is correctly positioned and balanced. It has already been stated that the vice jaws should be at elbow height for convenience when fitting. This is particularly true when filing. Figure 8.14(a) shows the correct height of the vice and Fig. 8.14(b)

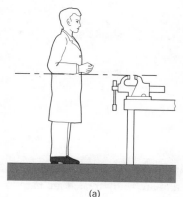

(a)

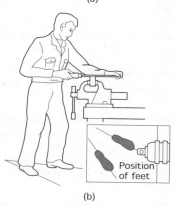

Position of feet

(b)

Figure 8.14 *Use of a file: (a) top of the vice should be in line with forearm held parallel to the ground; (b) position of feet and balance*

shows the correct position for your feet and the way your body should be balanced.

Equally important is the way the file is held. During each stroke, the weight must be gradually transferred from the front hand to the hand gripping the file handle. If this is not done correctly the file will rock and a flat surface will not be produced. Figure 8.15 shows how a file should be held for various operations.

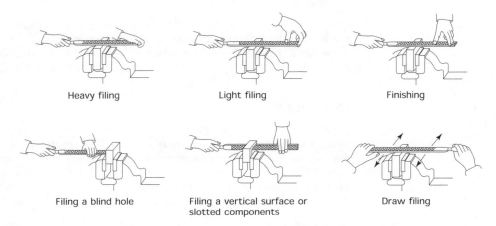

| Heavy filing | Light filing | Finishing |

| Filing a blind hole | Filing a vertical surface or slotted components | Draw filing |

Figure 8.15 *Correct grip for different file applications*

8.8.4 Care of files

Files should be treated with care. Files that are badly treated are hard to use and leave a poor finish and poor accuracy.

- Keep all files in a suitable rack. Do not jumble them up in a draw or keep them with other tools as this will chip and damage the teeth.

- Keep your files clean with a special wire brush called a *file card*. Bits of metal trapped in the teeth reduce the rate of metal removal and score the surface of the work.

- Never use new files on steel. This will chip the teeth and make the file useless. Always 'break in' a new file on softer and weaker metals such as brass or bronze.

- Never file quickly, this only wears out the file and the user. Slow, even strokes using the full length of the file are best.

- Files cut only on the forward stroke. The downward pressure should be eased on the return stroke to reduce wear on the teeth. Do not lift the file off the work on the return stroke. Keeping the file in contact with the work helps to remove the particles of metal that lie between the teeth and also maintains your balance and rhythm that are essential to the production of a flat surface.

8.8.5 Safety when filing

When filing:

- Always ensure that the file is fitted with the correct size of handle and that the handle is secured to the file. Never use a file without a handle. The tang can easily stab into your wrist causing serious damage leading to the paralysis of your fingers.

- A badly fitted handle or the wrong size of handle reduces your control over the file causing you to slip and have an accident.

- A split handle does not protect you from the tang of the file.

8.9 The hacksaw

Figure 8.16(a) shows a typical engineer's hacksaw with an adjustable frame that will accept a range of blade sizes. For the best results the blade should be carefully selected for the work in hand. It must be correctly fitted and correctly used.

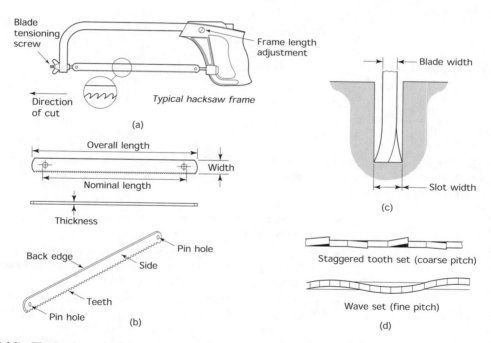

Figure 8.16 *The hacksaw and its blades: (a) engineer's hacksaw showing typical hacksaw frame; (b) hacksaw blade; (c) the effect of set; (d) types of set*

Figure 8.16(b) shows the main features and dimensions of a hacksaw blade. The essential cutting angles have already been discussed in Section 8.5.3. To prevent the blade jamming in the slot that it is cutting, side clearance must be provided by giving the teeth of the blade a *set* as shown in Fig. 8.16(c).

There are two ways in which set may be applied. For coarse pitch blades for general workshop use, the teeth are bent alternatively to the left and right with each intermediate tooth left straight to clear the slot of swarf. Some blades leave every third tooth straight. For fine tooth blades used for cutting sheet metal and thin walled tubes, the edge of the blade is given a 'wave' set. Both types of set are shown in Fig. 8.16(d).

8.9.1 Hints when sawing

- The coarser the pitch of the teeth the greater will be the rate of metal removal and the quicker the metal will be cut. However, there must always be a minimum of three teeth in contact with the metal as shown in Fig. 8.17(a).

Material	Pitch (mm) solid metal	Pitch (mm) tube and sheet
Ferrous metal	1.4–1.6	0.8
Non-ferrous metal	1.8–2.1	1.0–1.2

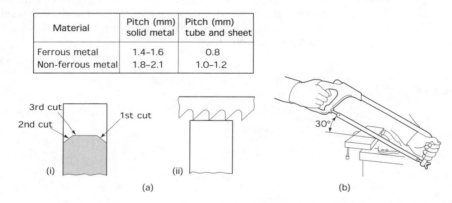

Figure 8.17 *The hacksaw blade: (a) blade selection – (i) a wide component should be broken down in a series of short cuts; (ii) the pitch of the blade should be chosen so that at least three teeth are in contact with the workpiece all the time; (b) use of a hacksaw*

- Thick material should be broken down into shorter surfaces as shown in Fig. 8.17(b).
- 'Rigid' or 'all-hard' high-speed steel blades give the best results but tend to break easily in unskilled hands. 'Flexible' or 'soft-back' blades are best for persons who are not yet fully skilled.
- The teeth of the blade should face the direction of cut and the blade should be correctly tensioned. After the slack has been taken up, the wingnut should be given at least another full turn.
- The rate of sawing should not exceed 50 to 60 strokes per minute.
- The correct way to hold and use a hacksaw is shown in Fig. 8.17(b).
- With use, the blade gradually loses its set and the slot cut will become narrower. For this reason never use a new blade in the slot started by an old blade. It will jam and break. Always start a new cut with a new blade.

8.9.2 Sawing sheet metal

The depth to which a hacksaw can cut is limited to the depth of the frame. Long narrow cuts are often required in sheet metal and, for this purpose, the blade can be turned through 90° as shown in Fig. 8.18(a). It is not so easy to exert downward force on the blade with the saw in this position, but this is not so important when cutting sheet material of limited thickness.

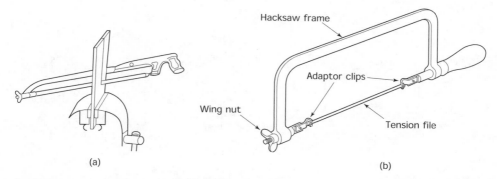

(a)   (b)

Figure 8.18   *Cutting sheet metal: (a) the blade turned through 90° to cut sheet metal; (b) tension file – when the wingnut is tightened, the frame distorts and is put in a state of stress; in trying to spring back to its original shape it exerts a tensile (pulling) force on the blade or file, which is now in a state of tension*

An ordinary hacksaw blade is useless for cutting profiles and, for this purpose, a tension file should be used. This is a long, thin, round file that is kept in tension by the saw frame as shown in Fig. 8.18(b). It is held in the frame by means of adapter clips.

8.10 Screw thread applications

In this book we are concerned only with threads with a V-form. Figure 8.19 shows a typical screw thread and names its more important features.

- The *major diameter* of the thread is the maximum diameter measured over the tops of the threads.

- The *nominal diameter* of the thread is the diameter by which it is known and specified. For most practical purposes it can also be considered to be the same as the major diameter.

- The *pitch (simple effective) diameter* is, as its name suggests, the diameter at which the pitch of the thread is measured. It is also the diameter at which the thickness of the external thread and the thickness of the internal thread are equal.

- The *pitch* is the distance from a point on one thread to an identical point on the next thread.

- The *thread angle* is the angle of the 'V' that gives the thread its form.

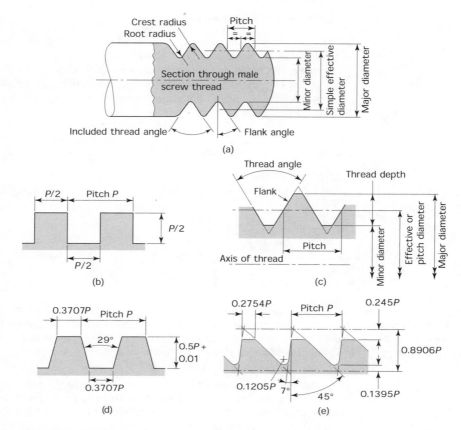

Figure 8.19 *Screw thread elements*

- The *root* is the bottom of the thread – usually radiused.

- The *crest* is the top of the thread – it may be radiused or it may be flat.

- The *flank* is the side of the thread. Only the flanks of the threads should make contact.

8.10.1 Specifying screw threads

To identify a screw thread the following information must be specified.

- *The nominal diameter*. This is stated in metric or inch units.

- *The pitch or the TPI*. For metric threads the actual pitch size is stated in millimetres. For inch units the number of *threads per inch* (TPI) is stated.

- *The type of thread form*. There are various types of thread form and, although metric screw threads should be specified for all new equipment, the older thread forms are still widely used mainly for maintenance purposes.

Let's now consider the V-thread forms that are available to us.

Unified thread form

This has a 60° thread angle and is dimensioned in inch units. It is the basis of unified coarse threads (UNC) and unified fine threads (UNF); these threads originated in the USA but are also used in the UK. A typical example would be specified as 3/8-24 UNF indicating that the thread is unified fine, 3/8″ nominal diameter, 24 threads per inch.

ISO metric thread form

This is the same as the *unified form* but is dimensioned in millimetres. A typical example would be M10 × 1.50 indicating that the thread has a metric form (M), that its nominal diameter is 10 mm and that the pitch of the thread is 1.50 mm.

British Association (BA) thread form

This was originally introduced for the small threaded fasteners used in instruments and later was widely used in electrical equipment. It has a $47\frac{1}{2}°$ thread angle and is dimensioned in millimetres. The largest thread is 0 BA which has a nominal diameter of 6.00 mm and a pitch of 1 mm. The smallest is 25 BA which has a nominal diameter of 0.25 mm and a pitch 0.07 mm. For new equipment this thread system should be replaced with the ISO miniature thread system.

Whitworth thread form

This has a 55° thread angle and is dimensioned in inch units. It is the basis of British Standard Whitworth (BSW), British Standard Fine (BSF), and British Standard Pipe (BSP) threads. A typical example would be specified as $1/2″ \times 12$ BSW indicating that the thread is to British Standard Whitworth form, with a nominal diameter of 1/2 inch, there are 12 threads per inch (TPI). Although the first standardized screw thread system in the world, it is now obsolete.

8.10.2 Screw thread applications

Some typical threaded fasteners and their applications are shown in Fig. 8.20. Note how the joint line of a bolted joint lies across the plain shank of the bolt. It should never lie across the threads. Normal nuts and bolts have *right-hand* threads. With right-handed threads the bolt moves into the nut when it is rotated in a *clockwise* direction. With *left-handed* threads, the bolt moves into the nut when rotated in an *anticlockwise* direction. An example is the double-ended off-hand grinding machine. The nut securing the right-hand grinding wheel has a right-hand thread.

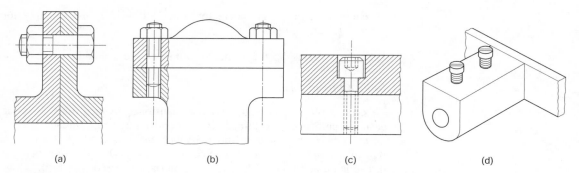

(a)   (b)   (c)   (d)

Figure 8.20 *Use of screwed fastenings: (a) section through a bolted joint – plain shank extends beyond joint face; (b) stud and nut fixing for an inspection cover – this type of fixing is used where a joint has to be regularly dismantled; the bulk of the wear comes on the stud, which can be eventually replaced cheaply which prevents the wear falling on the expensive casting or forging; (c) cap head socket screw – although much more expensive than an ordinary hexagon head bolt, the socket screw is made from high tensile alloy steel, heat treated to make it very strong, tough and wear resistant; socket screws are widely used in the manufacture of machine tools and this example shows how the head may be sunk into a counterbore to provide a flush surface; (d) cheese head brass screws – these are used in small electrical appliances for clamping cables into terminals*

The nut securing the left-hand grinding wheel should have a left-hand thread. This is so that the sudden snatch that occurs when the machine is turned on does not loosen the retaining nuts. Think about it!

As well as fastening things together, screw threads are used to change rotary motion into linear motion and this was discussed earlier (see square threads and acme threads). Screw threads can also provide dimensional control. The micrometer caliper uses a screw and nut as a measuring device. The micrometer dials on machine tool handwheels work in conjunction with their respective lead screws and nuts to provide dimensional control.

8.11 Cutting internal screw threads (use of taps)

Figure 8.21(a) shows a section through a thread-cutting tap and how rake and clearance angles are applied to a thread-cutting tap. Since the 'teeth' are *form relieved*, the clearance face is curved and the *clearance angle* is formed by the tangent to the clearance face at the cutting edge. The rake angle is formed by the flute, so we still have our metal-cutting wedge. Figure 8.21(b) shows a typical thread-cutting tap and names its more important features. Figure 8.21(c) shows a set of three taps.

- The *taper* tap is tapered off for the first 8 to 10 threads and is used first. The taper helps to guide the tap into the previously drilled tapping size hole with its axis parallel to the axis of the hole. The taper also helps to increase the depth of cut gradually and helps to prevent overloading the teeth.

- The *intermediate* or *second* tap has only 3 to 4 threads tapered to guide it into the threaded hole started by the taper tap. This tap can

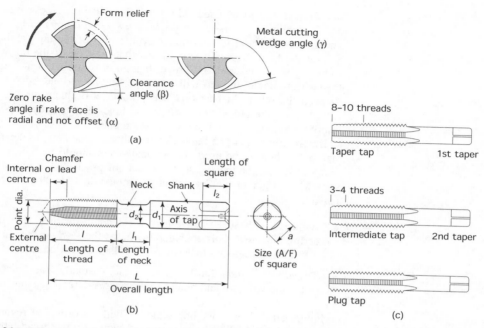

Figure 8.21 *Screw thread taps: (a) cutting angles applied to a thread cutting tap; (b) nomenclature for taps; (c) set of thread cutting taps*

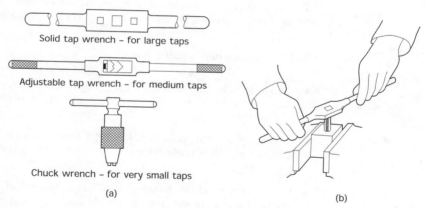

Figure 8.22 *Tap wrenches: (a) types of tap wrench; (b) use of tap wrench*

be used to finish threading a through hole. It also helps to cut full threads near to the bottom of a blind hole.

- The *plug* tap does not have any tapered threads and is used for cutting a full thread to the bottom of a blind hole.

Thread-cutting taps are rotated by means of a tap wrench. Various types of tap wrench are shown in Fig. 8.22(a) and Fig. 8.22(b) shows how a tap wrench should be used. The tap is rotated in a clockwise direction and it should be reversed every one or two revolutions to break up the swarf. It is essential to start and keep the axis of the tap parallel to the axis of the hole. Normally this means that the axis of the tap will be at right angles to the work as shown. If the tap is started at an angle other than a right angle, the tap will cut more heavily on one side of the hole than on the other. At best this will produce a drunken thread, at worst it will cause the tap to break off in the hole. It is usually impossible to remove a broken tap and the work is scrapped.

Before you can cut an internal screw thread, you have to decide on the size of the hole to be used. Theoretically this should be the same as the *minor diameter* of the thread to be cut. In practice, the hole is always somewhat larger in diameter than the minor diameter for the following reasons.

- A thread with 80% engagement is adequate for most general engineering purposes. This considerably eases the load on the tap which is a fragile cutting tool that is easily broken if overloaded.

- The nearest standard drill size available. A smaller one cannot be used or the tap will jam and break, so the nearest larger size has to be used.

Published sets of workshop tables provide information regarding tapping drill sizes. Table 8.1 shows part of such a screw thread table. To cut an M10 × 1.5 metric thread the table recommends the use of an 8.50 mm diameter drill to give the 80% engagement or an 8.60 mm diameter drill if 70% engagement would be adequate. Compare these sizes with the minor diameter of this thread which is 8.376 mm (minimum).

8.11.1 Hints when tapping holes

- Make sure the taps are sharp and in good condition (no chipped or missing teeth) or they will jam and break off in the hole scrapping the job.

- Use a cutting compound that has been formulated for thread cutting. Lubricating oil is useless since it cannot withstand the cutting forces involved.

- Select the correct size of tap wrench to suit the size of the tap you are using. The wrong size will inevitably lead to a broken tap. A range of tap wrenches should be available.

- Make sure the tap is at right angles to the surface of the component. Figure 8.23(a) shows a large tap being checked with a try-square. Figure 8.23(b) shows a method of ensuring a small tap is started in line with the hole. Unfortunately you will need to make a guide bush for each size of tap. However, you will most likely find that you keep using a small range of sizes on a regular basis. The hole through the bush is not threaded but is a precision clearance fit on the tap simply to give guidance.

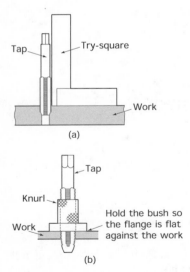

Figure 8.23 *Starting the tap: (a) checking a tap with a try-square to ensure it is aligned with the hole; (b) use of a bush to start a small tap*

TABLE 8.1 *Screw thread data*

ISO metric tapping and clearance drills, coarse thread series

Nominal size	Tapping drill size (mm)		Clearance drill size (mm)		
	Recommended 80% engagement	Alternative 70% engagement	Close fit	Medium fit	Free fit
M1.6	1.25	1.30	1.7	1.8	2.0
M2	1.60	1.65	2.2	2.4	2.6
M2.5	2.05	2.10	2.7	2.9	3.1
M3	2.50	2.55	3.2	3.4	3.6
M4	3.30	3.40	4.3	4.5	4.8
M5	4.20	4.30	5.3	5.5	5.8
M6	5.00	5.10	6.4	6.6	7.0
M8	6.80	6.90	8.4	9.0	10.0
M10	8.50	8.60	10.5	11.0	12.0
M12	10.20	10.40	13.0	14.0	15.0
M14	12.00	12.20	15.0	16.0	17.0
M16	14.00	14.25	17.0	18.0	19.0
M18	15.50	15.75	19.0	20.0	21.0
M20	17.50	17.75	21.0	22.0	24.0
M22	19.50	19.75	23.0	24.0	26.0
M24	21.00	21.25	25.0	26.0	28.0
M27	24.00	24.25	28.0	30.0	32.0
M30	26.50	26.75	31.0	33.0	35.0
M33	29.50	29.75	34.0	36.0	38.0
M36	32.00	–	37.0	39.0	42.0
M39	35.00	–	40.0	42.0	45.0
M42	37.50	–	43.0	45.0	48.0
M45	40.50	–	46.0	48.0	52.0
M48	43.00	–	50.0	52.0	56.0
M52	47.00	–	54.0	56.0	62.0

8.12 Cutting external screw threads (use of dies)

Figure 8.24(a) shows how the basic cutting angles are applied to a thread-cutting button die. You can see that a die has rake, clearance and wedge angles like any other cutting tool. Figure 8.24(b) shows the main features of a button die, whilst Fig. 8.24(c) shows a typical diestock that is used to rotate the die. Figure 8.24(d) shows how the die is positioned in the diestock.

Screw thread dies are used to cut external threads on engineering components. The split button die shown in Fig. 8.24 is the type most widely used by a fitter. The diestock has three adjusting screws. The centre screw engages the slot in the die and spreads the die to reduce the depth of cut. The other two screws close the die and increase the depth of cut. As for a tap the die must be started square with the work axis as shown in Fig. 8.25(a). It is difficult to control a screw-cutting die and any attempt to cut a full thread in one pass will result in a 'drunken' thread. It is better

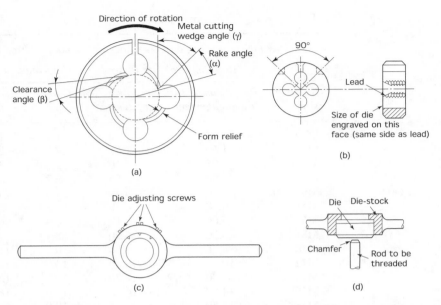

Figure 8.24 *Split button dies: (a) cutting angles applied to a thread-cutting die; (b) split die; (c) diestock; (d) positioning of die in stock – the engraved face of the die is visible, ensuring that the lead of the die is in the correct position*

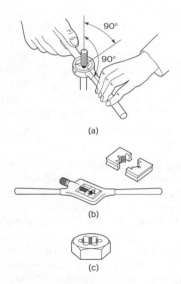

Figure 8.25 *Screw thread dies: alignment and further types: (a) diestock must be aligned with the axis of the work; (b) rectangular split dies; (c) solid die nut*

to open up the die to its fullest extent for the first cut. (This will also produce a better finish on the thread.) Then close the die down in stages for the subsequent cuts until the thread is the required size. The thread size can be checked with a nut. The diestock is rotated in a clockwise direction and should be reversed after every one or two revolutions to break up the swarf. A thread-cutting lubricant must be used.

8.12.1 Miscellaneous thread-cutting devices

Rectangular loose dies

These dies are also used but are less common than button dies. They have a bigger range of adjustment but require a special type of diestock – an example is shown in Fig. 8.25(b).

Die nut

Die nuts, as shown in Fig. 8.25(c), are used for cleaning up bruised threads on existing bolts and studs when carrying out maintenance work. They are not adjustable.

8.12.2 Hints when using screw-cutting dies

- The die has its size and the manufacturer's name on one face only. This is the face that should show when the die is in the stock. This will ensure that the taper lead of the die will engage with the end of the work.

- A chamfer on the end of the work will help to locate the die.

- Start with the die fully open and gradually close it down to the required size in successive cuts.

- Select the correct size of stock for the die. This is largely controlled by the diameter of the die. A range of diestocks should be available.

- Use a cutting compound that has been formulated for thread cutting.

8.13 Hand reamers and reaming

When producing a hole with a twist drill, that hole will invariably have a poor finish, be out-of-round and be oversize. These faults can be overcome by drilling the hole very slightly undersize and correcting it for finish, roundness and size by *reaming*. This can be done by hand at the bench using a hand reamer rotated by a tap wrench or in a drilling machine or lathe using taper shank machine reamers. Reamed holes are usually used for fitting dowels when building up assemblies. Note that dowels only provide location, they are not fasteners.

Figure 8.26 shows a typical parallel hand reamer and names its main features. Hand reamers are rotated by means of a tap wrench and they are rotated in a clockwise direction. When withdrawing the reamer it must continue to be turned in the same direction. *It must not be reversed.* A reamer will always follow the original hole. It *cannot* be used to correct the *position* of a hole. An adjustable reamer is used when a hole of non-standard diameter has to be sized.

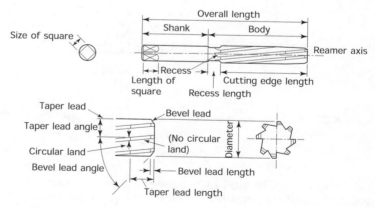

Figure 8.26   *Hand reamer*

8.13.1   Hints when reaming

- Use a suitably formulated cutting compound, lubricating oils are not suitable for reaming.

- Always turn the reamer clockwise. Never reverse it.

- Reamed dowel holes should always be 'through' holes so that the dowel can be knocked out from the reverse side when the assembly has to be dismantled.

- Leave the minimum of metal in the drilled hole to be removed by the reamer. A reamer is only a finishing tool.

- The dowel should be a light drive fit. There is a saying: 'Never use the biggest hammer in the shop to drive a dowel in, since you may need an even bigger one to knock it out.'

8.13.2 Taper pin reamers

Figure 8.27(a) shows typical taper pin reamers. These are used for producing tapered holes in components that require to be locked in place by a tapered pin as shown in Fig. 8.27(b). For this purpose a tapered pin is preferable to a parallel dowel since it locks up tight as it is driven home and is retained by its wedging action. However, it is immediately released when driven back in the opposite direction. Any wear in the hole caused by repeated dismantling and assembly is compensated for by the pin merely having to be driven into the hole a little deeper.

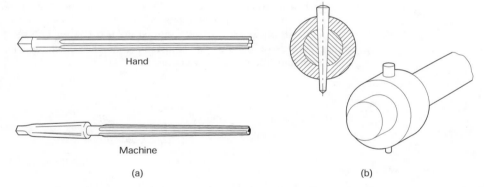

Hand

Machine

(a)   (b)

Figure 8.27 *Taper pin reamers and their use: (a) taper pin reamers; (b) a collar secured to a shaft by means of a taper pin*

8.14 Tools used in assembly and dismantling

Another and very important aspect of the fitter's work is the assembly and dismantling of engineering equipment.

8.14.1 Screwed fastenings

Screwed fastenings are most widely used by bench fitters during the assembly or the dismantling of engineering equipment. Examples of joining techniques using threaded (screwed) fastenings were shown previously in Fig. 8.20.

8.14.2   Locking devices for screwed fastenings

Locking devices are employed to prevent threaded fastenings from slacking off in use as a result of vibration. Some examples of locking devices are shown in Fig. 8.28. You will see that they are divided into two categories. Those which depend upon friction and those where the locking action is positive. Positive locking devices are more time consuming to fit, so they are used only for critical joints where failure could cause serious accidents, for example the control systems of vehicles and aircraft.

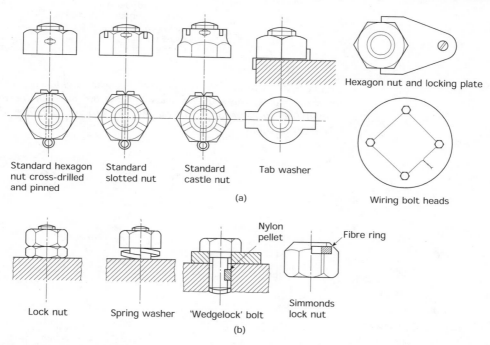

Standard hexagon nut cross-drilled and pinned   Standard slotted nut   Standard castle nut   Tab washer   Hexagon nut and locking plate   Wiring bolt heads

(a)

Lock nut   Spring washer   'Wedgelock' bolt   Nylon pellet   Fibre ring   Simmonds lock nut

(b)

Figure 8.28   *Locking devices for screwed fastenings: (a) positive locking devices; (b) friction locking devices*

8.14.3   Spanners and keys

To turn the nut or the bolt you have to use various types of spanners, keys and wrenches. Spanners are proportioned so that the length of the spanner provides sufficient leverage for a person of average strength to be able to tighten the fastening correctly. A spanner must not be extended to get more leverage. Extending the spanner will overstress the fastening and weaken it. Further, it will also damage the spanner jaws so that they will not fit properly and this can give rise to injuries. Figure 8.29 shows the correct way to use spanners.

8.14.4   Screwdrivers

Screwdrivers must also be chosen with care so that they fit the head of the screw correctly. A variety of screwdrivers and their correct application are shown in Fig. 8.30.

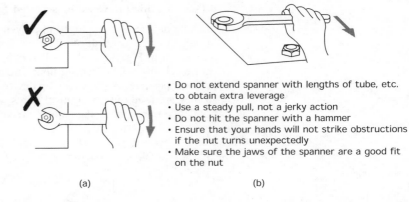

- Do not extend spanner with lengths of tube, etc. to obtain extra leverage
- Use a steady pull, not a jerky action
- Do not hit the spanner with a hammer
- Ensure that your hands will not strike obstructions if the nut turns unexpectedly
- Make sure the jaws of the spanner are a good fit on the nut

(a)   (b)

Figure 8.29 *Correct use of spanners: (a) when tightened correctly, the force exerted on the spanner tends to keep the jaws on the nut; used wrongly, the jaws tend to slip off the nut; (b) pull towards your body whenever possible*

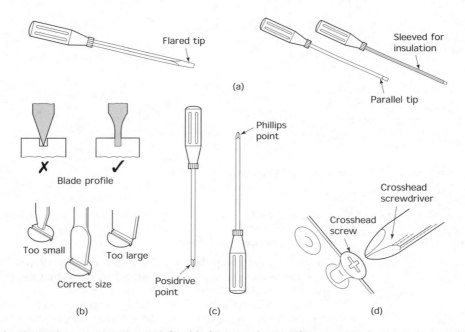

Figure 8.30 *Screwdrivers: (a) types of flat blade screwdriver; (b) correct selection of screwdriver blade; (c) types of crosshead screwdriver; (d) the correct size and type of crosshead screwdriver must always be used for crosshead (recessed head) screws*

8.14.5 Pliers

Pliers are also used for assembly and dismantling operations where they are useful for holding small components and for inserting and removing split pins. Pliers with special jaws are used for removing circlip type fastenings. A selection of pliers and their uses are shown in Fig. 8.31. On no account should pliers be used for tightening or loosening hexagon nuts and bolts.

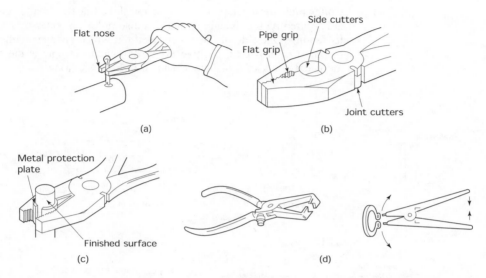

Figure 8.31 *Pliers: (a) flat nose pliers; (b) combination pliers; (c) protecting finished surfaces; (d) circlip pliers*

8.14.6 Miscellaneous fixing and locating devices

Dowels

Threaded fastenings such as screws, bolts and nuts are usually inserted through clearance holes. The exception being 'fitted' bolts which have turned or ground shanks and are inserted through reamed holes. Where clearance holes are used it is necessary to use parallel dowels to provide a positive location between two components. The dowel is manufactured to be a light drive fit in a reamed hole. It is given a slight taper lead so that as it is driven into the hole the metal of the component expands slightly and that of the dowel compresses slightly. The elastic 'spring-back' holds the dowel rigidly in place and ensures positive location. Dowels are case hardened and ground, not only for precision, but to prevent them 'picking up' as they are driven into their holes.

Taper pins

Taper pins are used for fastening components such as collars or handles onto shafts. When the collar or handle has been correctly located on the shaft, a parallel hole is drilled through the component and the shaft. This hole is then opened up using a taper pin reamer of the appropriate size.

The taper pin is then driven home in the tapered hole. A typical example was shown in Section 8.13.2.

Cotter pins

Cotter pins are taper pins with a screw thread at the smaller end. They are secured by the thread and nut that also pulls the cotter tightly against its seating. One side of the cotter has a flat which engages with a flat on the shaft to provide a positive drive. A typical example is the fixing of the pedal crank of a bicycle as shown in Fig. 8.32(a).

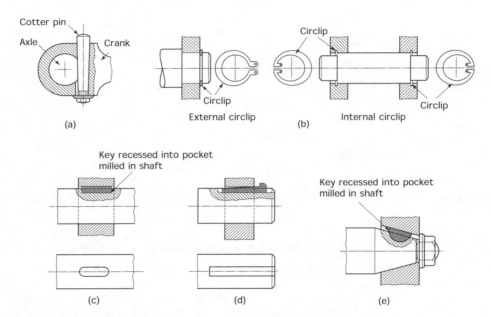

Figure 8.32 *Miscellaneous fixings: (a) cotter pins; (b) circlips; (c) feather key; (d) gib-head key; (e) Woodruff key*

Circlips

These are spring steel clips used for locating components against a shoulder as shown in Fig. 8.32(b). The clips can be opened or closed for fitting by specially shaped pliers that fit into the holes in the lugs at the end of the clips.

Feather key

This type of key fits into a pocket milled into a shaft. It transmits rotational movement between the shaft and the wheel. Generally the pocket is end milled as shown in Fig. 8.32(c). This enables the key and the wheel or other device it is driving to be positioned at any point along a shaft. The key is fitted only on its width and is clearance on its depth. It drives only the wheel or other device and these have to be secured to the shaft positionally by some arrangement such as a set screw.

Gib-head (tapered) key

This type of key is driven into a slot that is cut half into the wheel and half into the shaft. It transmits rotational movement between the shaft and the wheel. Being tapered, the key can be driven in tight and is secured by the spring-back of the metal to form a mechanical compression joint. The wheel, or other device, is secured by friction only, although the drive is positive. For safety, a positive fixing device is also provided. An example of a gib-head key is shown in Fig. 8.32(d) and it can be seen that such a key can be fitted only when the wheel it is driving is mounted on the end of a shaft. The key can be removed by driving a wedge between the wheel hub and the gib-head of the key.

Woodruff key

This is fitted into a segmental socket that is milled into the shaft. It transmits rotational movement between the shaft and the wheel. Since the key can 'float' it is self-aligning and is widely used in conjunction with tapered mountings as shown in Fig. 8.32(e). A special milling cutter is used to cut the pocket in the shaft. The key is used to provide a positive drive. It does not secure the wheel or other device on the shaft. In the example shown, you can see that a nut is used to secure the wheel in place.

8.14.7 Levers and supports

Levers in the form of crowbars (pinch bars) are widely used for raising heavy objects manually (Fig. 8.33(a)). Levers depend upon the *principle of moments* for their force magnification as shown in Fig. 8.33(b). The greater the distance of the effort from the pivot point (fulcrum), the greater will be the lifting force applied to the load. Similarly, the smaller the distance between the load and the pivot point the greater will be the force applied to the load.

Figure 8.33(c) shows two types of pinch bar (crowbar) and their correct use. *Never* use a brittle packing material, such as a brick, for the fulcrum. This can collapse without warning leading to an accident. Wood is the best material since the bar will bite into the wood and this prevents the bar from slipping. Also, if the load is too great, you can see the bar starting to sink into the wood and you can release the load in a controlled manner so as to prevent an accident. Metal is the strongest packing but there is always the danger of the bar slipping on it.

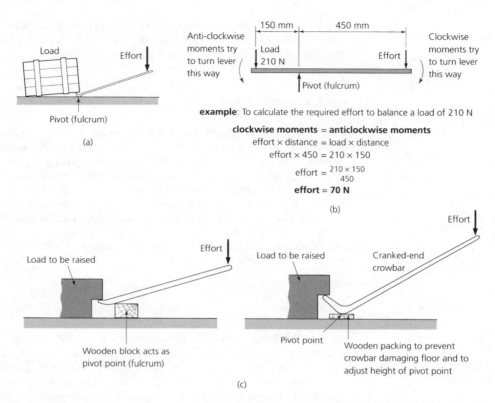

Figure 8.33 *Levers (crowbars) and supports: (a) crowbar; (b) principle of moments applied to a lever – if the effort is less than 70 N the lever will rotate in an anticlockwise direction; if the effort is greater than 70 N the lever will rotate in a clockwise direction; (c) use of crowbars*

Press down on the bar with the flat of your hand. Never wrap your fingers round it. If the bar slipped, your fingers would be trapped between the bar and the floor and your fingers would be broken and crushed.

Never work under equipment that is suspended from a hoist. Always lower the equipment onto suitable supports before commencing work as was shown in Fig. 1.25.

8.15 Preparation of hand tools

Before using hand tools they should be checked to see if they are fit and safe for use.

- Files should be checked to see if the handle is properly fitted on the tang, that the handle is not split, and that the handle is a suitable size for the file.

- Files should be checked to see if the teeth are clean. If there are particles of metal between the teeth they should be removed with a file card. If the teeth have a glazed or shiny appearance, the file will be blunt and should be exchanged for one in better condition.

- Hacksaw blades should be checked for missing teeth and lack of set; they should be securely mounted in the saw frame and correctly tensioned. There should be no twist in the blade.

- Hammer heads must be secure and undamaged. They must not be cracked or chipped. The shaft of a hammer must not be split or damaged.

- Chisels must have sharp cutting edges and be correctly ground. The head of the chisel must not be 'mushroomed'. If it is 'mushroomed' the head of the chisel must be dressed on an off-hand grinding machine to restore its correct shape before use.

- Never use defective equipment: report it immediately to the appropriate person.

Note: The double-ended off-hand grinding machine and its use will be discussed in Chapter 12.

8.16 Making a link

Let's now consider the manufacture of the link previously introduced in Section 7.6 when discussing marking-out techniques. This time we are going to consider its manufacture. Table 8.2 lists the operations for two alternative ways of producing this link.

TABLE 8.2 *Making the link*

Method 1	Method 2
1. Set up for drilling whilst sides of blank are still parallel	1. Set up for drilling whilst sides of blank are still parallel
2. Drill pilot holes	2. Drill pilot holes
3. Drill for reaming	3. Drill for reaming
4. Ream to size	4. Ream to size
5. Remove surplus metal with hacksaw or band saw leaving minimum metal to clean up	5. Remove surplus metal by chain drilling and chiselling
6. File smooth	6. File smooth
7. Deburr	7. Deburr
8. Check	8. Check
9. Grease up	9. Grease up

Note: The marking out of the link has already been described in *Fundamentals of Engineering*. This table is concerned with the manufacture of the link.

A common mistake is to rush into cutting out the component from the stock material as the first operation. A little thought will show that once this component is cut out, it will be very difficult to hold in a vice for drilling the holes. That is why the operation sequence given in Table 8.2

recommends that all drilling operations are done first. Figure 8.34 shows a suitable drilling set-up. Since the link is relatively thin compared with the diameter of the holes it is advisable to drill a 6 mm diameter pilot hole and then open up the hole in two steps to the required 18 mm diameter, and three steps for the 25 mm diameter hole. Further, because the plate is relatively thin compared with the diameter of the holes, there will be a tendency for the larger drills to chatter and leave a rough finish and a hole that is not truly round. Therefore it is advisable to drill the holes 0.5 mm under size and finish them with a reamer using a suitable cutting fluid. Drilling and machine reaming operations are considered in detail in Chapter 9.

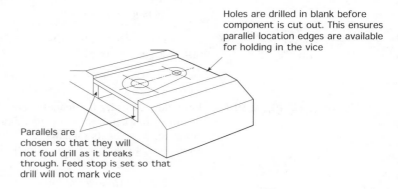

Holes are drilled in blank before component is cut out. This ensures parallel location edges are available for holding in the vice

Parallels are chosen so that they will not foul drill as it breaks through. Feed stop is set so that drill will not mark vice

Figure 8.34 *Drilling the link*

Table 8.2 gives the options of:

- Sawing away the surplus material round the blank.
- Chain drilling and chiselling.

For a component of this size and shape there is little to choose between the two methods. However, had the material been thicker, then chain drilling and chiselling would have been the better way. Figure 8.35 shows the additional holes that would have had to be drilled whilst the blank was still set up for drilling and reaming the two large holes.

Figure 8.36(a) shows how the surplus metal is removed by using a chisel to break through the webs between the drilled holes. Note that as for any chipping operations the following precautions must be observed.

- Wear safety glasses or goggles.
- Do note chip towards another person.
- Place a chipping screen in front of your vice.

Figure 8.36(b) shows the problems that can occur when the material is thick and shows how the problems can be overcome by using a special chisel made from a piece of worn-out power hacksaw blade.

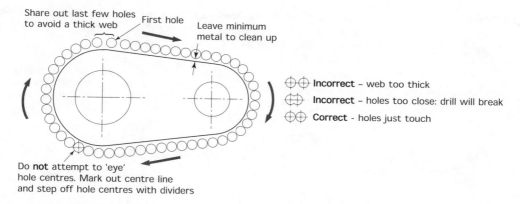

Share out last few holes to avoid a thick web

First hole

Leave minimum metal to clean up

Incorrect – web too thick

Incorrect – holes too close: drill will break

Correct - holes just touch

Do **not** attempt to 'eye' hole centres. Mark out centre line and step off hole centres with dividers

Figure 8.35 *Chain drilling*

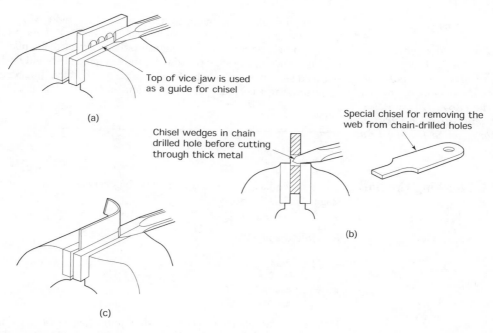

Top of vice jaw is used as a guide for chisel

(a)

Chisel wedges in chain drilled hole before cutting through thick metal

Special chisel for removing the web from chain-drilled holes

(b)

(c)

Figure 8.36 *(a) Use of the chisel to remove surplus material; (b) problem when chiselling through thick metal – a chisel made from an old piece of HSS power hacksaw blade (right) will not wedge; note the cutting edge is ground off square; not a chisel edge; (c) cutting thin sheet metal using a cold chisel*

Figure 8.36(c) shows how sheet metal can be cut using the shearing effect of the chisel used in conjunction with the vice jaws.

The roughed-out link is now ready for finishing by filing away the rough edges left by sawing or chain drilling and chiselling. Until you are more practised, filing the sides flat and straight can best be achieved by

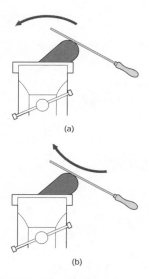

(a)

(b)

Figure 8.38 *Filing: generation of a curve: (a) incorrect – filing up and over a radius requires an unnatural arm action; this results in a untrue curve; (b) correct – filing in this direction gives a natural arm action leading to a true curve*

using a piece of old hard-back hacksaw blade as a guide as shown in Fig. 8.37.

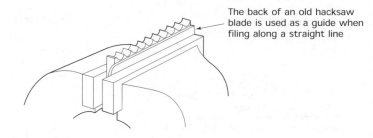

The back of an old hacksaw blade is used as a guide when filing along a straight line

Figure 8.37 *Filing to a straight line*

Some difficulty is often encountered when filing radii. Many beginners try to file over the radius as shown in Fig. 8.38(a). This produces an unnatural arm action and a poor result. The correct technique for filing radii is shown in Fig. 8.38(b). Finally the component should be deburred; sharp edges removed and checked for size. After which, it can be greased up to prevent it corroding and stored until required.

8.17 Checking the link

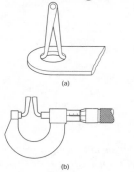

(a)

(b)

Figure 8.39 *Link: checking the hole diameters: (a) inside calipers are set to the hole diameter; (b) taking care not to disturb the calipers, they are checked with a micrometer to determine the diameter of the hole*

The link we have just made must now be checked. This is done in three stages.

- Hole diameters.

- Hole centres.

- Profile.

Hole diameters can be checked using plug gauges or standard workshop measuring equipment. For example, Fig. 8.39 shows the use of inside calipers and a micrometer. For holes of this size it might be better to use a vernier caliper since the pressure of the micrometer anvils may change the setting of the inside caliper. Great care would need to be taken.

There are several possibilities for measuring the hole centres and two alternatives are shown in Fig. 8.40. If dowels are not available, pieces of silver steel of the correct diameter would be suitable for the accuracy of this component. Finally the profile is checked as shown in Fig. 8.41 and marked with the inspector's stamp.

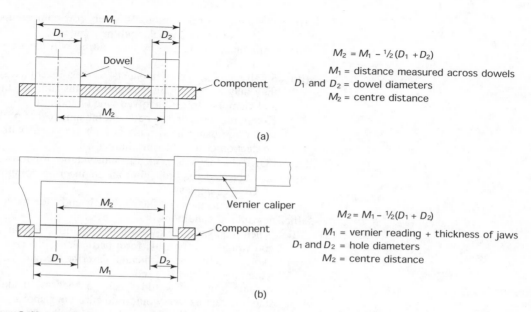

$$M_2 = M_1 - \tfrac{1}{2}(D_1 + D_2)$$

M_1 = distance measured across dowels
D_1 and D_2 = dowel diameters
M_2 = centre distance

(a)

$$M_2 = M_1 - \tfrac{1}{2}(D_1 + D_2)$$

M_1 = vernier reading + thickness of jaws
D_1 and D_2 = hole diameters
M_2 = centre distance

(b)

Figure 8.40 *Link: checking hole centres: (a) checking across dowels; (b) checking with a vernier caliper – always check to outside of holes to obtain line contact*

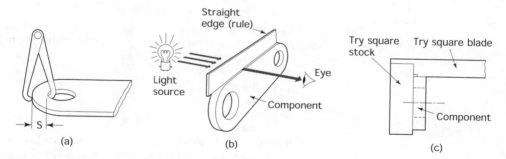

Figure 8.41 *Link: checking profile: checking end radii – knowing the hole diameters, the end radii can be checked with outside calipers using the formula $S = R - \tfrac{1}{2}D$, where S = caliper setting, R = end radius and D = hole diameter; (b) checking straight lines – light will be visible between straight edge and component where any hollows exist in the profile of the component; (c) checking edges for perpendicularity (also check against light source as in (b))*

Exercises   **8.1**   *Selecting suitable hand tools*

(a)   Indicate whether the following statements are TRUE or FALSE, giving the reason for your choice.

(i)   Bench fitting, using hand tools, is suitable for the mass production of engineering components.

(ii) The initial cost of hand tools is very low compared with the cost of machine tools and their cutters.

(iii) Components produced by hand fitting will have a poor finish and low accuracy.

(iv) Small and delicate components are best machined since they may not be strong enough to withstand the cutting and clamping forces involved when hand fitting.

(v) Except for some prototype work, the unit cost of production when using hand tools is high compared with the production costs when machining.

(b) State FOUR factors that will affect the choice of tools and equipment selected for producing an engineering component by hand. Give examples.

(c) List the requirements of a fitter's bench and vice to ensure efficient working conditions.

(d) (i) When requisitioning a file from the stores, explain how you would specify a file for a particular job.

(ii) Sketch FOUR types of file and describe the purposes for which they would be used.

(iii) Explain how you would specify a hacksaw blade and state the factors that would influence your choice.

(iv) Sketch two typical cold chisels and describe the purposes for which they would be used.

(v) Describe the hazards associated with chipping and the safety precautions that should be taken for this operation.

8.2 *Preparation of hand tools*

(a) Name the faults you would look for before using the following items of equipment:
(i) hammer;
(ii) chisel;
(iii) file;
(iv) spanner;
(v) screwdriver.

(b) Briefly describe the five principal precautions that should be taken when storing and using files to ensure that they are maintained in good condition.

(c) Briefly explain why spanners should not be extended to provide additional leverage.

8.3 *Principles of material removal*

(a) Name the three fundamental cutting angles of cutting tools.

(b) Explain briefly how the properties of the workpiece material can influence these angles.

(c) With the aid of a sketch show how the cutting angles are applied to a cold chisel, a scraper and the teeth of a hacksaw blade.

(d) Explain why a hacksaw blade has to have a 'set' and, with the aid of a sketch, show how this 'set' can be applied to the teeth of the blade.

8.4 *Screw threads and fastenings*

(a) (i) Name the type of thread form used on the majority of nuts and bolts.

  (ii) A detail drawing specifies a screw thread as M12 × 1.25. What does this signify?

(b) With the aid of sketches describe how you would cut an internal thread specified as M8 × 1.00. How would you select a suitable tapping size drill? What size would you use?

(c) State why a diestock has three screws around the die pocket and explain how these screws are used.

(d) With the aid of sketches describe two positive and two frictional locking devices for screwed fastenings.

8.5 *Reamers and reaming*

(a) Indicate whether the following statements are TRUE or FALSE, giving the reason for your choice.

  (i) Hand reamers are used to correct the position of hole centres.

  (ii) Hand reamers are used to improve the accuracy and roundness of drilled holes.

  (iii) Taper reamers are used to correct holes that have become tapered.

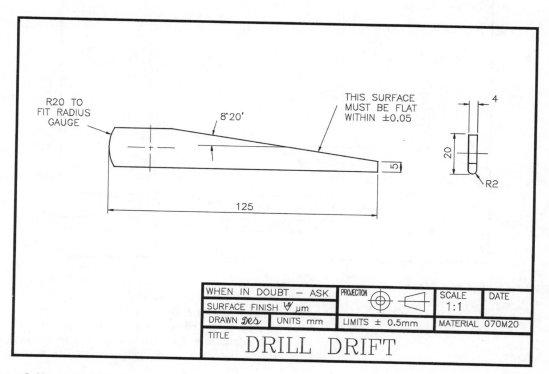

Figure 8.42 *Exercise 8.6(a)*

(iv) Reamers are only finishing tools and can remove only small amounts of metal compared with drills.

(b) Briefly describe FOUR precautions that should be taken when reaming to ensure that an accurate hole of good finish is obtained.

8.6 *Workshop applications*

(a) Figure 8.42 shows a simple drift for removing taper shank drills. Draw up an operation schedule for its manufacture listing the tools and measuring equipment required.

(b) The design of the drift is modified to allow a 4 mm diameter hole to be drilled through the wider end so that it can be hung up on a hook when not in use. The hole is to lie on the centre line 8 mm from the wide end.

 (i) Describe how the hole position should be marked out prior to manufacture and list the equipment required.

 (ii) Explain how the modification will affect the operation schedule previously described if the blank is to be held in a machine vice whilst the hole is drilled.

(c) Figure 8.43 shows the jaws for a toolmaker's clamp.

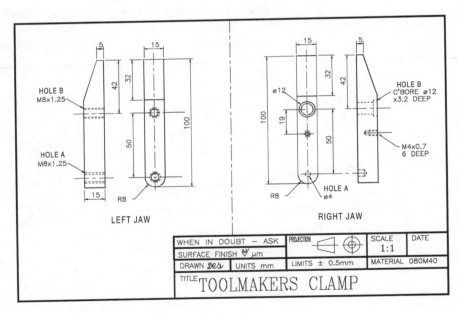

Figure 8.43 *Exercise 8.6(c)*

(d) (i) Draw up an operation schedule for manufacturing these jaws. Refer to Chapter 9 for advice on drilling the holes.

 (ii) With reference to Chapter 4, describe how the jaws can be case hardened and suggest a method of keeping the screw threads soft.

9 Drilling techniques and drilling machines

When you have read this chapter you should understand the:

- Application of cutting principles as applied to twist drills.
- Application of cutting angles as applied to twist drills.
- Types of drills that are normally available.
- Application of cutting angles to hand tools.
- Techniques for drilling, reaming, countersinking and counterboring holes in workpieces.
- The basic construction and use of bench and pillar drilling machines.

9.1 The twist drill

A twist drill does not produce a precision hole. Its sole purpose is to remove the maximum volume of metal in the minimum period of time. The hole drilled is never smaller than the diameter of the drill, but it is often slightly larger. Dimensional inaccuracy of the hole is brought about by incorrect grinding of the drill point causing the drill to flex. The hole is often out of round, especially when opening up an existing hole with a two flute drill. The finish is often rough and the sides of the hole scored. Thus a twist drill should be used only as a roughing-out tool and, if a hole of accurate size, roundness and good finish is required the hole should be finished by reaming or by single point boring.

The modern twist drill is made from a cylindrical blank by machining two helical grooves into it to form the *flutes*. The flutes run the full length of the body of the drill and have several functions:

- They provide the rake angle.
- They form the cutting edge.
- They provide a passage for any coolant/cutting lubricant.
- They provide a passage for the swarf to leave the hole.

The flutes are not parallel to the axis of the drill but are slightly tapered, becoming shallower towards the shank of the drill as shown in Fig. 9.1(a). This allows the web to be thicker at the shank than at the point of the drill and provides a compromise between the strength and cutting efficiency. A thick web would give maximum strength, but a thin web is required at the point of the drill to give an efficient 'chisel edge' for drilling from the solid. Thus a drill that has been reduced in length by repeated sharpening requires 'point thinning' to compensate for the thickening of the web.

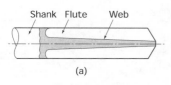

Shank   Flute   Web

(a)

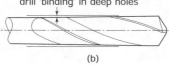

Body clearance to prevent drill 'binding' in deep holes

(b)

Figure 9.1 *Taper in the twist drill body: (a) web thickness – to give strength to the drill the web thickens towards the shank and the flutes become shallower; point thinning becomes necessary as the drill is ground back; (b) body clearance – the body of the drill is tapered towards the shank to give clearance in the drilled hole*

The *lands* are also ground with a slight taper so that the overall diameter of the drill is less at the shank end than at the point as shown in Fig. 9.1(b). This increases the life of the drill and increases its cutting efficiency by preventing the drill from binding in the hole, with a consequent increase in drill life and efficiency. The tapers of the core and the drill body are shown in Fig. 9.1 where they have been exaggerated for clarity.

Figure 9.2 shows a typical twist drill and names its more important features. Although a taper shank drill is shown, the same names apply to parallel shank drills.

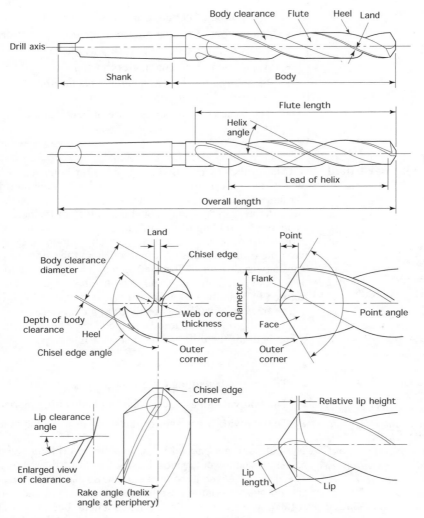

Figure 9.2 *Twist drill elements*

9.2 Twist drill cutting angles

Like any other cutting tool the twist drill must be compared with the correct cutting angles. Figure 9.3(a) shows how the basic metal cutting wedge is applied to this cutting tool. Because the rake angle is formed by a helical groove (one of the flutes), the rake angle varies from point to point along the lip of the drill as shown in Fig. 9.3(b). You can see that it varies from a positive rake angle at the outer corner of the drill to a negative rake angle near the centre of the drill. The fact that the cutting conditions are poor at the point of the drill does not affect the quality of the hole produced by the outer corner where the cutting conditions are relatively good.

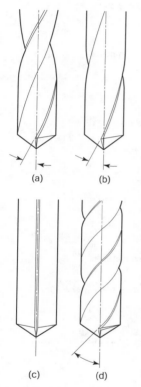

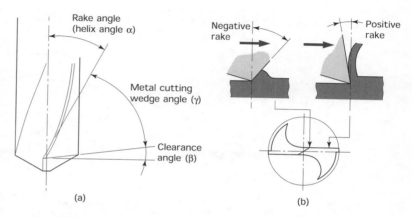

Figure 9.3 *Twist drill cutting angles: (a) cutting angles applied to a twist drill; (b) variation in rake angle along lip of drill – note that the rake angle at the periphery is equal to the helix angle of the flute*

The poor cutting conditions at the chisel point of the drill resist its penetration into the metal being cut. This is why, when drilling a large diameter hole, it is often preferable to drill a pilot hole first using a smaller diameter drill. This will have a smaller chisel point and will penetrate the metal more easily, reducing the feed force required and putting less of a load on the drilling machine.

As has already been stated, the *rake angle* of a twist drill is controlled by the helix angle of the flutes. This is fixed at the time of manufacture and can be only slightly modified during regrinding. Some control of the rake angle is possible by choosing drills with the correct rake angle for the material being cut. Figure 9.4 shows some various types available. These are rarely stock items and are only available to order for production purposes where a quantity of any one size can be ordered.

The *clearance angle* of a twist drill can be adjusted during grinding of the drill point. Insufficient clearance leads to rubbing and overheating of the cutting edge. This, in turn, leads to softening and early drill failure. Excessive clearance, on the other hand, reduces the strength of the cutting edge leading to chipping and early drill failure. Excessive clearance also causes the drill to dig in and 'chatter'.

Figure 9.4 *Helix angles: (a) normal helix angle for drilling low and medium tensile materials; (b) reduced or 'slow' helix angle for high tensile materials; (c) straight flute for drilling free-cutting brass – to prevent drill trying to draw in; (d) increased helix angle or 'quick' helix for drilling light alloy materials*

As well as varying the clearance and rake angle of the drill, its performance can also sometimes be improved by modifying the point angle from the standard 118° for certain materials. Where a large number of drills of the same size are being purchased, the *web* and *land* can also be varied by the manufacturer with advantage. Figure 9.5 shows how the point angle, web and land should be varied for the materials being cut.

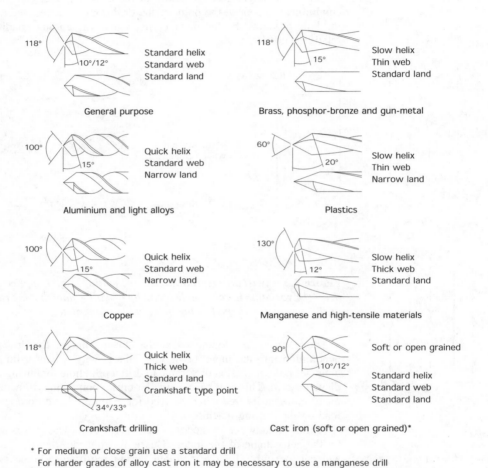

118° 10°/12°
Standard helix
Standard web
Standard land

General purpose

118° 15°
Slow helix
Thin web
Standard land

Brass, phosphor-bronze and gun-metal

100° 15°
Quick helix
Standard web
Narrow land

Aluminium and light alloys

60° 20°
Slow helix
Thin web
Narrow land

Plastics

100° 15°
Quick helix
Standard web
Narrow land

Copper

130° 12°
Slow helix
Thick web
Standard land

Manganese and high-tensile materials

118° 34°/33°
Quick helix
Thick web
Standard land
Crankshaft type point

Crankshaft drilling

90° 10°/12°
Soft or open grained

Standard helix
Standard web
Standard land

Cast iron (soft or open grained)*

* For medium or close grain use a standard drill
For harder grades of alloy cast iron it may be necessary to use a manganese drill

Figure 9.5 *Point angles*

9.3 Twist drill cutting speeds and feeds

For a drill to give a satisfactory performance it must operate at the correct speed and rate of feed. The conditions upon which the cutting speeds and feed rates given in this chapter are based assume:

- The work is rigidly clamped to the machine table.

- The machine is sufficiently robust and in good condition.

- The work is sufficiently robust to withstand the cutting forces.

- A coolant is used if necessary.

- The drill is correctly selected and ground for the material being cut.

The rates of feed and cutting speeds for twist drills are lower than for most other machining operations. This is because:

- A twist drill is relatively weak compared with other cutting tools such as lathe tools and milling cutters. In a twist drill the cutting forces are resisted only by the slender web. Further, the point of cutting is remote from the point of support (the shank) resulting in a tendency to flex and vibrate.

- In deep holes it is relatively difficult for the drill to eject the chips (swarf).

- It is difficult to keep the cutting edges cool when they are enclosed by the hole. Even when a coolant is used, it is difficult to apply it to the cutting edge. This is because, not only are the flutes obstructed by the chips that are being ejected, but the helix of the flutes tends to 'pump' the coolant out of the hole when the drill is rotating.

Table 9.1 lists a range of cutting speeds for jobbing work using standard high-speed steel twist drills under reasonably controlled conditions. Table 9.2 lists the corresponding rates of feed. If the recommended speed and feeds are not available on the drilling machine being used, always select the nearest alternative feed and speed that is *less* than the recommended rate.

TABLE 9.1 *Cutting speeds for high-speed steel (HSS) twist drills*

Material being drilled	Cutting speed (m/min)
Aluminium	70–100
Brass	35–50
Bronze (phosphor)	20–35
Cast iron (grey)	25–40
Copper	35–45
Steel (mild)	30–40
Steel (medium carbon)	20–30
Steel (alloy – high tensile)	5–8
Thermosetting plastic*	20–30

*Low speed due to abrasive properties of the material.

TABLE 9.2   *Feeds for HSS twist drills*

Drill diameter (mm)	Rate of feed (mm/rev)
1.0–2.5	0.040–0.060
2.6–4.5	0.050–0.100
4.6–6.0	0.075–0.150
6.1–9.0	0.100–0.200
9.1–12.0	0.150–0.250
12.1–15.0	0.200–0.300
15.1–18.0	0.230–0.330
18.1–21.0	0.260–0.360
21.1–25.0	0.280–0.380

Example 9.1   *Calculate the spindle speed in rev/min for a high speed steel drill 12 mm diameter, cutting mild steel.*

$$N = \frac{1000S}{\pi d}$$

where: N = spindle speed in rev/min
S = cutting speed in m/min
d = drill diameter (mm)
π = 3.14

From Table 9.1, a suitable cutting speed (S) for mild steel is 30 m/min, thus:

$$N = \frac{1000 \times 30}{3.14 \times 12} = \textbf{796.2 rev/min}$$

In practice a spindle speed between 750 and 800 rev/min would be satisfactory with a preference for the lower speed.

Example 9.2   *Calculate the time taken in seconds for the drill in Example 9.1 to penetrate a 15 mm thick steel plate.*

- From Example 9.1, the spindle speed has been calculated as 796 rev/min (to nearest whole number).

- From Table 9.2, it will be seen that a suitable feed for a 12 mm diameter drill is 0.2 mm/rev.

$$t = \frac{60P}{NF}$$

$$= \frac{60 \times 15}{796 \times 0.2}$$

where: t = time in seconds
P = depth of penetration (mm)
N = spindle speed (rev/min)
F = feed (mm/rev)

$$= \textbf{5.7 seconds} \text{ (to one decimal place)}$$

The calculation of speeds and feeds for drilling is rarely necessary as tables of speeds and feeds for different sizes of drill and material combinations are published in workshop pocketbooks and by drill manufacturers in both book and wall chart form.

9.4 Twist drill failures and faults

Twist drills suffer early failure or produce holes that are dimensionally inaccurate, out of round and of poor finish for the following general reasons:

- Incorrect regrinding of the drill point.
- Selection of incorrect speeds and feeds.
- Abuse and mishandling.

Table 9.3 summarizes the more common causes of twist drill failures and faults and suggests probable causes and remedies. Most cutting tools receive guidance from the machine tool via their shanks or spindles. Unfortunately, twist drills are too flexible to rely on this alone, and derive their guidance from the forces acting on their cutting edges. If these forces are balanced by correct point grinding the drill will cut a true hole of the correct size. However, if these forces are unbalanced due to faulty point grinding, the hole may be oversize, or the drill may wander and follow a curved path, or only one lip may do all the work and be overloaded, or all of these.

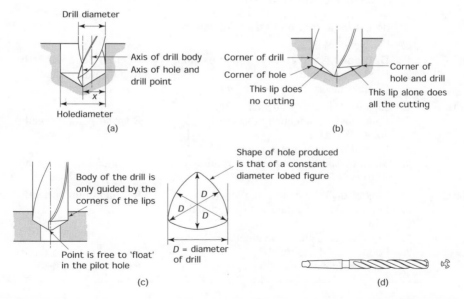

Figure 9.6 *Hole faults: (a) effect of unequal lip length – diameter of hole drilled = 2x, where x = greatest distance from drill point to a corner; oversize hole is caused by drill being ground off centre; (b) unequal angles – only one lip cuts; (c) out of roundness resulting from opening up a pilot hole with a two-flute drill; (d) three-flute core drill will open up an existing hole without loss of roundness*

TABLE 9.3 *Twist drill fault-finding chart*

Failure		Probable cause	Remedy
Chipped lips	1.	Lip clearance angle too large	Regrind point
	2.	Feed too great	Reduce rate of feed
Damaged corners	1.	Cutting speed too high, drill 'blues' at outer corners	Reduce spindle speed
	2.	Coolant insufficient or incorrect	Check coolant
	3.	Hard spot, scale, or inclusions in material being drilled	Inspect material
Broken tang	1.	Drill not correctly fitted into spindle so that it slips	Ensure shank and spindle are clean and undamaged before inserting
	2.	Drill jams in hole and slips	Reduce rate of feed
Broken drill	1.	Drill is blunt	Regrind point
	2.	Lip clearance angle too small	
	3.	Drill point incorrectly ground	
	4.	Rate of feed too great	Reduce rate of feed
	5.	Work insecurely clamped	Re-clamp more securely
	6.	Drill jams in hole due to worn corners	Regrind point
	7.	Flutes choked with chips when drilling deep holes	Withdraw drill periodically and clean
Damaged point	1.	Do not use a hard-faced hammer when inserting the drill in the spindle	Do not abuse the drill point
	2.	When removing the drill from the spindle, do not let it drop on to the hard surface of the machine table	
Rough hole	1.	Drill point is incorrectly ground or blunt	Regrind point correctly
	2.	Feed is too rapid	Reduce rate of feed
	3.	Coolant incorrect or insufficient	Check coolant
Oversize hole	1.	Lips of drill are of unequal length	Regrind point correctly
	2.	Point angle is unequally disposed about drill axis	
	3.	Point thinning is not central	
	4.	Machine spindle is worn and running out of true	Recondition the machine
Unequal chips	1.	Lips of drill are of unequal length	Regrind point correctly
	2.	Point angle is unequally disposed about drill axis	
Split web (core)	1.	Lip clearance angle too small	
	2.	Point thinned too much	Regrind point correctly
	3.	Feed too great	Reduce rate of feed

Figure 9.6(a) shows that, when drilling from the solid, the drill is controlled by the chisel point. If the chisel point is offset – the lips of the drill are of unequal length – the hole may be round but it will be oversize as shown. Figure 9.6(b) shows a drill point where the two lips are

of equal length but the point angle is not symmetrical. In this case the lip with the shallower angle will do all the work and the imbalance in the cutting forces will cause the drill to 'wander' and follow a curved path. Figure 9.6(c) shows a hole that has been opened up using a two flute drill. In this example the point of the drill is floating in the pilot hole and the drill is controlled only by the outer corners of the cutting edge. The diameter of the hole will be correct (the distance between the two corners) but the shape of the hole will be a *constant diameter lobed* figure as shown. This fault can be overcome by using a multi-flute (core) drill as shown in Fig. 9.6(d). This drill usually has three flutes and gets its name from the fact that it is used for opening up cored holes in castings. Since it has more than two corners for guidance it will produce a more truly round hole. Core drills cannot be used for drilling from the solid. They can be used only for opening up previously drilled pilot holes.

9.5   Blind hole drilling

A 'blind' hole is one that stops part way through the workpiece. The difference between drilling a 'through' hole and drilling a 'blind' hole is that, in the latter case, a means must be found of stopping the in-feed of the drill when it has reached the required depth.

Most drilling machines are provided with adjustable stops attached to the quill as shown in Fig. 9.7(a). You can see that the depth stop is engraved with a rule type scale graduated in millimetre or in inch units on its front face. This scale is used as shown in Fig. 9.7(b). Touch the drill onto the work and note the reading on the scale. Then use the scale to set the stop nut and lock nut. Figure 9.7(c) shows how these nuts stop

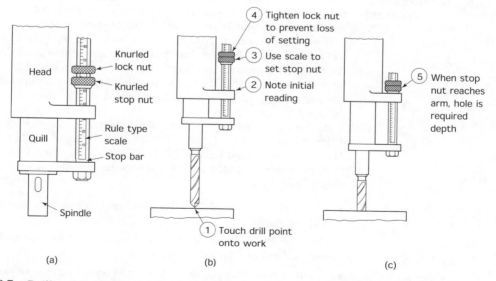

Figure 9.7   *Drilling blind holes: (a) depth stop attachment; (b) setting depth stop (setting = initial reading + depth of hole); (c) drill hole to depth; (d) precision depth setting*

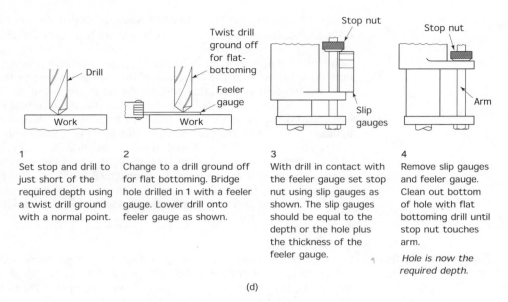

1

Set stop and drill to just short of the required depth using a twist drill ground with a normal point.

2

Change to a drill ground off for flat bottoming. Bridge hole drilled in 1 with a feeler gauge. Lower drill onto feeler gauge as shown.

3

With drill in contact with the feeler gauge set stop nut using slip gauges as shown. The slip gauges should be equal to the depth or the hole plus the thickness of the feeler gauge.

4

Remove slip gauges and feeler gauge. Clean out bottom of hole with flat bottoming drill until stop nut touches arm.

Hole is now the required depth.

(d)

Figure 9.7 *(continued)*

the in-feed of the drill when the set depth has been reached. For precision depth setting, slip gauges can be used as shown in Fig. 9.7(d).

9.6 Reamers and reaming

Reamers have many more flutes than a core drill and are designed as a finishing tool. They will remove only a very small amount of metal, but will leave an accurately sized, round hole of good finish.

Hand reamers were introduced in Section 8.13. They have a taper lead and a bevel lead. The taper lead provides guidance into the hole, whilst the bevel lead removes any excess metal. Cutting takes place on both the bevel and the taper leads. The parallel flutes have a radial land that prevents cutting but imparts a burnishing action to improve the finish of the hole.

Reamers intended for use in drilling machines and lathes have a rather different cutting action. Figure 9.8 shows three types of machine reamer. They differ from hand reamers in several ways. They have a taper shank to fit the machine spindle and they do not have a taper lead. They have only a bevel lead.

- Reamers that cut only on the bevel lead are said to have a *fluted* cutting action.

- Reamers that also cut on the periphery of the flutes (no radial land) are said to have a *rose* cutting action.

- Hand reamers that cut on the bevel and on the tapered section of the flutes but retain a radial land on the parallel section of the flutes are said to have both a fluted and a rose cutting action.

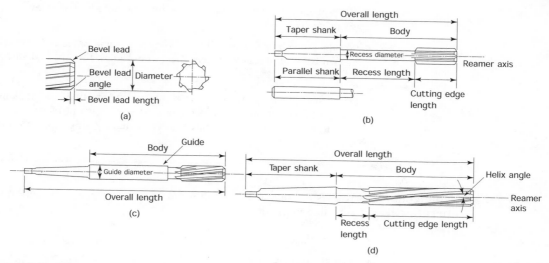

Figure 9.8 *Types of machine reamer: (a) entering end of parallel machine reamer (long fluted machine reamer); (b) machine (chucking) reamer with Morse taper or parallel shank; (c) machine jig reamer; (d) long fluted machine reamer with Morse taper shank, right-hand cutting with left-hand helical flutes*

Long fluted machine reamers

These cut only on the bevel lead where they have a rose cutting action. The flutes have a radial land and are parallel.

Machine chucking reamers and jig reamers

These may have either a rose cutting action or a fluted cutting action. The recessed diameter of the chucking reamer allows it to operate in deep holes without rubbing and also allows room for the swarf so that no scoring of the previously reamed hole can take place. The guide diameter of the jig reamer allows it to be located by the bush in the jig and ensures that it follows the axis of the previously drilled holes. It is sometimes thought that this can lead to ovality of the finished hole and that it is better to let the reamer float and follow the hole itself. There are no hard and fast rules about this.

Fluted reamers give the best results with steels and similar ductile materials, whereas rose-action reamers are best for cast iron, brass and bronze materials. This latter group of materials tends to spring back and close on the reamer. The peripheral cutting edges of the flutes of a reamer with a rose cutting action remove additional metal as the hole shrinks back on the reamer preventing seizure and broken tooling. Similarly, rose-action reamers are preferable when reaming plastic materials as these also tend to close on the reamer.

Although standard reamers are made for right-hand cutting (clockwise rotation of the reamer), they have flutes that are straight or have a left-hand helix. This serves two purposes:

- To prevent the reamer being drawn into the hole by the screw action of the helix.

- To eject the chips (swarf) ahead of the reamer and prevent them being drawn back up the hole, where they would mark the finished surface of the hole.

The reamer always tries to follow the axis of the existing hole: it cannot correct positional errors. If the original drilled hole is out of position or out of alignment, these errors must be corrected by single point boring (see Section 10.16.3).

9.7 Miscellaneous operations

As well as drilling holes the following operations can also be performed on a drilling machine:

- Trepanning.
- Countersinking.
- Counterboring.
- Spot facing.

9.7.1 Trepanning

Not only is it dangerous to try to cut large holes in sheet metal with a twist drill, but the resulting hole will not be satisfactory. Sheet metal and thin plate have insufficient thickness to guide the drill point and resist the cutting forces. This will result in the drill 'grabbing', resulting in a hole that has torn, jagged edges and which is out of round. The metal in which the hole is drilled will also be buckled and twisted round the hole.

One way of overcoming this problem is to use a *trepanning cutter*. Instead of cutting all the metal in the hole into swarf, the trapping cutter merely removes a thin annulus of metal. This leaves a clean hole in the stock and a disc of metal slightly smaller than the hole. The principle of trepanning is shown in Fig. 9.9(a). The simplest type of trepanning cutter is the adjustable 'tank cutter' shown in Fig. 9.9(b). It gets its name from the similar type of cutter used by plumbers for cutting holes in sheet metal water tanks for pipe fittings. The central pilot locates the cutter in a previously drilled hole of small diameter. The one-sided, unbalanced cutting action of this device has a number of disadvantages, and the *hole saw* shown in Fig. 9.9(c) is to be preferred if a number of holes of the same size are to be cut.

9.7.2 Countersinking

Figure 9.10(a) shows a typical countersink bit. This is called a *rose* bit since it cuts on its bevel edges (see the cutting action of reamers: Section 9.6). Since the bit is conical in form it is self-centring and does not require a pilot to ensure axial alignment.

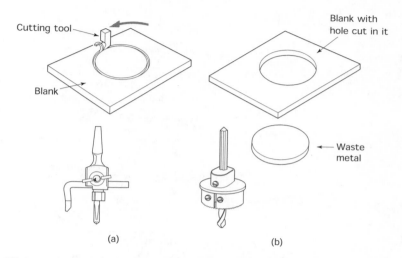

Figure 9.9 *Trepanning large holes: (a) tank cutter; (b) hole saw*

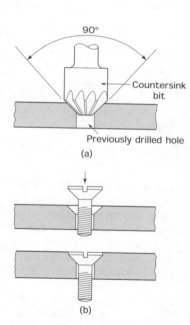

Figure 9.10 *Countersinking: (a) cutting a countersink; (b) the countersink allows head of the screw to be recessed*

Countersinking is mainly used for providing the recess for counter-sunk screws as shown in Fig. 9.10(b). Less deep countersinking is used to chamfer the sharp edges of previously drilled holes to facilitate the insertion of a bolt, to remove sharp edges and burrs that could lead to cuts, and to reduce the risk of cracking when a component has to be hardened.

9.7.3 Counterboring

Counterboring produces a cylindrical recess for housing the head of a cheese-head screw or a socket-head cap screw flush with the surface of a component. Figure 9.11(a) shows a typical counterbore cutter; Fig. 9.11(b) shows a cap head screw within the recess. The type of cutter used is called a *piloted counterbore* and is similar in appearance to a short, stubby end mill with a pilot. The purpose of the pilot is to ensure that the counterbored hole is concentric with the previously drilled hole. (*Concentric* means that both holes have a *common axis*.)

9.7.4 Spot facing

The purpose of spot facing is to produce a local flat surface as shown in Fig. 9.12(a). This provides a seat for a bolt head or a nut. Bolt heads and nuts must always seat on a surface that is square to the axis of the bolt hole so that the shank of the bolt does not become bent. The type of cutter used is similar to a counterbore cutter but with a larger cutter diameter relative to the diameter of the pilot that fits the previously drilled hole. This is because the spot face has to be slightly larger in diameter than the distance across the corners of the hexagon head of the bolt or nut as shown in Fig. 9.12(b).

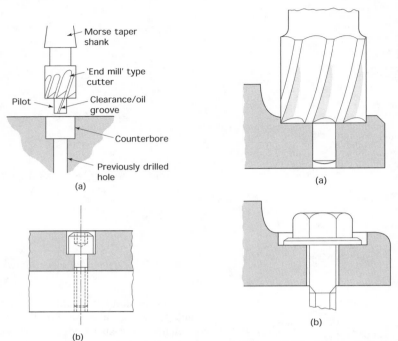

Figure 9.11 *Counterboring: (a) cutting a counterbore; (b) cap head screw recessed into a counterbore*

Figure 9.12 *Spot facing: (a) cutting a spot facing on a casting; (b) spot facing provides a seating for the bolt head*

9.8 Toolholding

The various cutting tools described previously in this chapter have either a *parallel* (cylindrical) shank or a *taper* shank. Figure 9.13(a) shows a drilling machine spindle suitable for locating and driving taper shank tooling. The tool shanks and the bore of the spindle have matching tapers. These are normally *morse tapers*. The morse taper system provides for tapers that are 'self-securing'. That is, the wedging action of the taper prevents the drill, or other tool, from falling out and it also drives the tool.

Table 9.4 lists the range of drill diameters associated with various morse taper shanks. Figure 9.13(b) shows a typical adapter sleeve for use when the taper of the drill shank is smaller than the taper of the spindle. It also shows an adapter socket for use when the taper shank of the drill is larger than the spindle taper or when converting from one taper system to another. Care must be taken not to overload the machine. The tang on the end of the drill shank is only for removing the drill from the taper in the machine spindle. It is *not* for driving the drill. Figure 9.13(c) shows how a drift is used to remove the drill. *On no account must the drill be overloaded so that it slips in the machine spindle.* This damages the taper shank and the taper bore of the machine spindle. This damage (scoring) would prevent the

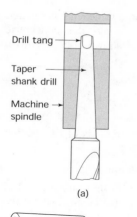

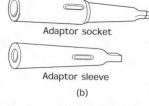

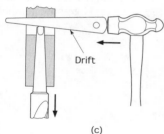

Figure 9.13 *Tool holding: taper shank drills*

TABLE 9.4 *Morse taper shank sizes for twist drills*

Morse taper	Drill diameters for normal taper shanks (mm)	Drill diameters for oversize taper shanks (mm)
MT1	3.00–14.00 (inc.)	–
MT2	14.25–22.75 (inc.)	12.00–18.00 (inc.)
MT3	23.00–31.50 (inc.)	18.25–23.00 (inc.)
MT4	32.00–50.50 (inc.)	26.75–31.75 (inc.)
MT5	51.00–76.00 (inc.)	40.50–50.50 (inc.)
MT6	77.00–100.00 (inc.)	64.00–76.00 (inc.)

taper from holding the drill in position and in alignment with the spindle axis. Further, it would no longer be capable of driving the drill.

Figure 9.14(a) shows a drill chuck used for holding and driving tools with a parallel shank together with its chuck key for tightening and loosening the chuck and a chuck arbor. Some small drilling machines have a spindle nose with an external taper to fit directly into the chuck arbor hole. Such machines cannot be used with taper shank drills and tools. For larger drilling machines the chuck arbor is used. It is permanently inserted into the arbor hole of the chuck and is inserted into the spindle of the drilling machine when parallel shank tools are to be used. It can be removed by means of a drift when taper shank tools are to be used.

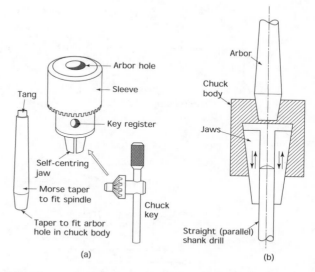

Figure 9.14 *The drill chuck: (a) typical drill chuck and accessories; (b) principle of the drill chuck – this drawing shows how a series of concentric tapers are used to maintain axial alignment between the arbor, the chuck and the drill, jaws are shown at 180° for clarity, and the mechanism for moving the jaws is omitted*

The chuck itself is self-centring and consists of jaws moving in tapered slots. Therefore, because the system consists of a series of concentric tapers, axial alignment is maintained at all times as shown in Fig. 9.14(b).

9.9 Workholding

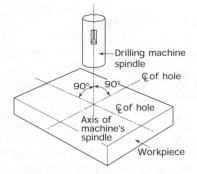

Figure 9.15 *Basic drilling alignments*

To successfully drill a hole in the correct position four basic conditions must be satisfied.

- The axis of the drill must be concentric with the axis of the drilling machine spindle.
- The drill and spindle must rotate together without slip.
- The workpiece must be located so that the axis of the spindle and drill combination passes through the intersection of the centre lines of the hole to be drilled as shown in Fig. 9.15.
- The workpiece must be restrained so that it is not dragged round by the action of the drill.

9.9.1 Rectangular and similar workpieces

These can be bolted directly to the machine table as shown in Fig. 9.16(a) or they can be held in a vice as shown in Fig. 9.16(b). Note how parallel

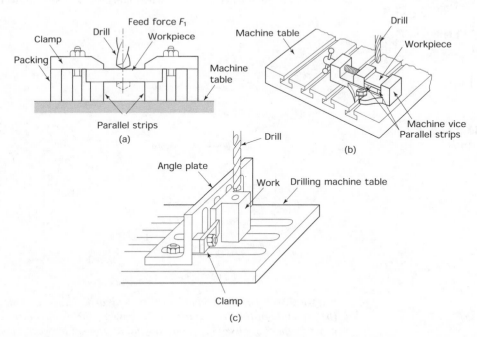

Figure 9.16 *Workholding – rectangular workpieces: (a) direct clamping to the machine table; (b) use of a machine vice; (c) use of an angle plate*

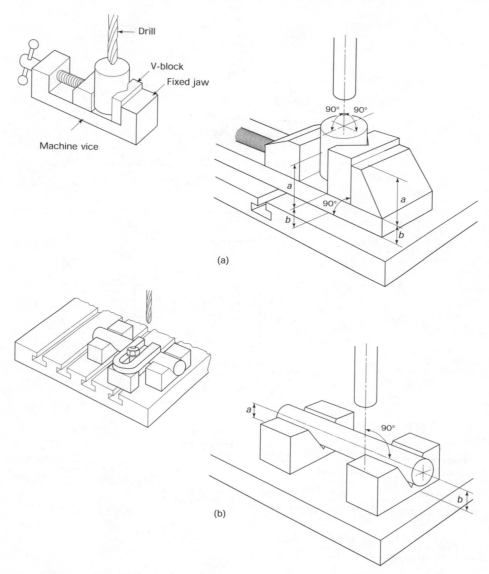

Figure 9.17 *Workholding – cylindrical workpieces: (a) holding cylindrical work in a machine vice – to ensure that the spindle axis is parallel to the workpiece axis (i.e. perpendicular to the end face) the following alignments must be checked:* **1** *– the Vee block must be seated on the vice slide so that its end face is parallel to the slide (a–a);* **2** *– the vice slide must be parallel to the machine table (b–b);* **3** *– the fixed jaw must be perpendicular to the machine table; (b) clamping cylindrical work directly to the machine table – to ensure that the axis of the spindle is perpendicular to the axis of the workpiece, the Vee blocks must be a matched pair so that the workpiece axis is parallel to the machine table (a–a)*

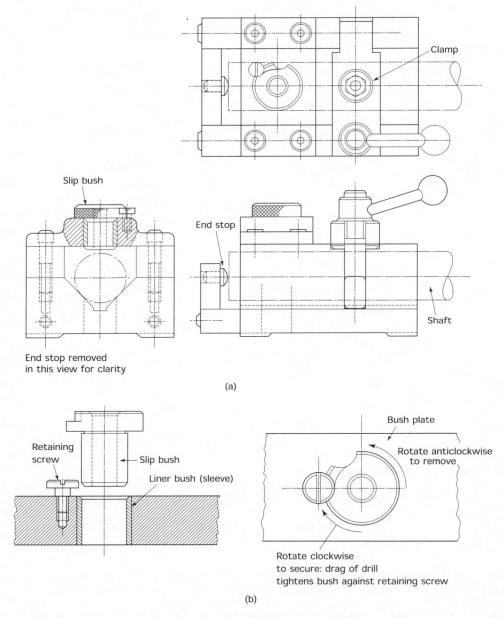

Figure 9.18 *Workholding: drilling jig: (a) simple drill for drilling a hole through a shaft at right angles to the axis of the shaft; (b) removable bush and liner sleeve*

packing strips are used to support the work so as to prevent the drill from damaging the machine table or the vice as the drill breaks through the underside of the workpiece. Sometimes an angle plate is used when the hole is to be drilled parallel to the datum surface of the work as shown in Fig. 9.16(c).

9.9.2 Cylindrical workpieces

Cylindrical workpieces are more difficult to hold since only a line contact exists between a cylindrical surface and a flat surface. It is advisable to insert a Vee block between a cylindrical component and the fixed jaw of a machine vice to provide a three-point location as shown in Fig. 9.17(a). When the cylindrical component is to be mounted in a horizontal position as shown in Fig. 9.17(b) two vee blocks should be used as shown. Vee blocks are always manufactured in matched pairs for situations such as this and they should always be kept as matched pairs.

9.9.3 Drill jigs

These are used where a number of identical components are to be drilled. The jig is bolted or clamped to the machine table so that it locates and restrains every component that is put into it in exactly the same position relative to the axis of the machine spindle. Thus all the components will have their holes in exactly the same position.

The jig also has a drill bush (or bushes if there is more than one hole) to guide the drill so that it does not wander when the hole is being started. Remember that for this sort of work there is no centre punch mark to guide the drill point. The use of jigs eliminates the expensive process of marking out the components individually. Figure 9.18(a) shows a simple drill jig and names its more important parts. Figure 9.18(b) shows details of the removable bush and its liner sleeve. The bush is inserted in the liner sleeve whilst the hole is drilled in the workpiece. The bush is then removed whilst the hole is reamed at the same setting of the workpiece. This allows the reamer to follow the axis of the previously drilled hole. Also the reamer is larger than the drill and would not pass through the drill bush. Sometimes two different size bushes are used: one for drilling a pilot hole and one for drilling out the hole to the finished size.

9.10 The basic alignments of drilling machines

Let's now refer back to Fig. 9.16, which shows the basic alignments of the spindle axis and the workpiece and see how this is achieved.

- The geometry of a drilling machine must ensure that these basic alignments are achieved.

- The machine must be robust enough to maintain these alignments when subjected to the cutting forces resulting from drilling operations.

- The machine must be robust enough to maintain these alignments when subjected to the load of the workpiece on the machine table.

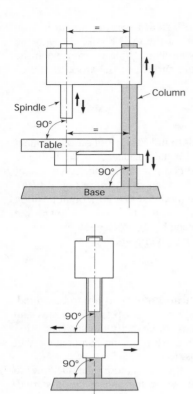

Figure 9.19 *The drilling machine: basic alignments*

The *spindle* of the drilling machine locates and rotates the drill. It is itself located in precision bearings in a *sleeve* that can move in the body of the drilling machine. The sleeve complete with its spindle is called the *quill*, which can move up or down, without losing its axial alignment. This enables the drill to be fed into the workpiece which is supported on the machine table.

The following basic requirements build up into the skeleton of a drilling machine as shown in Fig. 9.19. This figure also shows the geometrical alignments and movements to be described.

● The spindle axis is perpendicular to the surface of the worktable.

● The worktable is adjustable up and down the column to allow for work of different thicknesses and drills of different lengths. It must also be possible to swing the table from side to side on the column to allow for positioning the work.

● The head of the machine can itself be moved up or down the column to provide further height adjustment.

● After making any of the above movements there must be provision for locking the machine elements in position so that the settings will not move whilst drilling is taking place.

● The column is perpendicular to the base.

● The spindle and sleeve (quill) can move up or down to provide in-feed for the drill when cutting, and allow the drill to be withdrawn from the hole when cutting is finished.

● The axes of the column and the spindle are parallel to each other to maintain the alignments as these movements take place.

9.11 The bench (sensitive) drilling machine

This simplest type of drilling machine is the bench drilling machine as shown in Fig. 9.20(a). It is capable of accepting drills up to 12.5 mm (0.5 inch) diameter. Generally these machines have the chuck mounted directly onto the spindle nose taper. However, some have a spindle with a taper bore to accept either a drill chuck or taper shank tooling in the smaller sizes. Variation in spindle speed is achieved by altering the belt position on the stepped pulleys.

Safety. The machine must be stopped and the electrical supply isolated before removing the guard and changing the belt position.

For normal drilling the spindle axis must be perpendicular to the working surface of the worktable. However, if the hole is to be drilled at an

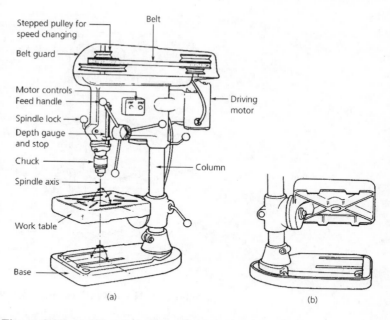

Stepped pulley for
speed changing

Belt

Belt guard

Motor controls

Feed handle

Spindle lock

Depth gauge
and stop

Chuck

Spindle axis

Work table

Base

Driving
motor

Column

(a)

(b)

Figure 9.20 *(a) Bench drilling machine; (b) table tilted*

angle to the workpiece, the table can be tilted as shown in Fig. 9.20(b). Always leave the table horizontal for the next user.

The feed is operated by hand through a rack and pinion mechanism. This type of feed enables the operator to 'feel' the progress of the drill through the material being cut so that the operator can adjust the feed rate to suit the cutting conditions. It is from this close control that the operator has over the feed of the drill, that this type of drilling machine gets its name of a *sensitive drilling machine*. Some sensitive drilling machines have an elongated column so that they can be floor standing instead of bench mounted. Otherwise they are essentially the same machine.

9.12 The pillar drilling machine

Figure 9.21(a) shows a typical pillar drilling machine. It can be seen that it is an enlarged and more powerful version of the machine just described. It is floor mounted and much more ruggedly constructed. The spindle is driven by a more powerful motor and speed changing is accomplished through a gearbox instead of belt changing. Sensitive rack and pinion feed is provided for setting up and starting the drill. Power feed is provided for the actual drilling operation. The feed rate can also be changed through an auxiliary gearbox. The spindle is always bored with a morse taper to accept taper shank tooling as well as a drill chuck.

Figure 9.21(b) shows that the circular worktable can be rotated as well as swung about the column of the machine. This allows work clamped to any part of the machine table to be brought under the drill by a combination of swing and rotation. This enables all the holes to be drilled

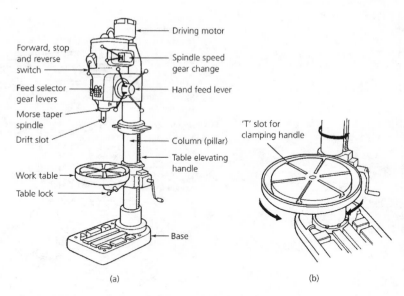

Figure 9.21 *(a) Pillar drilling machine; (b) circular worktable*

in a component without having to unclamp it and reposition it on the worktable. Holes up to 50 mm diameter can be drilled from the solid on this type of machine.

Exercises   **9.1**   *Cutting principles and cutting angles as applied to twist drills*
   (a)   Indicate whether the following statements are TRUE or FALSE giving the reason for your choice.
       (i)   The drilled hole may be larger than the nominal diameter of a twist drill but never smaller.
       (ii)   A twist drill is a single-point cutting tool.
       (iii)   A twist drill provides a hole that is accurate in size and roundness with a good finish.
       (iv)   The web of a twist drill tapers in thickness, increasing towards the shank.
       (v)   The diameter of a twist drill decreases slightly towards the shank.
   (b)   (i)   State the purposes of the flutes of a twist drill.
       (ii)   Sketch a 'D' bit, and briefly describe the advantages and limitations of such a drill and state when it would be used in preference to a twist drill. You will have to research this for yourself.
   (c)   (i)   With the aid of a sketch show how the basic cutting angles of rake, clearance and wedge angle can be applied to a twist drill.
       (ii)   Name a material for which you would require a straight flute drill.

      (iii) Name a material for which you would require a drill whose flutes have a 'slow' helix.

      (iv) Name a material for which you would require a drill whose flutes have a 'quick' helix.

(d) An 8 mm diameter twist drill is to be used at a cutting speed of 40 m/min and a feed rate of 0.15 mm/rev.

    (i) Calculate the required spindle speed in rev/min.

    (ii) Calculate the time taken from the point of contact for the drill to penetrate 12 mm into a component.

9.2 *Twist drill failures and faults*

(a) When drilling a hole, what is indicated by the swarf only being ejected from one flute? Does this matter?

(b) With the aid of sketches show the probable point errors that could result in a drill cutting oversize.

(c) What damage to the drill will result from:

    (i) too high a cutting speed;

    (ii) too high a feed rate.

(d) What are the most likely causes of a rough finish to the hole?

(e) What are the most likely causes of a drill requiring an excessive downward force to make it penetrate into the work?

9.3 *Reamers and reaming*

(a) The use of hand reamers was introduced in Chapter 8. With the aid of sketches show the essential differences between:

    (i) a hand reamer;

    (ii) a long flute machine reamer;

    (iii) a chucking reamer.

(b) (i) In what way do the cutting conditions vary for reaming compared with drilling?

    (ii) Although most reamers are designed for right-hand (clockwise) cutting, they have straight flutes or left-hand helical flutes. Why is this?

9.4 *Miscellaneous drilling operations*

(a) (i) With the aid of sketches show the differences between countersinking, counterboring and spot facing.

    (ii) Explain briefly where the above operations are used and why.

(b) With the aid of sketches show the difference between trepanning and hole sawing. Under what circumstances is hole sawing preferable to trepanning?

9.5 *Tool holding and workholding*

(a) Describe, with the aid of sketches, the two most common methods of holding drills in drilling machines.

(b) Describe, with the aid of sketches:

    (i) TWO methods of holding rectangular work on a drilling machine;

    (ii) TWO methods of holding cylindrical work on a drilling machine.

(c) Large work often has to be clamped directly to the drilling machine table. How can the work be positioned under the drill when using a pillar drill to drill a number of holes, *without* unclamping and resetting the work on the machine table.

9.6 *Drilling machines*
(a) A sensitive drilling machine is often bench mounted and is used for drilling holes of 12 mm diameter or less.
    (i) Explain why it is called a 'sensitive' drilling machine.
    (ii) Explain why it is suitable for drilling small diameter holes.
(b) Describe how a pillar type milling machine differs from a sensitive drilling machine.
(c) With the aid of a sketch show how a DTI can be used to check that the worktable of a drilling machine is perpendicular to the axis of the machine spindle.
(d) Sketch a suitable guard for a sensitive drilling machine.

9.7 *Drilling operations*
Draw up an operation schedule for manufacturing the depth gauge component shown in Fig. 9.22 as a single prototype. List the equipment required. Note that the 9 mm radii would be produced by drilling and reaming to 18 mm diameter before cutting out. You may assume that the blank has been squared up and marked out in readiness for manufacture.

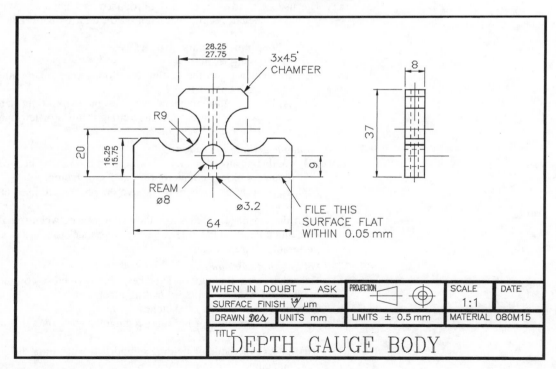

Figure 9.22 *Exercise 9.7*

10 Centre lathe and turning techniques

When you have read this chapter you should be able to:

- Identify the main features of a centre lathe.
- Identify the main movements and alignments of a centre lathe.
- Identify the surfaces produced by the main movements of a centre lathe.
- Identify the types of spindle nose and chuck mounting for centre lathes and appreciate the advantages and limitations of each system.
- Understand the correct procedures for starting up and closing down the machine.
- Identify and select the type of chucks and chuck mountings normally used.
- Understand and use the methods of setting and holding work in various types of chucks.
- Understand and use the methods of holding work between centres.
- Understand and use the normal methods of tool holding.
- Select cutting tools appropriate to the job in hand.
- Select and use drills and reamers appropriate to the job in hand.
- Calculate the speeds and feeds appropriate to the job in hand and set the machine accordingly.
- Produce screw threads in the centre lathe using taps and dies.
- Produce knurled surfaces.
- Apply the above techniques to typical workpieces.

10.1 The safe use of machine tools

10.1.1 Personal safety

- Do not use a machine unless you have received instruction in its operation.
- Do not use a machine without the permission of your instructor or supervisor.
- Do not lift heavy workpieces or workholding devices onto a machine without assistance or without using the mechanical lifting equipment supplied.

- Do not lean on a machine whilst it is working.
- Do not wear rings on your fingers whilst operating a machine. They may get caught in it.
- Do not place tools and measuring equipment on the headstock of a lathe where they may fall into the revolving chuck.
- Do not attempt to remove swarf with your bare hands – use the rake provided.
- Always wear overalls in good condition and keep them buttoned up so as to prevent any loose clothing becoming caught in any moving machinery. Keep your sleeves rolled up or keep the cuffs closely buttoned at your wrists.
- Always wear safety goggles when cutting is in progress.
- Always wear safety boots or shoes.
- Always adopt a short hairstyle or keep your hair covered in a suitable industrial cap.
- Always use a barrier cream to protect your skin.
- Always report accidents no matter how small.

10.1.2 Machine safety

- Do not attempt to change tools on a lathe whilst the work is revolving.
- Do not remove stops, guards or safety equipment or adjust such devices unless, as part of your training, you do so under the direct supervision of your instructor.
- Do not change the spindle speed whilst the machine is operating as this will cause considerable damage to the gearbox.
- Do not change the direction of rotation of a machine whilst it is running.
- Do not leave your machine unattended whilst it is running.
- Always keep the area around your machine clean and tidy and clear up oil and coolant spills immediately.
- Always clean down your machine when you have finished using it.
- Always make sure you know how to stop a machine.
- Always isolate a machine when changing cutters and workholding devices and loading or unloading work.
- Always stop the machine and isolate it when anything goes wrong.
- Always switch off the machine and isolate it before leaving it at the end of your shift.
- Always check oil levels before starting the machine.
- Always check that workholding devices are correctly mounted and secured before cutting commences.

- Always check that the work is securely restrained in the workholding devices before cutting commences.

- Always make sure the machine is set to rotate in the correct direction before setting it in motion.

- Always make sure any automatic feed facilities are turned off before setting the machine in motion.

- Always clean and return tools and accessories to their storage racks or to the stores immediately after use.

- Always use the correct tools, cutters and workholding devices for the job in hand, never 'make do' with a makeshift set-up.

- Always check that the cutting zone is clear of loose tools, clamps, spanners and measuring equipment before starting the machine.

- Always stop the machine and report any mechanical or electrical defect immediately to your instructor.

Safety is largely a matter of common sense. Never become complacent and take risks to save time. Safety should become a way of life at home and at work. Accidents are always waiting to happen to the inattentive, the careless and the unwary.

This chapter is concerned with centre lathes. There are a number of guards on a lathe; some of these are installed to prevent you coming into contact with the transmission components such as gears and belts. These only have to be removed for maintenance and repairs and, apart from making sure they are in place, you should not have to concern yourself with them. In addition, there are two guards that do concern you.

10.1.3 Chuck guard

This is mounted on the headstock of the lathe and a typical example of a chuck guard is shown in Fig. 10.1. The guard is opened to change the chuck and to load and unload the work. It should be closed before starting the machine and during cutting. Its purposes are as follows:

- To prevent you coming into contact with the rapidly revolving chuck and suffering severe injuries.

- To prevent loose objects placed on the headstock – where they shouldn't be – falling into the revolving chuck and being thrown out with considerable force.

- To prevent the lathe being started up with the chuck key still in place. This used to be a common source of accidents and damage to the machine before chuck guards became commonplace.

- To prevent coolant being thrown out over the floor and the operator when working close to the chuck.

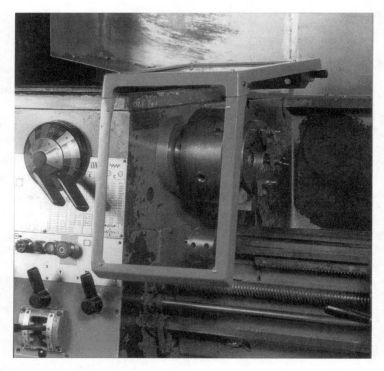

Figure 10.1 *Chuck guard*

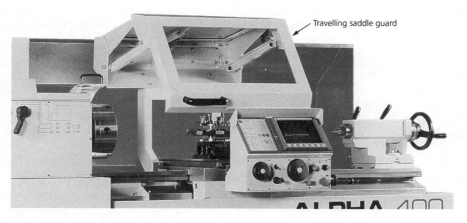

Travelling saddle guard

Figure 10.2 *Travelling guard*

10.1.4 Travelling guard

This type of guard is mounted on the saddle as shown in Fig. 10.2. The guard consists of a metal frame fitted with transparent panels so that you can visually monitor the cutting process. The purpose of this guard is to:

- Protect the operator from being sprayed with coolant.

- Protect the operator from chips (swarf) as they fly from the cutting tool. When cutting at high speeds with carbide-tipped tools the chips can be very hot and sharp, particularly if the tool incorporates a chip-breaker.

10.2 Constructional features of the centre lathe

A centre lathe is a machine tool designed and manufactured to produce cylindrical, conical (tapered) and plain (flat) surfaces. It produces these surfaces using a single point tool. It can also be used to cut screw threads. Figure 10.3 shows a typical centre lathe and names the more important features. You can see that it is built up from a number of basic units that have to be accurately aligned during manufacture in order that precision turned components may be produced.

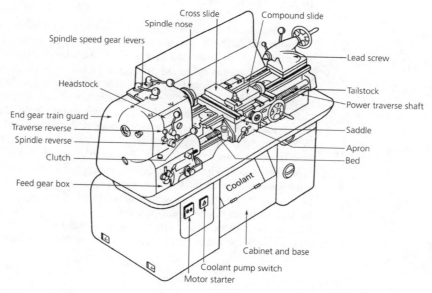

Figure 10.3 *Centre lathe*

10.2.1 The bed

A typical lathe bed is a strong, bridge-like member, made of high grade cast iron and is heavily ribbed to give it rigidity. Its upper surface carries the main slideways that are sometimes referred to as the 'shears'. Since these slideways locate, directly or indirectly, most of the remaining units, they are responsible for the fundamental alignments of the machine. For this reason the bed slideways must be manufactured to high dimensional and geometrical tolerances. Further, the lathe must be installed with care to avoid distortion of the bed.

10.2.2 The headstock

The headstock, or 'fast-head' as it is sometimes called, is a box-like casting supporting the *spindle* and containing a gearbox through which the spindle is driven and its speed adjusted to suit the work being turned.

The spindle is machined from a massive, hollow, alloy-steel forging and its purpose is to carry and drive various workholding devices and the work itself. The spindle is hollow to accept bar stock and its nose is bored internally to a morse taper to accept an adapter sleeve that, in turn, accepts the smaller morse taper of the live centre (turning between centres will be described in Section 10.6). The spindle nose is machined externally to carry various workholding devices such as chucks and faceplates. There are a number of different types of spindle nose in current use and these are described in Section 10.4.

10.2.3 The tailstock

The tailstock, or loose head as it is sometimes called, is located at the opposite end of the bed to the headstock. It can be moved back and forth along its slideways on the bed and can be clamped in any convenient position. It consists of a cast iron body in which is located the *barrel* or *poppet*. The barrel is hollow and is bored with a morse taper. This taper locates the taper shank of the dead centre and it can also locate the taper shanks of tooling such as drill chuck, taper shank drills, die holders, etc. The bore is *coaxial* with the taper bore and nose of the spindle. That is, they have a *common axis* that is parallel to the bed slideways. This is a basic alignment of a lathe. Figure 10.4 shows a section through a typical tailstock. The barrel is given a longitudinal movement within the tailstock body by means of a screw and handwheel. The screw also acts as an ejector for any device inserted in the taper of the barrel. The barrel can be locked in any convenient position within its range of movement. The base of the tailstock has adjusting screws that provide lateral movement. This enables the tailstock to be offset for taper turning (see Section 10.4).

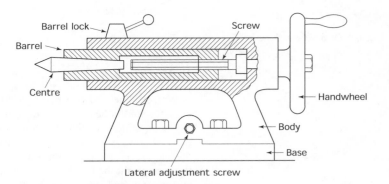

Figure 10.4 *Centre lathe tailstock*

10.2.4 The carriage

A typical lathe carriage is shown in Fig. 10.5. This consists of a *saddle* that lies across the bed of the lathe and an *apron* that hangs down in front of the saddle and carries most of the carriage controls.

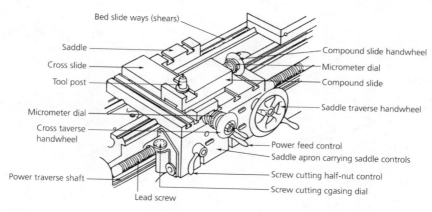

Figure 10.5 *Carriage*

- The *carriage* moves along the bed of the lathe on the bed slide-ways. Its movement is parallel to the common axis of the headstock spindle and the tailstock barrel. This movement is used when turning cylindrical components.

- The *cross-slide* is situated on top of the saddle and its movement is perpendicular (at right angles) to the common axis of the headstock spindle and tailstock barrel. This movement is used to provide 'in-feed' for the cutting tool when turning cylindrical components. It is also used to face across the ends (faces) of components to provide plain (flat) surfaces.

- The *compound slide*, which is also called the *top-slide*, is mounted on top of the cross-slide. It is used to control the 'in-feed' of the cutting tool when facing. It also has a swivel base and can be set at an angle when turning short, steep tapers such as chamfers.

- The cross-slide and compound slides are provided with micrometer dials on their screws so that their movements can be accurately controlled (see also Section 10.3).

- The *apron* carries the controls for engaging and disengaging the power traverse for the carriage and the power cross-feed for the cross-slide. It also carries the control for engaging and disengaging the half-nut when screw cutting from the lead screw.

10.2.5 The tool post

The tool post is mounted on top of the compound slide and carries the cutting tool. Figure 10.6 shows the four types most commonly used. The tool post shown in Fig. 10.6(a) is simple and robust but not much used

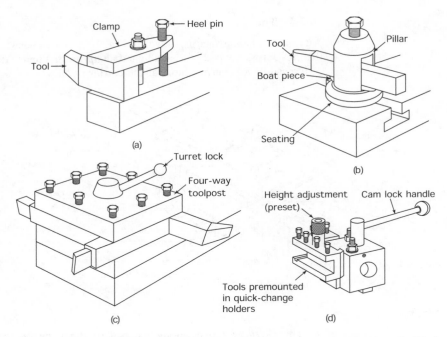

Figure 10.6 *Centre lathe toolposts: (a) English (clamp) type toolpost; (b) American (pillar) type toolpost; (c) turret (fourway) type toolpost; (d) quick release type toolpost*

nowadays other than on small, low-cost lathes. The height of the tool can be adjusted only by adding or removing packing and shims until the tool is at the correct height. The tool post shown in Fig. 10.6(b) is commonly used on light-duty lathes. The tool height is quickly and easily adjusted by rocking the boat-piece in its spherical seating. Unfortunately this type of tool post lacks rigidity due to the overhang of the tool. Further, tilting the tool to adjust its height alters the effective cutting angles. The four-way turret tool post shown in Fig. 10.6(c) saves time when making a batch of components. All the tools required are mounted in the tool post and each can be swung into position as required by rotating (indexing) the turret. This limits the number of tools that can be used to four. Also the only way to adjust the tool height is by the use of packing. Tools with only relatively small shanks can be held in this type of tool post.

The quick release tool post shown in Fig. 10.6(d) is increasingly used. An unlimited number of tools can be preset in the holders ready for use. Tool height is quickly and easily adjusted by means of a screw. Also the tools can be preset for height in a setting fixture away from the lathe. The tool holder complete with tool is slipped over the dovetail slide of the tool post and locked in position by a lever-operated cam. It is just as easily and quickly removed.

10.2.6 The feed gearbox

It has already been said that the carriage apron has controls for screw cutting from the lead screw and for power traverse for the carriage and cross-slide. The drive to the lead screw and the traverse shaft is through a variable speed gearbox. This feed gearbox is driven from the spindle of the lathe by an *end-train* of gears as shown in Fig. 10.7. The reason for driving the feed gearbox from the spindle is that once the feed has been set for a particular operation, the tool movement per revolution of the work must remain constant even if the spindle speed is changed. The feed gearbox has three functions.

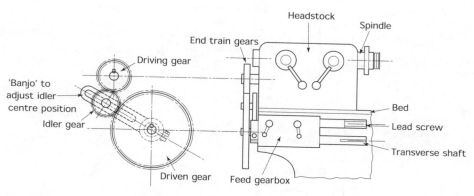

Figure 10.7 *Centre lathe end train gears*

- To control the speed at which the saddle is driven along the bed of the lathe when cylindrically turning with longitudinal power traverse.

- To control the speed at which the cross-slide moves across the saddle when power cross-traversing (facing).

- To control the speed of the lead screw relative to the rotational speed of the workpiece when screw cutting and thus control the lead of the screw being cut.

10.3 Main movements and alignments

Figure 10.8(a) shows the basic alignment of the headstock, tailstock, spindle and bed slideways. The common spindle and tailstock axis is parallel to the bed slideways in both the vertical and horizontal planes. This is the basic alignment of the lathe and all other alignments are referred to it. The movements of the carriage and the tailstock along the bed and the movement of the tailstock barrel within the tailstock body are parallel to the common axis in both the vertical and horizontal planes. These movements are shown in Fig. 10.8(b). These alignments and movements are fundamental to the accuracy of the machine and must be carefully preserved.

The cross-slide, which is mounted on the carriage, is aligned so that it is perpendicular (90°) to the common spindle and tailstock axis. This is shown in Fig. 10.9(a). The movement of the cross-slide is also at right angles to the common spindle and tailstock axis. Therefore this axis can be used for producing plane surfaces that are perpendicular to the common axis (facing) as shown in Fig. 10.9(b). This slide is also used for

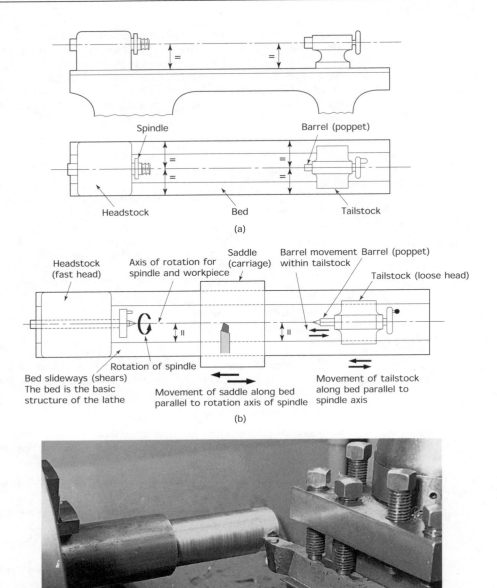

Figure 10.8 *Centre lathe: basic alignments: (a) basic alignment; (b) the carriage or saddle provides the basic movement of the cutting tool parallel to the work axis; (c) cylindrical (parallel) turning*

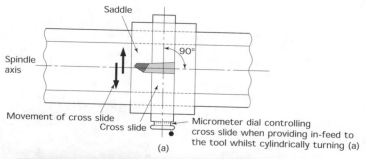

(a)

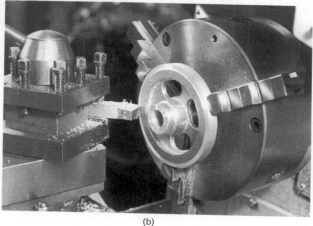

(b)

Figure 10.9 *The cross-slide (a), facing (surfacing) (b)*

providing and controlling the in-feed of the cutting tool when turning cylindrical workpieces. For this purpose its traverse screw is fitted with a micrometer dial.

The compound slide (top slide) is located on top of the cross-slide and can be set parallel to the common headstock and tailstock axis. In

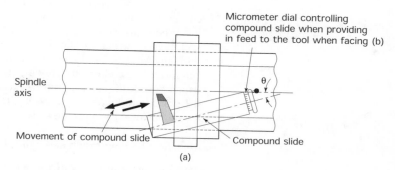

(a)

Figure 10.10 *The compound (top) slide (a), taper turning (b)*

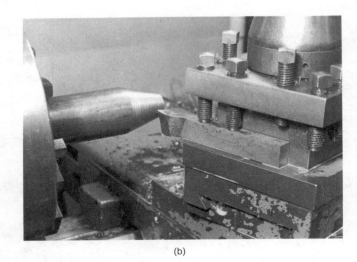

(b)

Figure 10.10   *(continued)*

this position it can be used for providing and controlling the in-feed of the cutting tool when facing across plane surfaces. For this purpose its traverse screw is fitted with a micrometer dial.

The compound slide can also be set at an angle to the common axis when short tapers, such as chamfers, are to be produced. The movement of this slide when taper turning is shown in Figs 10.10(a) and 10.10(b).

10.4   Types of spindle nose

Figure 10.11 shows three types of spindle nose in common use. To ensure that the workholding device mounted on the spindle nose runs true, *always* clean the plain or tapered spindle mountings and the corresponding internal registers of the workholding devices carefully before mounting them on the spindle.

10.4.1   Plain nose spindle

The *plain nose spindle*, as shown in Fig. 10.11(a), is the simplest and cheapest to manufacture but is the least effective. There is no way that it can be adjusted to compensate for wear. After heavy cutting the chuck will have tightened on the thread to such an extent as to make removal difficult. Any attempt to stop the lathe quickly using an emergency brake can result in the chuck unscrewing itself and spinning off which is highly dangerous. If the lathe is run in reverse to cut a left-hand thread, again the chuck will tend to unscrew itself. Plain nose spindles are found only on small low-cost lathes nowadays.

10.4.2   The long taper nose spindle

The *long taper nose spindle*, as shown in Fig. 10.11(b), provides a taper location that is much more accurate than the plain nose. Also as wear takes

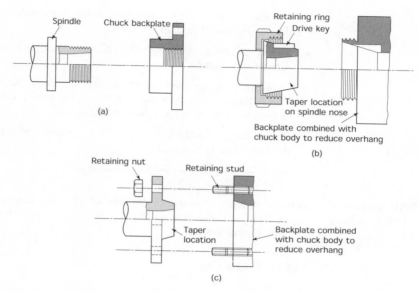

Figure 10.11 *Spindle nose mountings: (a) plain nose spindle; (b) long taper nose spindle; (c) short taper nose spindle*

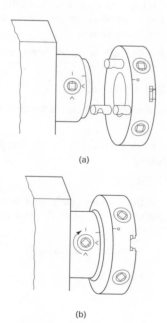

(a)

(b)

Figure 10.12 *Cam lock spindle mounting: (a) locate pegs in holes on spindle nose; (b) turn clockwise to lock chuck*

place the chuck or other workholding device simply seats more deeply on the taper and no accuracy of alignment is lost. The drive is positive and via a key and keyway. The chuck or other workholding device is retained on the spindle and pulled tight against the taper nose by a threaded ring. There is no way in which the chuck can spin off the spindle nose or work loose under any cutting conditions.

10.4.3 The short taper nose spindle

The *short taper nose spindle* is used with workholding devices retained by studs and nuts on older machines as shown in Fig. 10.11(c). The short nose taper has the advantage of reducing the overhang of the mounting, resulting in increased rigidity.

10.4.4 The camlock spindle

The *camlock spindle* is shown in Fig. 10.12. It also has a short taper but, in place of the studs and nuts of the previous example, it has a cam locking system that is quicker and easier to use when changing workholding devices. It is the most widely used mounting on modern industrial size lathes. To fit a workholding device to a camlock spindle:

- Clean the tapered spigot and face on the machine spindle.

- Clean the tapered register, face and pins on the back of the chuck.

- Use the square ended key provided to turn the camlock device so that the setting marks line up.

- Mount the chuck on the spindle, engaging the pins in the holes in the spindle nose flange.

- Using the key, turn the camlock devices clockwise until they are tight. The setting mark must now be between the two V marks. These are at 90° and 180° to the original setting mark.

- Repeat for all camlock devices. To remove the workholding device the procedure is reversed.

10.5 Starting up and closing down the machine

Before considering the use of the lathe to produce components, it is necessary to understand how to start up and close down the machine in a safe and proper manner.

10.5.1 Starting up

- Check that the isolating switch is in the *off* position.

- Visually inspect to ensure all controls are in the *off* or *neutral* positions, the key has not been left in the chuck, and no tools, measuring instruments, or workpieces have been left lying about on the machine. Check that the machine is clean and free from swarf.

- Fit the appropriate workholding device for the work in hand and ensure it is securely fastened.

- Mount the workpiece in the workholding device securely.

- Select and set an appropriate tool in the tool post and check for centre height.

- With the gearbox in neutral, rotate the work by hand to ensure that it does not foul on the machine or the cutting tool.

- Select the required spindle speed and feed rate.

- Turn on the isolating switch, switch on the coolant pump if it is to be used, switch on the low voltage lighting if it is required. Start the main drive motor.

- Engage the clutch gradually to see that the work rotates safely.

- Commence the cutting operation.

10.5.2 Shutting down

- Stop the machine and turn off the isolating switch.

- Ensure all controls are left in a safe position.

- Remove the work, the cutting tools and the workholding device.

- Return all tools, measuring instruments and other ancillary equipment to the stores or the cabinet at the side of the machine as appropriate.

- Remove swarf from the coolant tray and clean the machine.

- Remove any spilt oil or coolant and swarf from the floor around the machine and leave the floor safe.

Leave the machine as you would wish to find it.

10.6 Workholding devices (centres)

Holding work between centres is the traditional method of workholding from which the centre lathe gets its name. This method of workholding is shown in Fig. 10.13. The *centres* locate the work in line with the common axis, and the work is driven by the *catchplate* on the spindle nose and a *carrier* on the workpiece. The centres are located in morse tapers to ensure concentricity with the bores of the spindle nose and the tailstock barrel.

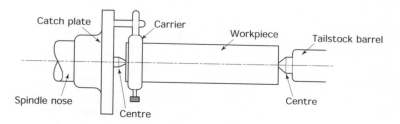

Figure 10.13 *Workholding between centres*

To ensure true running of the workpiece, the centres and the bores must be carefully cleaned before the centres are inserted. The tailstock centre does not rotate so it is made from hardened steel to prevent wear. It must be suitably lubricated. The headstock centre rotates with the spindle so there should be no wear and a hard centre is not necessary. Despite this, a hard centre is usually used in the spindle. It should be checked with a dial gauge (DTI) for true running. If after cleaning it still cannot be made to run true, a soft centre can be used and it is turned to the 60° taper position in the machine spindle to ensure true running.

It is also essential to drill the centre holes in the workpiece correctly. Figure 10.14(a) shows the preparation of a workpiece for holding between centres. The work is held in a three-jaw, self-centring chuck whilst the end of the work is faced off smooth and the centre hole is drilled (chucks will be considered in Sections 10.8 to 10.10 inclusive). The centre drill is held in a drill chuck. The drill chuck has a morse taper mandrel that fits in the barrel of the tailstock. A centre drill is designed and manufactured to produce a pilot hole and the taper location in one operation.

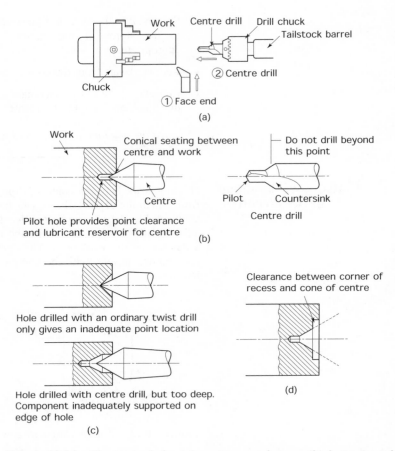

Figure 10.14 *The centre hole: (a) centring workpiece; (b) formation of the centre hole; (c) typical centre hole faults; (d) recessed or protected centre*

Figure 10.14(b) shows a correctly formed centre hole with the centre in position. Location should be on the flanks of the taper and not on the point of the taper. The pilot hole not only provides point clearance, it also provides a reservoir for lubricant. The essential features of a centre drill are also shown. These are usually double ended.

Figure 10.14(c) shows typical centre hole faults. If the centre hole becomes damaged, then the work will not run true. To stop the edges of the centre hole becoming bruised during handling, it can be recessed as shown in Fig. 10.14(d). This is called a *protected centre hole*.

Sometimes a rotating tailstock centre is used; an example is shown in Fig. 10.15. The centre is supported in ball bearings or in roller bearings that are designed to resist the radial and axial forces. Rotating centres are used where high spindle speeds are required, as when carbide-tipped tools are used, and for supporting heavy workpieces.

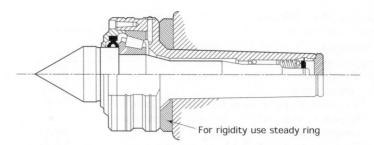

For rigidity use steady ring

Figure 10.15 *Revolving tailstock centre (reproduced courtesy of Jones and Shipman plc)*

For parallel turning, the common axis of the spindle and the tailstock barrel must be parallel to the main bed slideways. The tailstock is provided with lateral (sideways) adjustment to achieve this end. When turning between centres a trial cut should be taken along the work. The diameter of the work is then checked at each end with a micrometer caliper. If the readings are the same, then the work is a true cylinder and the roughing and finishing cuts can be taken. If the readings are different, then the tailstock needs to be adjusted as shown in Fig. 10.16. Further trial cuts are taken after each adjustment until the diameter is constant along its whole length. The advantages and limitations of workholding between centres are listed in Table 10.1.

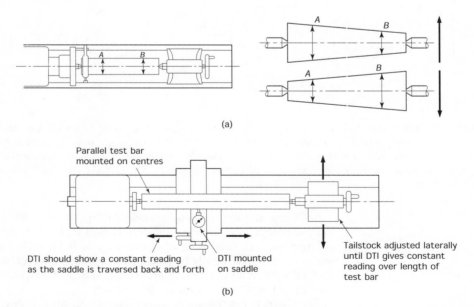

(a)

Parallel test bar
mounted on centres

DTI should show a constant reading
as the saddle is traversed back and forth

DTI mounted
on saddle

Tailstock adjusted laterally
until DTI gives constant
reading over length of
test bar

(b)

Figure 10.16 *Parallel cylindrical turning: (a) the axis of the headstock spindle must be in alignment with the tailstock barrel axis; if this is so the diameter A will be the same as diameter B; (b) use of test bar*

TABLE 10.1 *Workholding between centres*

Advantages	Limitations
1. Work can be easily reversed without loss of concentricity	1. Centre holes have to be drilled before work can be set up
2. Work can be taken from the machine for inspection and easily re-set without loss of concentricity	2. Only limited work can be performed on the end of the bar
3. Work can be transferred between machines (e.g. lathe and cylindrical grinder) without loss of concentricity	3. Boring operations cannot be performed
	4. There is lack of rigidity
4. Long work (full length of bed) can be accommodated	5. Cutting speeds are limited unless a revolving centre is used. This reduces accuracy and accessibility
	6. Skill in setting is required to obtain the correct fit between centres and work

10.7 Workholding devices (taper mandrel)

Taper mandrels enable hollow components to be turned so that the external diameter runs true with the bore (that is, they are concentric) as shown in Fig. 10.17(a). A mandrel press, as shown in Fig. 10.17(b), is used to insert and remove the mandrel.

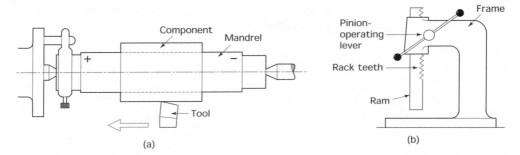

(a) (b)

Figure 10.17 *The taper mandrel: (a) turning on the mandrel – the component is rough turned, bored and reamed to size, it is then pressed onto a mandrel set up between centres and the outside diameter is finished turned concentric with the bore, the mandrel is tapered so that the further the component is forced on, the more firmly it is held in place – therefore the direction of cutting should be towards the plus end of the mandrel; (b) the mandrel press*

Let's consider the component shown in Fig. 10.18(a). We could hold the component in a three-jaw chuck and drill it. If we want a hole of accurate size and roundness we could ream it. If the drilled hole 'runs out' we can correct it only by single point boring. However, it would be very difficult to make a boring tool that is sufficiently rigid, yet is long enough and small enough for the hole shown.

The alternative technique is shown in Fig. 10.18(b). Instead of trying to bore the hole true with the outside diameter, we make the hole first and then turn the outside diameter true with the bore as shown.

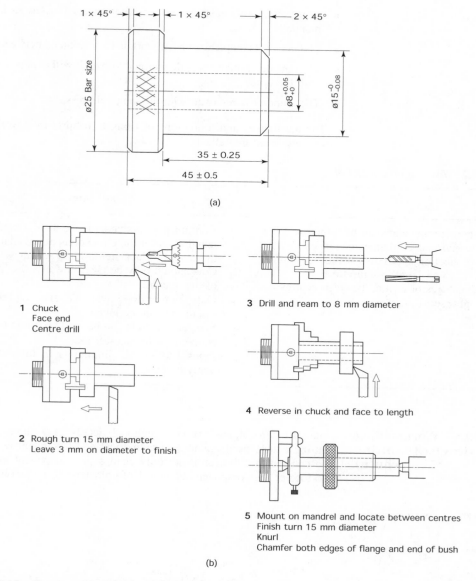

Figure 10.18 *Turning a bush: (a) bush with small diameter bore; (b) turning on a mandrel*

- First drill and ream the hole.

- Then mount the work on a *taper mandrel*. This is hardened and ground with a slight taper. The work is mounted so that the direction of the cutting forces tends to push the work towards the large end of the mandrel.

- A mandrel press (also called an arbor press) is used to insert the mandrel.

- The mandrel complete with the work is then mounted between centres.

- The outside of the work is then turned to size. It will then be concentric with the bore.

- The mandrel is removed with the mandrel press.

The advantages and limitations of using a mandrel as a workholding device are listed in Table 10.2.

TABLE 10.2 *Turning on a mandrel*

Advantages	Limitations
1. Small-bore components can be turned with the bore and outside diameters concentric	1. Bore must be a standard size to fit a taper mandrel. Adjustable mandrels are available but these tend to lack rigidity and accuracy
2. Batch production is possible without loss of concentricity or lengthy setup time	2. Cuts should only be taken towards the 'plus' end of the mandrel
3. The advantages of turning between centres also apply (see Table 4.1)	3. Only friction drive available, and this limits size of cut that can be taken
	4. Special mandrels can be made but this is not economical for one-off jobs
	5. Items 2 to 5 of the limitations in Table 4.1 also apply here

10.8 Workholding devices (self-centring chuck)

Figure 10.19(a) shows the constructional details of a three-jaw, self-centring chuck, used for holding cylindrical and hexagonal workpieces. You can see that the scroll not only clamps the component in place, it also locates the component as well. Unfortunately, if the scroll becomes

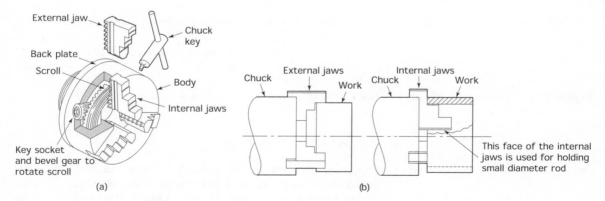

Figure 10.19 *The three-jaw, self-centring chuck: (a) construction; (b) external and internal jaws*

worn or damaged the chuck loses its accuracy. However, modern chucks are very accurate and maintain their accuracy over a long period of time provided they are used correctly and kept clean.

- *Never* try to hammer the work true if it is running out.

- *Never* hold work that is not round, such as hot-rolled (black) bar. Being out of round it will strain the jaws and the highly abrasive scale may also get into the scroll causing early wear.

- *Never* hold work on the tips of the jaws. This not only strains the jaws but the work is not held securely and safely.

The jaws for this type of chuck are *not* reversible. Separate internal and external jaws have to be used as shown in Fig. 10.19(b). When changing jaws the following points must be observed.

- Check that each jaw in the set carries the same serial number as the number on the chuck body.

- Make sure the jaws are numbered 1 to 3.

- Insert the jaws sequentially starting with number 1.

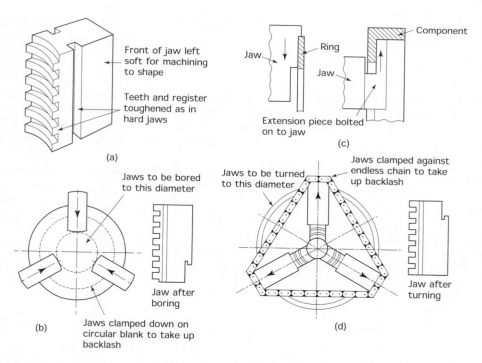

Figure 10.20 *Use of soft jaws: (a) soft jaw; (b) boring soft jaws; (c) applications – (left) jaw bored to give maximum support to a thin ring whilst it is being bored and faced, (right) jaw fitted with extension piece to avoid holding onto and damaging the flange; (d) turning soft jaws*

10.8.1 Soft jaws

When awkward components – such as thin discs – have to be held, or where greater accuracy is required from a three-jaw chuck, *soft jaws* can be used. These are inserted like any other jaws and the same rules apply. These jaws are not hardened but can be turned to the shape required whilst in position in the chuck. Figure 10.20 shows how they should be machined in order to eliminate backlash errors, and also shows a typical component where soft jaws are an advantage. The advantages and limitations of the self-centring chuck are listed in Table 10.3.

TABLE 10.3 *The self-centring chuck*

Advantages	Limitations
1. Ease of work setting	1. Accuracy decreases as chuck becomes worn
2. A wide range of cylindrical and hexagonal work can be held	2. Accuracy of concentricity is limited when work is reversed in the chuck
3. Internal and external jaws are available	3. 'Run out' cannot be corrected
4. Work can be readily performed on the end face of the job	4. Soft jaws can be turned up for second operation work, but this is seldom economical for one-off jobs
5. The work can be bored	5. Only round and hexagonal components can be held

10.9 Workholding devices (collets)

Collets of the type as shown in Fig. 10.21(a) are located in the taper bore of the spindle nose either directly or in a tapered adapter sleeve. The range of movement is very small and a separate collet is required for each bar size. The collets can be either pushed into the taper by a collar

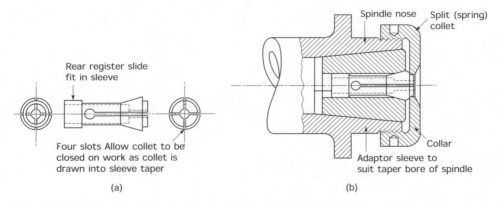

(a)

(b)

Figure 10.21 *The split-collet chuck: (a) split (spring) collet; (b) collet chuck for a simple plain nose spindle (typical of small instrument lathes) tightening the collar forces the collet back into the taper bore of the sleeve which closes the collet down onto the workpiece; (c) draw-bar collet chuck for taper nose spindles*

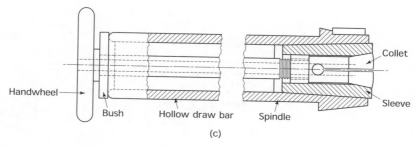

Figure 10.21 *(continued)*

as shown in Fig. 10.21(b). This system can be used only with plain nose spindles as found on some small bench lathes or alternatively, collets can be drawn into the taper by a hollow draw bar as shown in Fig. 10.21(c). This system can be used with taper nose spindles. The advantages and limitations of split collets mounted directly into the spindle bore are listed in Table 10.4.

TABLE 10.4 *The split-collet chuck*

Advantages	Limitations
1. Very high accuracy of concentricity 2. Accuracy maintained over long periods of use 3. Simple, compact and reliable 4. Very quickly loaded 5. Considerable gripping power 6. Unlikely to mark or damage work 7. Work can be removed and replaced without loss of accuracy 8. Work can be turned externally, internally (bored) and end faced 9. No overhang from spindle nose reduces chatter and geometrical inaccuracy. Very useful where work has to be parted off	1. Only accurately turned, ground or drawn rod can be held in a collet 2. Separate collets have to be used for each size of rod. Range of adjustment very small 3. Although simple, initial cost is high due to the large number of collets that have to be bought 4. Range of sizes that can be held limited by bore of spindle 5. Work can only be held on external surfaces 6. Only collets with circular or hexagonal jaws are available from stock. Other sections have to be made to special order (costly) 7. Special adaptor sleeve required to suit bore of spindle nose

10.10 Workholding devices (four-jaw, independent chuck)

Figure 10.22 shows the constructional details of this type of chuck. It is more heavily constructed than the self-centring chuck and has much greater holding power. Each jaw is moved independently by a square thread screw and the jaws are reversible. These chucks are used for holding:

- Irregularly shaped work.

- Work that must be set to run concentrically.

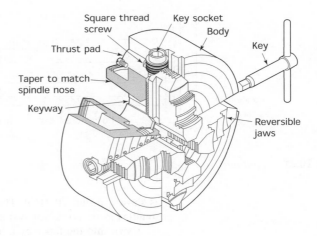

Figure 10.22 *The four-jaw chuck*

- Work that must be deliberately offset to run eccentrically. Eccentrically mounted work must be balanced to prevent vibration.

Since the jaws of a four-jaw chuck *can be reversed*, there is no need for separate internal and external jaws. Since the jaws move independently in this type of chuck, the component has to be set to run concentrically with the spindle axis by the operator. This is done when the work is mounted in the chuck.

- Figure 10.23(a) shows how a floating centre can be used to set the work concentrically with the intersection of previously scribed lines.

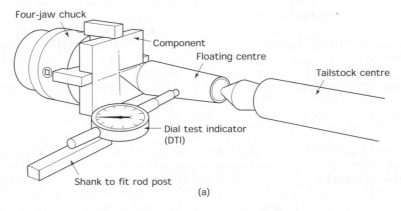

Figure 10.23 *The four-jaw chuck: work setting: (a) the chuck is adjusted until the DTI maintains a constant reading whilst the chuck is revolved; (b) the chuck is adjusted until the scriber point just touches each opposite edge or corner as the chuck is revolved; (c) dial test indicator will show a constant reading when component is set to run true*

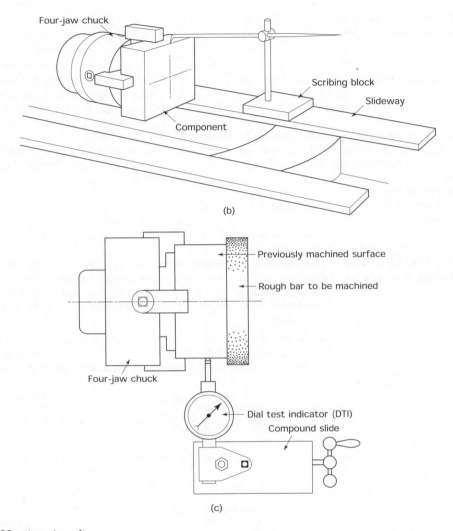

Four-jaw chuck

Scribing block

Slideway

Component

(b)

Previously machined surface

Rough bar to be machined

Four-jaw chuck

Dial test indicator (DTI)

Compound slide

(c)

Figure 10.23 *(continued)*

Note that the setting will only be as accurate as the positioning of the centre punch mark.

- Figure 10.23(b) shows how work of lower accuracy can be set using a scribing block.

- Figure 10.23(c) shows how work may be set using a DTI to register on a previously machined surface. When correctly set the DTI should show a constant reading. All diameters turned at this setting will be concentric with the original diameter used for setting the workpiece.

The advantages and limitations of a four-jaw chuck are listed in Table 10.5.

TABLE 10.5 *The four-jaw chuck*

Advantages	Limitations
1. A wide range of regular and irregular shapes can be held	1. Chuck is heavy to handle on to the lathe
2. Work can be set to run concentrically or eccentrically at will	2. Chuck is slow to set up. A dial test indicator (DTI) has to be used for accurate setting
3. Considerable gripping power. Heavy cuts can be taken	3. Chuck is bulky
4. Jaws are reversible for internal and external work	4. The gripping power is so great that fine work can be easily damaged during setting
5. Work can readily be performed on the end face of the job	
6. The work can be bored	
7. There is no loss of accuracy as the chuck becomes worn	

10.11 Workholding devices (faceplate)

The workholding devices previously described are designed so that a diameter may be machined true to another existing diameter. However, the faceplate enables a component to be mounted so that the workpiece may be turned either *parallel* or *perpendicular* to a previously machined flat surface.

- In Fig. 10.24(a) the axis of the bore will be *perpendicular* to the datum surface of the workpiece. That is, to the previously machined flat base of the component which is clamped directly to the faceplate.

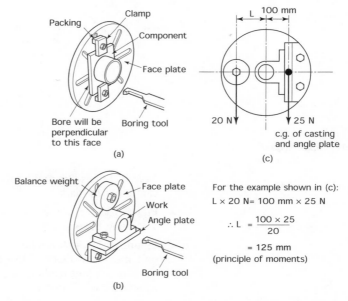

For the example shown in (c):

$L \times 20\ N = 100\ mm \times 25\ N$

$$\therefore L = \frac{100 \times 25}{20}$$

$= 125\ mm$
(principle of moments)

Figure 10.24 *The faceplate: (a) balanced work; (b) unbalanced work; (c) positioning the balance weight*

- In Fig. 10.24(b) the axis of the bore will be *parallel* to the datum surface. That is, to the previously machined flat base of this component that is mounted on an angle plate bolted to the faceplate.

In the example shown in Fig. 10.24(a), the work is symmetrical about the spindle centre line and no balance weight is required. However, in Fig. 10.24(b), the work is offset and unbalanced so a balance weight has had to be added to ensure the smooth running of the set-up at the machining speed required. This is to prevent out-of-balance forces from causing vibrations that could damage the spindle bearings of the machine or, in extreme cases, cause the machine to rock dangerously on its mountings. Offset components in a four-jaw chuck must also be balanced in a similar manner. Figure 10.24(c) shows how the balance weight is positioned. The advantages and limitations of using a faceplate are listed in Table 10.6.

TABLE 10.6   *The faceplate*

Advantages	Limitations
1. A wide range of regular and irregular shapes can be held	1. The face plate is slow and tedious to set up. Not only must the workpiece be clocked up to run true, clamps must also be set up on the face plate to retain the component
2. Work can be set to a datum surface. If the datum surface is parallel to the workpiece axis, it is set on an angle plate mounted on the face plate. If the datum surface is perpendicular to the workpiece axis, the workpiece is set directly on to the face plate	2. Considerable skill is required to clamp the component so that it is rigid enough to resist both the cutting forces, and those forces that will try to dislodge the work as it spins rapidly round
3. Work on the end face of the job is possible	3. Considerable skill is required to avoid distorting the workpiece by the clamps
4. The work can be bored	4. Irregular jobs have to be carefully balanced to prevent vibration, and the job rolling back on the operator
5. The work can be set to run concentrically or eccentrically at will	5. The clamps can limit the work that can be performed on the end face
6. There are no moving parts to lose their accuracy with wear	
7. The work can be rigidly clamped to resist heavy cuts	

10.12   Use of steadies

The workholding devices discussed so far assume that the workpiece is sufficiently rigid to be self-supporting. However, this is sometimes not the case, and additional support has to be provided. If the workpiece is long and slender it will visibly deflect and either climb over the cutting tool or spring out of the centres, or both, resulting in damage to the workpiece, damage to the cutting tool and, possibly, serious injury to the machine operator.

10.12.1   Travelling steady

To balance the cutting forces and prevent the component from deflecting a *travelling steady* is used. An example of such a steady is shown in Fig. 10.25(a). The steady is mounted on the carriage of the lathe opposite

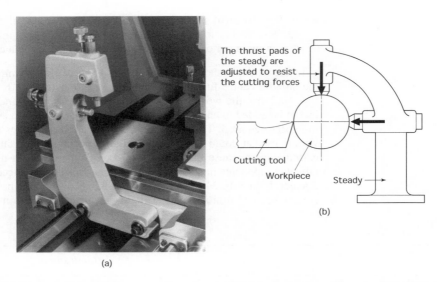

Figure 10.25 *The travelling steady mounted on the saddle (a); the action of the steady (b) (photograph reproduced courtesy of Colchester Lathe Co.)*

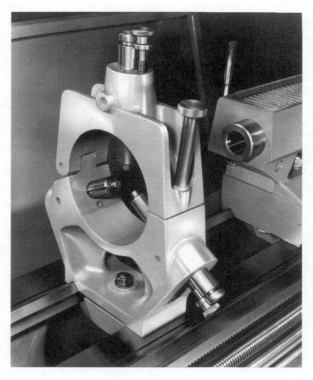

Figure 10.26 *The fixed steady (photograph reproduced courtesy of Colchester Lathe Co.)*

the cutting tool. As the saddle traverses along the bed of the lathe the steady moves with it, hence its name. Figure 10.25(b) shows how the adjustable, bronze thrust pads of the steady are positioned so that the work cannot deflect away from the cutting edge of the tool.

10.12.2 Fixed steady

The *fixed steady*, as its name implies, is fixed to the bed of the lathe. A typical fixed steady is shown in Fig. 10.26. It is used for two purposes:

- To support the end of long workpieces that cannot be held on a centre, for example if the end of the component has to be faced and bored.

- As a safety precaution when large and heavy components are supported on a tailstock centre. In this latter case the centre supports and locates the work, and the thrust pads of the steady are set to *just clear* of the work so as not to interfere with the alignment. However, if the centre fails under the load, the work merely drops a fraction of a millimetre and rests in the fixed steady. Otherwise it would break free from the lathe, doing considerable damage to the machine and causing serious injury to the operator.

10.13 Lathe tool profiles

The profile of a lathe tool is the shape of the tool when viewed from above. Figure 10.27 shows a selection of lathe tools and states their typical applications. A lathe tool is selected to suit the job to be done. The rake angle is indicated by the letter R and the direction of the rake is indicated by the associated arrow. Chip formation and the geometry of lathe tools will be considered in Section 10.20.

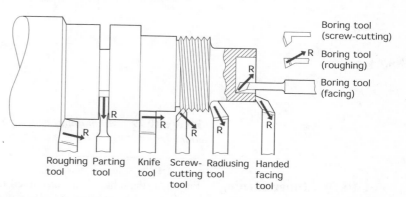

Figure 10.27 *Lathe tool profiles: these tools are right handed; left-hand tools cut towards the tailstock; the arrows indicate the rake angle (R) of each tool*

10.14 Concentricity

When a component is being turned it is usual to try to keep the various diameters *concentric*. That is, we try to ensure that all the diameters of a component *have a common axis*. The meanings of concentricity and eccentricity are shown in Fig. 10.28.

In Fig. 10.28(a) the two diameters A and B are *concentric*. They have the same centre of rotation and lie on the same axis. In Fig. 10.28(b) the two diameters A and B are *eccentric*. They have different centres of rotation and do not lie on the same axis. The distance E between the two centres of rotation is the amount of 'offset' or eccentricity.

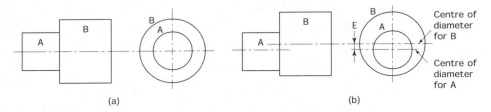

(a)   (b)

Figure 10.28 *Concentricity and eccentricity: (a) concentric diameters – both have the same centre; (b) eccentric diameters – each diameter has a different centre*

The easiest way to ensure concentricity is to turn as many diameters at the same setting as possible without removing the work from the lathe, as shown in Fig. 10.29. If the work does have to be removed from the lathe in order to turn it round, then it must be mounted in a four-jaw chuck and trued up using a dial test indicator on a previously machined diameter. Work held between centres can be removed and reversed as many times as is necessary without loss of concentricity.

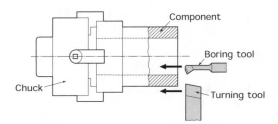

Figure 10.29 *Maintaining concentricity: both the bore and the outside diameter are turned at the same setting*

10.15 Taper turning

Earlier in this chapter we discussed the conditions necessary to produce a cylindrical component. Great emphasis was laid on the importance of maintaining the axial alignment of the headstock spindle and the tailstock barrel, together with the need for the cutting tool to move in a path parallel to this common axis.

Now we are going to consider the conditions for producing tapered (conical) components. Taper turning involves the controlled disturbance of the alignments previously described so that the tool moves in a path that is no longer parallel to the common headstock spindle and tailstock barrel axis but is inclined to it. This inclination is relative. The same effect is produced no matter whether the tool path is inclined to the axis, or whether the axis is inclined to the tool path. Three methods of taper turning will now be described.

10.15.1 Offset tailstock

Using the lateral adjusting screws, the body of the tailstock and, therefore, the tailstock centre can be offset. This inclines the axis of the workpiece relative to the path of the cutting tool when the workpiece is held between centres as shown in Fig. 10.30(a). The advantages and limitations of this technique are listed in Table 10.7.

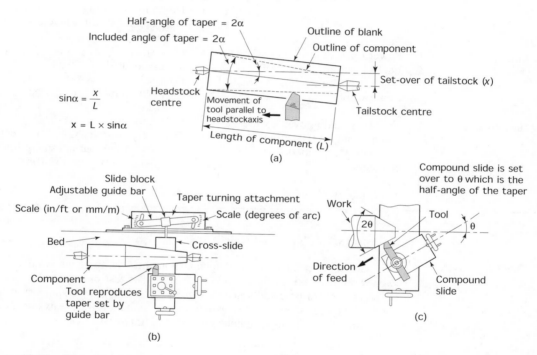

Figure 10.30 *Taper turning: (a) set over of centres; (b) the taper turning attachment; (c) compound slide*

10.15.2 Taper-turning attachment

Another way in which tapers may be produced is by the use of a taper-turning attachment. This is usually an 'optional extra' that can be purchased separately and bolted to the back of the lathe. Such attachments differ in detail from manufacturer to manufacturer but the principle remains the same. The movement of the cross-slide and, therefore, the tool path is controlled by the guide bar of the attachment as shown in Fig. 10.30(b). This can be set to the desired angle, and clamped in position. As the carriage traverses along the bed, the tool is moved into the workpiece or away from the workpiece according to the setting of the guide bar. In either case a taper is produced. If the work is supported between centres, then these are aligned as for cylindrical turning. The advantages and limitations of this technique are listed in Table 10.7.

TABLE 10.7 *Comparison of taper turning techniques*

Method	Advantages	Limitations
Set-over (offset) of tailstock	1. Power traverse can be used 2. The full length of the bed used	1. Only small angles can be accommodated 2. Damage to the centre holes can occur 3. Difficulty in setting up 4. Only applies to work held between centres
Taper turning attachments	1. Power traverse can be used 2. Ease of setting 3. Can be applied to chucking and centre work	1. Only small angles can be accommodated 2. Only short lengths can be cut (304–457 mm/12–18 in) depending on make
Compound slide	1. Very easy setting over a wide range of angles (Usually used for short, steep tapers and chamfers) 2. Can be applied to chucking, and centre work	1. Only hand traverse available 2. Only very short lengths can be cut. Varies with m/c but is usually limited to about 76–101 mm (3–4 in)

10.15.3 Compound slide

Setting over the compound slide also inclines the tool path relative to the workpiece axis as shown in Fig. 10.30(c). For ease of setting this slide has a protractor base calibrated in degrees of arc. This is the simplest method of turning tapers but it does have some limitations. The advantages and limitations of this technique are listed in Table 10.7.

10.16 Hole production

Hollow as well as solid components can be produced on a centre lathe. The hole will be concentric with the spindle axis. If the required hole is not in the centre of the job then the job has to be offset relative to the spindle axis. The holes may be produced by:

- Drilling.

- Reaming.

- Boring.

- A combination of the above processes.

10.16.1 Drilling

The drilling of centre holes in the ends of components prior to turning them between centres has already been considered. The drilling of deeper holes or the drilling of holes completely through the component is a similar process. For small diameter holes up to 12.5 mm (1/2 inch) diameter you should adopt the following procedure. The centre drill is held in a drill chuck fitted with a morse taper shank. The shank of the chuck is inserted sharply into the taper bore of the tailstock barrel so that it seats securely. It is important that:

- The shank of the chuck is clean and free from damage.

- The bore of the tailstock barrel is clean.

- The chuck is seated firmly so that it will not rotate and damage the bore of the tailstock barrel. Damage to this bore would destroy the basic accuracy of the machine.

The hole is started with a centre drill. The centre drill is replaced with a drill slightly smaller than the size of the hole required. The hole is drilled to the required depth. This is aided by a rule type scale engraved on the tailstock barrel. Having produced a *pilot hole*, the pilot drill is replaced by a drill of the required size. The hole is now opened up to the drawing size.

Where larger holes are required, the drills may be too large to fit into a drill chuck. In which case, after drilling the pilot hole, the hole is opened up as follows:

- Open up the pilot hole with the largest drill that can be held in the chuck.

- Wind the tailstock barrel (poppet) right back until the chuck is ejected.

- Insert *taper shank drills* directly in the tailstock barrel to enlarge the hole in stages until the required size is reached.

- Take care that the taper bore in the spindle is not damaged by the largest drill when drilling right through the component.

Producing holes with a twist drill is a convenient way of achieving rapid metal removal. However, a drill does not produce a precision hole. The limitations of drilled holes are:

- Poor finish compared with drilling and reaming.

- Lack of dimensional accuracy.

- Lack of 'roundness' or geometrical accuracy.

- Lack of positional accuracy as the drill tends to wander, especially when drilling deep holes in soft material such as brass.

10.16.2 Reaming

The finish and accuracy of a hole are greatly improved if it is drilled slightly undersize and finished with a reamer. Reamers and reaming techniques in drilling machines were discussed in Section 9.6 and the same comments apply to reaming in the centre lathe. The reamer should be held in a 'floating' reamer holder of the type shown in Fig. 10.31. This allows the reamer to follow the previously drilled hole without flexing. The ability of the reamer to float prevents ovality and 'bell-mouthing' in the reamed hole produced. Providing the correct speed has been used (less than for drilling), the reamer is fed into the work slowly, and as a coolant is used, a hole of good finish and roundness should be produced. However, the limitations of reaming are:

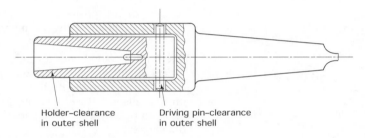

Holder–clearance   Driving pin–clearance
in outer shell   in outer shell

Figure 10.31 *Floating reamer holder*

- Lack of positional accuracy since the reamer follows the axis of the drilled hole and reproduces any 'wander' that may be present.

- Unless the quantities of components being produced warrants the cost of special tooling, only holes whose diameter is the same as standard reamer sizes can be produced.

Where a hole is too small to bore accurately, it is usual to drill and ream the hole to size than mount the component on a mandrel supported between centres. The outside of the component is then turned true with the hole (see Section 10.7). In this case the initial 'wander' of the drilled hole is unimportant.

10.16.3 Boring

Figures 10.32(a) and 10.32(b) show solid boring tools for use with small diameter holes, whilst Figs 10.32(c) and 10.32(d) show boring bars with inserted tool bits for larger diameter holes. Figure 10.32(e) shows the need for *secondary clearance* to prevent the heel of the tool from fouling the wall of small diameter bores. Holes produced by such tools are usually

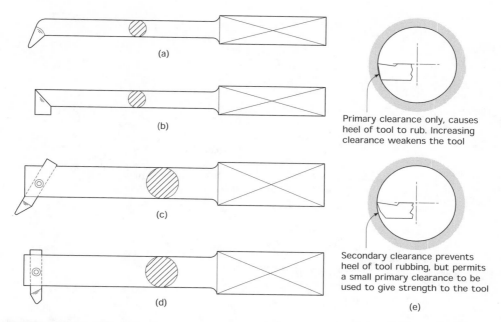

Figure 10.32 *Centre lathe boring tools: (a) solid bottoming tool for blind holes; (b) solid roughing tool for a through hole; (c) boring bar with inserted tool for bottoming a blind hole; (d) boring bar with inserted tool bit for roughing a through hole; (e) need for secondary clearance*

referred to as *bores*. Boring is the only way for correcting any axial wander in previously drilled pilot holes.

Because of the relatively slender shank of a boring tool and the long overhang of the tool point from the tool post, where the tool is secured, boring tools are prone to 'chatter' and leave a poor finish. Also the cut is liable to run off due to deflection of the tool shank. For this reason boring is a skilled operation compared with external turning. It requires careful grinding of the cutting tool to the correct shape, and careful selection of the speeds and feed rates.

10.17 Parting off

Where a number of small components have to be turned, such as the component shown in Fig. 10.33(a), it is easier to work from the bar than from previously sawn off blanks. The component is turned to shape on the end of the bar whilst being held in a three-jaw chuck. When finished the component is cut from the bar using a parting-off tool as shown in Fig. 10.33(b).

Figure 10.33(c) shows how a parting tool is ground. You can see that in addition to the usual rake and clearance angles, the tool also requires side clearance and plan (horizontal) clearance to prevent it rubbing on the sides of the groove. This is similar in effect to the set of a saw blade.

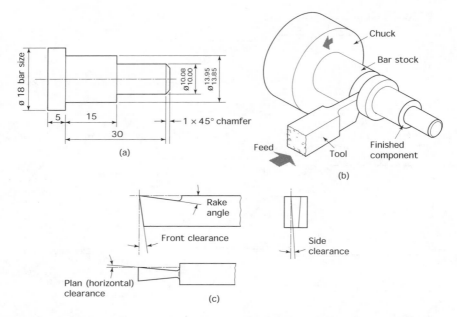

Figure 10.33 *Turning from the bar: (a) component – dimensions in millimetres; (b) parting component from the bar; (c) parting-off tool*

10.18 Cutting screw threads

The cutting of screw threads from the lead screw using single point tools is beyond the scope of this book.

10.18.1 External screw threads

The cutting of screw threads at the bench using a split button die in a diestock (dieholder) has already been considered. A similar technique can be used on a lathe with the added advantage that the thread will be true with the axis of the component.

Figure 10.34 shows a tailstock dieholder. The diestock body slides along a parallel mandrel mounted in the barrel of the tailstock. This ensures that the die is square with the work all the time it is cutting. The dieholder body is kept from rotating by the torque arm. Various diameter dies may be accommodated by changing the dieholder on the front of the body. The securing bolts are in clearance holes and should be only 'finger tight'. This allows the die to align itself axially with the work.

This arrangement is sufficiently rigid to allow threads to be cut with the lathe spindle rotating under power at a low speed. Before starting the machine ensure that the dieholder torque arm is safely engaged with the compound slide of the machine. The taking of roughing and finishing cuts and the use of a screw-cutting compound are as described previously. The lathe motor is switched to reverse for unscrewing the die. Again ensure that the torque arm is engaged with a suitable part of the carriage to

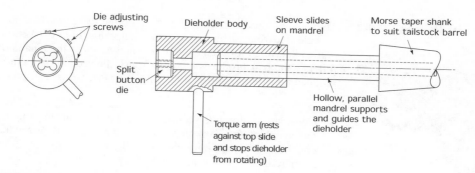

Figure 10.34 *Tailstock dieholder*

prevent reverse rotation, and is free to move along as the die unscrews, before starting the machine.

10.18.2 Internal screw threads

A tapping attachment similar to the tailstock dieholder previously described is shown in Fig. 10.35. The tap is held in the three-jaw chuck.

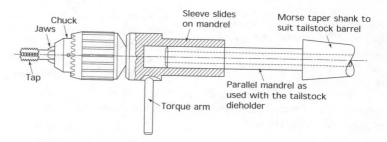

Figure 10.35 *Tailstock tapholder*

- Make sure the machine is turned off and put the gearbox into a neutral position.

- Hold the chuck from moving with your left hand and rotate the tap with your right hand using the torque arm of the tap holder.

- When you have rotated the tap as far as is convenient (about half a turn), rotate the chuck towards you, hold in position and rotate the tap again with the torque arm.

- Reverse the direction of rotation after every revolution or so to break up the chips and relieve the load on the tap. A screw-cutting compound should be used to lubricate the tap. There is a limit to the size of tap that can be held in the chuck without the tap slipping.

10.19   Knurling

This process produces a rough pattern on the turned surface so that it can be held and rotated by hand without slipping. Figure 10.36(a) shows a typical knurling tool. You can see that it consists of three pairs of grooved rollers. One pair produces a coarse knurl, the second pair can be used to produce a medium knurl and the third pair can be used to produce a fine knurl.

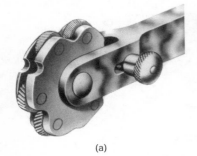

(a)

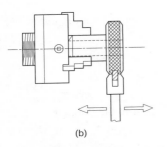

(b)

Figure 10.36 *Knurling: (a) knurling tool fitted with three pairs of knurls; coarse, medium and fine – the positive locking device is for use when single knurling only; (b) use of a knurling tool (photograph reproduced courtesy of Jones and Shipman plc)*

- Considerable force is required to make the knurling rollers bite into the metal of the workpiece, so the work should protrude from the chuck only for the minimum possible distance or it will need to be supported with a centre.

- Make sure the knurling tool is clean and free from swarf, select the pair of rolls for the coarseness of knurl required. (Rollers with alternative groove patterns are available for special purposes, but the usual pattern produces a diamond-shaped knurl.)

- Feed the knurling tool against the work gently with your right hand, using the cross-slide handwheel, whilst guiding the knurling head with your left hand until the rollers are firmly in contact with the work.

- Start up the lathe and, using a low spindle speed, traverse the knurling tool from side to side using the carriage traverse handwheel as shown in Fig. 10.36(b). At the same time increase the pressure on the rollers by means of the cross-slide handwheel.

- When the required pattern has been obtained, engage the power traverse (using a coarse rate of feed setting) and knurl along the work for the required distance. Use a flood of coolant not only to lubricate the rollers but also to wash away the swarf which might otherwise clog the rollers and spoil the pattern.

- When the required knurl has been achieved, wind off the cross-slide quickly and stop the traverse.

- Finally chamfer the end of the component to remove the ragged edge at the start of the knurl.

10.20   Chip formation and the geometry of lathe tools

There are three basic types of chip produced when cutting metals:

- Discontinuous chip.

- Continuous chip.

- Continuous chip with a built-up edge.

10.20.1   Chip formation

Discontinuous chip

The cutting action of a normal wedge-shaped cutting tool causes the metal to try to pile up ahead of the tool until the forces involved cause the piled-up metal to shear off from the workpiece along a shear plane as shown in Fig. 10.37(a). This is a continuous process of piling up and shearing off as shown. If the metal being cut is brittle, for example cast iron or free-cutting brass, the sheared-off pieces of metal will be quite separate and form the flaky or granular type of chip, called a *discontinuous chip*, as shown in Fig. 10.37(b).

Continuous chip

This type of chip is formed when ductile metals such as steel are being cut. Complete separation of the metal along the shear planes does not take place and a continuous ribbon type chip is formed as shown in Fig. 10.37(c). The outer face of the chip rubs against the rake face of the tool and is burnished smooth. The inside of the chip remains rough. Long, ribbon like chips may look spectacular as they coil away from the tool, but their razor sharp, ragged edges are extremely dangerous.

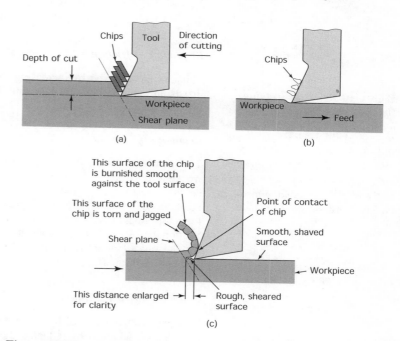

Figure 10.37 *Chip formation: (a) chip formation; (b) discontinuous chip; (c) continuous chip for ductile, low-strength metals*

Continuous chip with built-up edge

Under some conditions the friction between the chip and the rake face of the tool is very great. The combination of the contact pressure and the heat generated causes particles of metal from the chip to become pressure welded to the rake face of the tool as shown in Fig. 10.38(a). This makes the rake face of the tool rough at the cutting edge and increases the

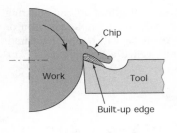

(a)

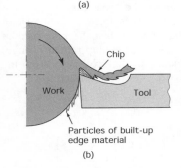

(b)

Figure 10.38 *Chip welding (built-up edge): (a) layers of chip material form on the rake face of the tool; (b) excessive chip welding produces an unstable built-up edge; particles of built-up edge material flake away and adhere to the workpiece, making it rough and spoiling the surface finish*

friction. This causes layer upon layer of metal to become built up, until a *built-up edge* is formed. A built-up edge masks the real cutting edge and the tool behaves as though it was blunt. Overheating occurs and the surface finish of the work is poor.

Eventually the amount of built-up metal increases to such an extent that it tends to become unstable and breaks down. The particles of built-up metal that flake away weld themselves to the chip and to the workpiece as shown in Fig. 10.38(b). This produces a dangerously jagged chip and a rough surface on the workpiece. The formation of a built-up edge is also referred to as *chip welding*.

10.20.2   Prevention of chip welding

Since chip welding has a considerable and adverse effect on tool life, power consumption, and surface finish, every attempt must be made to prevent it occurring. This is largely achieved by reversing the conditions that cause chip welding in the first place.

Reduction of friction

This can be achieved by increasing the rake angle, using a cutting fluid that is an extreme pressure lubricant as well as a coolant, and polishing the rake face.

Reducing the pressure

This can be achieved by increasing the rake angle. Remember this also weakens the tool and there is a limit to how far the rake angle can be increased for any given workpiece material. The pressure can also be reduced by increasing the approach angle of the tool. This reduces the chip thickness without reducing the rate of metal removal (see Section 10.23.1). Reducing the rate of feed and increasing the depth of cut the rate of metal removal whilst reducing the chip pressure on the tool (see Section 10.23.1).

Reducing the temperature

This can also be achieved by any of the above solutions. The temperature can also be achieved by reducing the spindle speed but this reduces the rate of metal removal.

Preventing metal to metal contact

This can be achieved by the use of a lubricant containing an extreme pressure additive. Such additives are usually sulphur or chlorine compounds. These additives tend to build up a non-metallic film on the surfaces of the tool and the chip. Since metal is not then in contact with metal chip welding cannot take place. Unfortunately active sulphur compounds attack copper and its alloys and should not be used on such metals. The use of non-metallic cutting tools such as tungsten carbide also helps to reduce the opportunity for a built-up edge to form.

10.20.3   Geometry of the lathe tool

The principles of cutting tool angles have already been discussed. These angles are applied to turning tools as shown in Fig. 10.39(a). In addition, we have to consider the *profile* of lathe tools. If the cutting edge is at *right angles* to the direction of feed, the tool is said to be cutting *orthogonally* as shown in Fig. 10.39(b). If the cutting edge is *inclined* so that it trails the direction of feed, it is said to be cutting *obliquely* as shown in Fig. 10.39(c). The purpose of an oblique *plan approach angle* is twofold:

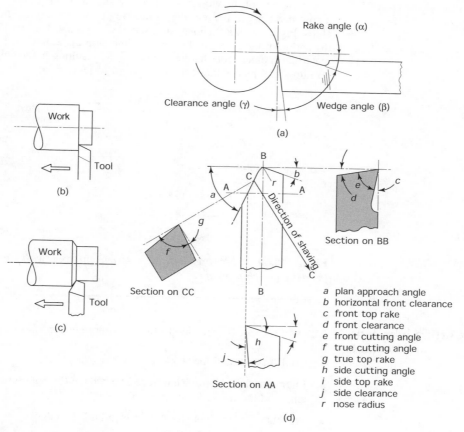

a plan approach angle
b horizontal front clearance
c front top rake
d front clearance
e front cutting angle
f true cutting angle
g true top rake
h side cutting angle
i side top rake
j side clearance
r nose radius

Figure 10.39   *Lathe tool angles: (a) cutting applied to an orthogonal turning tool; (b) orthogonal cutting – the cutting edge is perpendicular to the direction of feed, this is useful for producing a square shoulder; (c) oblique cutting – the cutting edge is inclined to the direction of feed, this is the most efficient form for rapid metal removal; (d) cutting angles applied to an oblique turning tool*

- To reduce the chip thickness, and therefore the load on the tool, whilst maintaining the same rate of material removal (see Section 10.23.1).

- To produce a back force on the tool. Wear of the cross-slide screw and nut results in 'backlash'. Without a back force on the tool, the forces acting on the rake face of the tool would result in the tool being drawn into the work, gradually increasing the depth of cut.

10.20.4 Chip-breaker

The dangers of continuous chips with their razor sharp jagged edges have already been discussed. Never remove these chips with your bare hands. Always use a chip rake. Stop the machine before removing the swarf. If it catches on the rapidly revolving job it can whip round and cause a serious accident. For the same reason the swarf must not be allowed to build up in the vicinity of the workholding device and the cutting zone. The use of a chip breaker can prevent the formation of dangerously long continuous chips. Figure 10.40(a) shows an inserted tip tool and Fig. 10.40(b) shows the action of the chip-breaker. It curls the chip up so tightly that the chip material becomes work hardened and brittle, resulting in the chip breaking up into small pieces that can be disposed of more easily and safely.

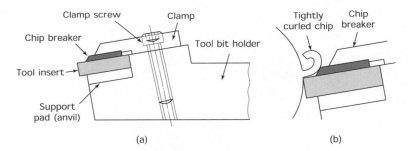

Figure 10.40 *Chip breaker: (a) inserted tip tool with chip breaker; (b) action of chip breaker*

10.21 Cutting lubricants and coolants

Cutting fluids are designed to fulfil one or more of the following functions:

- Cool the tool and the workpiece.

- Lubricate the chip/tool interface and reduce the friction between the chip and the rake face of the tool.

- Prevent chip welding (formation of a built-up edge).

- Improve the surface finish of the workpiece.

- Flush away the chips (swarf).

- Prevent corrosion of the work and the machine.

New compounds and synthetic additives and oils are being developed all the time. It is always best to consult the expert advisory service of the cutting fluid manufacturers. The selection and use of the correct cutting fluid can be the cheapest and most effective way of increasing the productivity of a machine shop. For general purpose machining a soluble oil is usually used.

10.21.1 Soluble oils

When water and oil are added together they refuse to mix but, if an emulsifier in the form of a detergent is added, the oil will break up into droplets and spread throughout the water to form an emulsion. This is what happens when the so-called 'soluble' cutting oils are added to water. The milky appearance of these emulsions is due to the light being refracted by the oil droplets. It is from this milky appearance that the emulsion gets its popular name of 'suds'.

The ratio of oil to water and the procedure for mixing will be recommended by the oil supplier. These conditions must be rigidly observed or

- the emulsion will break down on standing;

- the optimum cooling and lubrication properties of the emulsion will not be achieved.

The dilution of the oil with water greatly reduces the cost, but it also reduces the lubricating properties of the oil. This is why 'suds' are unsuitable for very severe machining operations such as gear cutting and broaching. Further, the high water content tends to cause corrosion of the work and the machine. Therefore, soluble oils should always contain a rust inhibitor.

Note that ordinary mineral oils are unsuitable as metal-cutting lubricants and coolants.

- Their viscosity is too high and their specific heat capacity is too low.

- They cannot withstand the very high pressures that exist between the chip and the tool. They give off noxious fumes when raised to the temperatures that exist in the cutting zone.

- They also represent a fire hazard.

10.22 Tool height

Figure 10.41 shows why it is essential to mount the tool at the centre height of the workpiece.

- Figure 10.41(a) shows the tool correctly set. You can see that the effective cutting angles are the same as those on the tool.

- Figure 10.41(b) shows the tool set below centre. You can see that, although the tool is ground to the same cutting angles, the rake angle

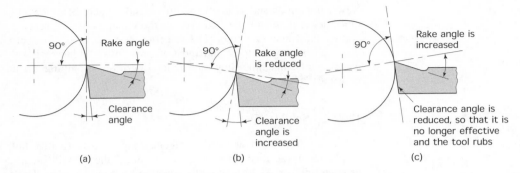

Figure 10.41 *Effect of tool height on lathe tool angles: (a) tool set correctly on centre height; (b) tool set below centre height; (c) tool set above centre height*

has been effectively reduced and the clearance has been effectively increased.

- Figure 10.41(c) shows the tool set above centre. You can see that once again the tool has been ground to the same cutting angles. This time the setting of the tool causes the rake angle to be effectively increased and the clearance angle to be effectively reduced, causing the tool to rub.

Figure 10.42 shows the effect of tool height on the effective cutting angles of a boring tool. You can see that this time the effects of the tool height on the effective cutting angles are reversed compared with those shown in the previous figure.

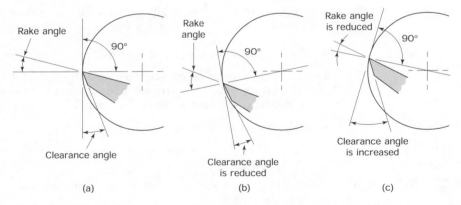

Figure 10.42 *Effect of tool height on boring tool angles: (a) tool set correctly on centre height; (b) tool set below centre height; (c) tool set above centre height*

The importance of setting a tool to the correct height when facing across the end of a workpiece is shown in Fig. 10.43.

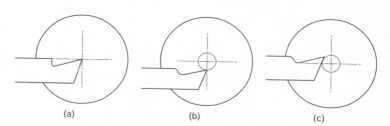

(a)   (b)   (c)

Figure 10.43 *Effect of tool height when facing: (a) tool setting correct – surface will be flat; (b) tool setting low – surface will not be flat; (c) tool setting high – surface will not clean up, and tool will be prevented from reaching centre of bar*

- In Fig. 10.43(a) the tool point is set to the centre height correctly and a smooth surface is produced.

- In Fig. 10.43(b) the tool is set below centre height and this time a 'pip' is left at the centre of the work. This is not only unsightly, but would produce difficulties if the end of the work needed to be centre drilled.

- In Fig. 10.43(c) the tool is set above centre height and this time it is impossible to face across the centre of the work.

- The tool can be set to the correct centre height by comparison with the point of the tailstock centre.

10.23 Relationship between depth of cut and feed rates as applied to turning operations

Orthogonal cutting and oblique cutting were introduced earlier in Fig. 10.39. Let's now investigate these techniques further as applied to parallel and perpendicular turning.

10.23.1 Cylindrical (parallel) turning

Figure 10.44(a) shows a cylindrical turning operation being performed by moving the tool parallel to the axis of the workpiece. Since the cutting edge of the tool is at right angles (perpendicular) to the direction of feed, the tool is said to be cutting orthogonally. The shaded area represents the cross-sectional area (shear area) of the chip. This area is calculated by multiplying the feed per revolution of the workpiece by the depth of cut ($A = f \times d$).

Figure 10.44(b) shows the same turning operation using a tool in which the cutting edge trails the direction of feed. Such a tool is said to be cutting obliquely. The cross-sectional area of the chip produced is the same as when cutting orthogonally since again $A = f \times d$. However, when cutting obliquely, the chip thickness (W) is reduced as shown in Fig. 10.44(c), where it can be seen that:

- The depth of cut d is constant in both examples.

- The feed/rev f is constant in both examples.

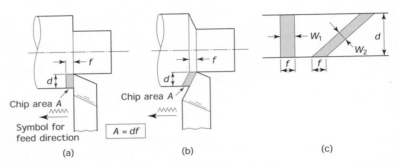

Figure 10.44 *Feed and depth of cut for parallel (cylindrical) turning: (a) orthogonal cutting; (b) oblique cutting; (c) chip width – depth of cut d, feed/rev f and chip area A (A = df) are constant for both figures; chip thickness W varies – oblique cutting reduces W without reducing A*

- The chip area ($A = f \times d$) is constant for both examples (parallelogram theory).
- The chip thickness is less when cutting obliquely because $W_1 > W_2$.

Since the chip is thinner when cutting obliquely the chip is more easily deflected over the rake face of the tool and the force it exerts on the tool is correspondingly less. This reduces wear on the tool and lessens the chance of chip welding without reducing the rate of material removal since the area of the cut is unaltered.

The same area of cut can be achieved using a shallow cut and a high rate of feed or by using a deep cut and a low rate of feed. Figure 10.45(a) shows what happens when a shallow cut at a high rate of feed is chosen. The chip is being bent across its deepest section. This not only requires considerable force, but the high feed rate will lead to a rough finish. In Fig. 10.45(b) a deep cut at a low rate of feed is being used. This time the chip is being bent across its thinnest section.

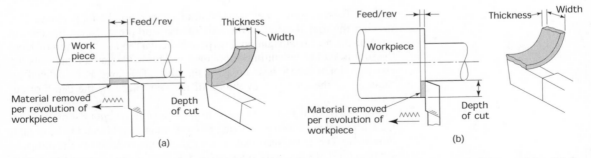

Figure 10.45 *Effects of feed rates and depth of cut: (a) coarse feed + shallow cut and effect on chip; (b) fine feed + deep cut and effect on chip*

Since the bending force varies as the cube (10^3) of the chip thickness, the force required to bend the chip is greatly reduced. For example, halving the chip thickness reduces the bending force to one-eighth of its previous value. Unfortunately a deep cut with a shallow feed can lead to chatter and a compromise has to be reached between depth of cut and rate of feed.

10.23.2 Perpendicular turning

Figure 10.46 shows examples of turning when the direction of feed is at right angles (perpendicular) to the axis of the workpiece. A parting-off operation is shown in Fig. 10.46(a), and the tool is cutting orthogonally since the cutting edge of the tool is at right angles to the direction of feed. You may find it strange that the depth of cut is controlled by the width of the tool, but look at it this way – Depth of cut is always at right angles to the direction of feed. Since the feed is perpendicular to the workpiece axis, it follows that the depth of cut must be parallel to the workpiece axis and this is the width of the tool.

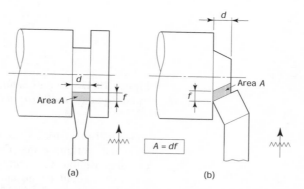

Figure 10.46 *Feed and depth of cut for perpendicular turning ($A = df$): (a) orthogonal cutting (grooving and parting off); (b) oblique cutting (sur-facing)*

A facing operation is shown in Fig. 10.46(b). This time the tool is cutting obliquely since the cutting edge is inclined to the direction of feed. In both examples the area of cut is the depth of cut multiplied by the feed per revolution ($A = d \times f$).

10.23.3 Cutting forces

Figure 10.47(a) shows the main cutting forces acting on a turning tool that is cutting orthogonally. Additional forces are present when the tool is cutting obliquely as shown in Fig. 10.47(b).

- The main cutting force F_c is a reaction force and is equal to but never greater than the downward force of the chip on the tool.

- The feed force F_f is also a reaction force and is caused by the resistance of the material being cut to the penetration of the cutting tool.

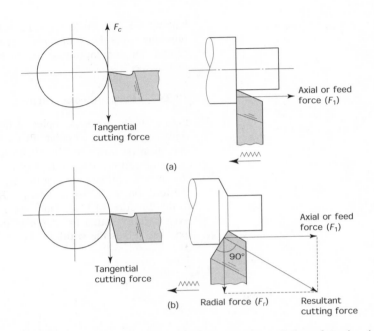

Figure 10.47 *Forces acting on turning tools: (a) orthogonal cutting (no radial force on tool); (b) oblique cutting*

We call these forces reaction forces because their magnitude depends upon the workpiece material and the cutting conditions. If the lathe is operated without the workpiece in place the tool would not be cutting and there would be no cutting force or feed force acting on the tool and, therefore, no reaction forces would be present. If the workpiece is a relatively weak material such as aluminium then modest cutting and feed forces would be exerted on the cutting tool. If a strong material such as alloy steel is cut with the same depth of cut and rate of feed then the forces acting on the tool would be very much greater. The limiting forces are those which are so great that the tool cannot withstand them and it breaks.

Let's now look at the remaining force. This is the radial force F_r in Fig. 10.47(b). This force exists only when the tool has an oblique cutting action. Figure 10.47(b) shows a roughing tool with a trailing approach angle. The radial force is trying to push the tool away from the work. Therefore, this force keeps the flanks of the cross-slide screw and nut in contact with each other and takes up any backlash due to wear. This prevents the tool being drawn into the work and producing undersize work.

10.24 Cutting speeds as applied to turning operations

To keep the cost of production to a minimum during a machining process, the rate of material removal must be kept as high as possible. It is usual to break down the component by means of a series of roughing cuts, leaving a small amount of metal on for a finishing cut to produce the finish and dimensional accuracy required. The factors controlling the rate of material removal are:

- Finish required.

- Depth of cut.

- Tool geometry.

- Properties and rigidity of the cutting tool and its mounting.

- Properties and rigidity of the workpiece.

- Rigidity of the work holding device.

- Power and rigidity of the machine tool.

Many of these factors have already been discussed but we still have to consider the cutting speed. Cutting speeds and feed rates depend upon the material being cut, the finish required and the type of tool material being used. Table 10.8 lists some typical values of cutting speeds for high-speed steel tools. These figures are only a guide and they may be

TABLE 10.8 *Cutting speeds and feeds (typical for HSS)*

Material being turned	Feed (mm/rev)	Cutting speed (m/min)
Aluminium	0.2–1.00	70–100
Brass (alpha) (ductile)	0.2–1.00	50–80
Brass (free-cutting)	0.2–1.5	70–100
Bronze (phosphor)	0.2–1.0	35–70
Cast iron (grey)	0.15–0.7	25–40
Copper	0.2–1.00	35–70
Steel (mild)	0.2–1.00	35–50
Steel (medium carbon)	0.15–0.7	30–35
Steel (alloy-high tensile)	0.08–0.3	5–10
Thermosetting plastic*	0.2–1.0	35–50

*Low speed due to abrasive properties.

increased or decreased as experience dictates. Much higher cutting speeds can be used when carbide-tipped tools are employed. When using tipped tools you should consult the manufacturers' literature for information on cutting speeds and feed to ensure that the tools are used efficiently.

Example 10.1 *Calculate the spindle speed, to the nearest rev/min, for turning a 25 mm diameter bar at a cutting speed of 30 m/min (take π as 3.14).*

$$N = \frac{1000S}{\pi D}$$

$$= \frac{1000 \times 30}{3.14 \times 25}$$

where: N = spindle speed
S = 30 m/min
π = 3.14
D = 25 mm

$$= \textbf{382 rev/min} \text{ (to nearest rev/min)}$$

Example 10.2 *Calculate the time taken to turn a brass component 49 mm diameter by 70 mm long if the cutting speed is 410 m/min and the feed rate is 0.5 mm/rev. Only one cut is taken (take π as 22/7).*

$$N = \frac{1000S}{\pi D}$$

$$= \frac{1000 \times 44 \times 7}{22 \times 49}$$

where: N = spindle speed
S = 44 m/min
π = 22/7
D = 49 mm

$$= \textbf{286 rev/min} \text{ (to nearest rev/min)}$$

Rate of feed (mm/rev) = 0.5 mm/rev

Rate of feed (mm/min) = 0.5 mm/rev × 286 rev/min

$$= 143 \text{ mm/min}$$

$$\left.\begin{array}{l} \text{Time in minutes taken} \\ \text{to traverse 70 mm} \end{array}\right\} = \frac{70 \text{ mm}}{143 \text{ mm/min}}$$

$$\left.\begin{array}{l} \text{Time in seconds taken} \\ \text{to traverse 70 mm} \end{array}\right\} = \frac{70 \times 60}{143} = \textbf{29.37 seconds}$$

10.25 The production of some typical turned components

10.25.1 Between centres

It has been stated earlier in this chapter that where two or more diameters are to be strictly concentric they must be turned at the same setting. Figure 10.48 shows a component with a number of concentric diameters. In this example, no matter what method of workholding is employed, it is impossible to turn all the diameters at the same time and at some stage the component has to be turned end for end. Since the component is not hollow it can be held between centres and this will ensure that the diameters turned at the second setting will be concentric with the diameters turned at the first setting.

The sequence of operations for the manufacture of this component is shown in Fig. 10.49. To ensure success it is essential to use a DTI to check that the headstock centre is running true. If it proves impossible to get the centre to run true then a soft centre must be used and turned *in situ*

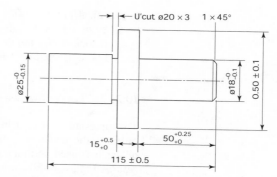

Figure 10.48 *Shaft: material free-cutting mild steel Ø 50 × 125 (dimensions in millimetres)*

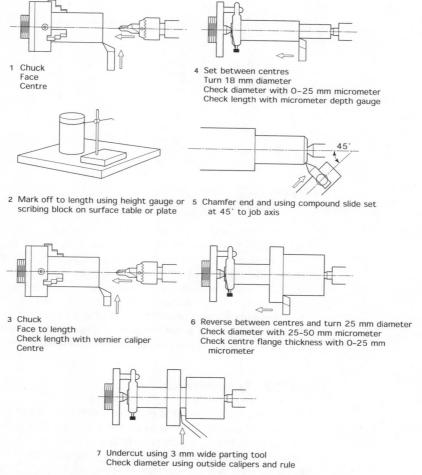

1 Chuck
  Face
  Centre

2 Mark off to length using height gauge or
  scribing block on surface table or plate

3 Chuck
  Face to length
  Check length with vernier caliper
  Centre

4 Set between centres
  Turn 18 mm diameter
  Check diameter with 0–25 mm micrometer
  Check length with micrometer depth gauge

5 Chamfer end and using compound slide set
  at 45° to job axis

6 Reverse between centres and turn 25 mm diameter
  Check diameter with 25–50 mm micrometer
  Check centre flange thickness with 0–25 mm
  micrometer

7 Undercut using 3 mm wide parting tool
  Check diameter using outside calipers and rule

Figure 10.49 *Turning shaft between centres*

to a conical point of 60° included angle of taper. A trial cut should then be taken along the length of the work to check that the headstock centre and tailstock centre are in alignment and that there is no taper. Any taper should be corrected by lateral adjustment of the tailstock.

10.25.2 Three-jaw, self-centring chuck

The three-jaw, self-centring chuck is the most popular workholding device on the lathe because of its ease and quickness in setting up. However, unless it is used and maintained with care it also gives the *least accurate results*. Figure 10.50 shows a typical component suitable for chuck work.

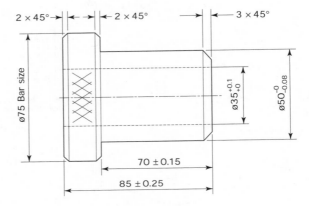

Figure 10.50 *Large bush*

In planning the operations for this component, it should be noted that only the 35 mm diameter and the 50 mm diameter have to be concentric. They must therefore be machined at the same setting. The knurled diameter of the collar does not require a greater degree of concentricity than is readily available with a three-jaw chuck. Therefore only the concentric diameters have to be turned at the same setting. Remember that a drilled hole has only limited accuracy and that it will be necessary to finish the 35 mm diameter by boring to remove any residual errors. Figure 10.51 shows a suitable operation sequence for this component.

10.25.3 Taper mandrel

If the bore of the bush had been too small to bore out with a substantial boring tool or boring bar, then an alternative method of production would be required. For example, after rough turning the external diameter, the hole could be drilled and reamed. The bush could then be pressed onto a taper mandrel and the external diameter finish turned between centres, as discussed earlier in this chapter, to ensure concentricity.

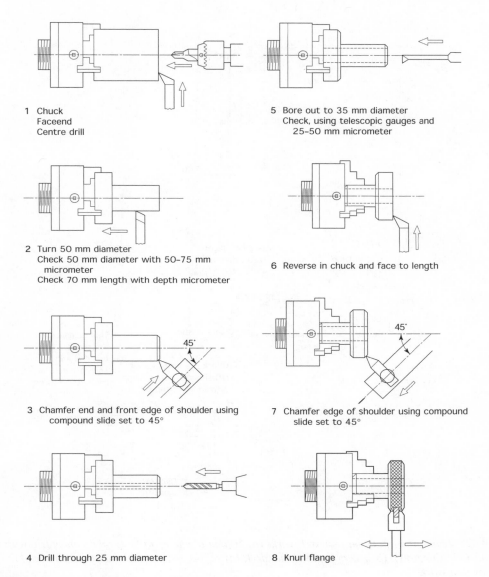

1 Chuck
   Faceend
   Centre drill

5 Bore out to 35 mm diameter
   Check, using telescopic gauges and
      25–50 mm micrometer

2 Turn 50 mm diameter
   Check 50 mm diameter with 50–75 mm
      micrometer
   Check 70 mm length with depth micrometer

6 Reverse in chuck and face to length

3 Chamfer end and front edge of shoulder using
      compound slide set to 45°

7 Chamfer edge of shoulder using compound
      slide set to 45°

4 Drill through 25 mm diameter

8 Knurl flange

Figure 10.51 *Turning the bush in a self-centring chuck*

10.25.4 Parallel mandrel (snug)

The component shown in Fig. 10.52(a) is too thin to mount on a taper mandrel; however, it can be held on a parallel mandrel or 'snug' as shown in Fig. 10.52(b). Should the mandrel have to be reused from time to time, it can be reset in a four-jaw chuck using a DTI as shown in Fig. 10.52(c) to ensure concentricity. This type of mandrel can also be

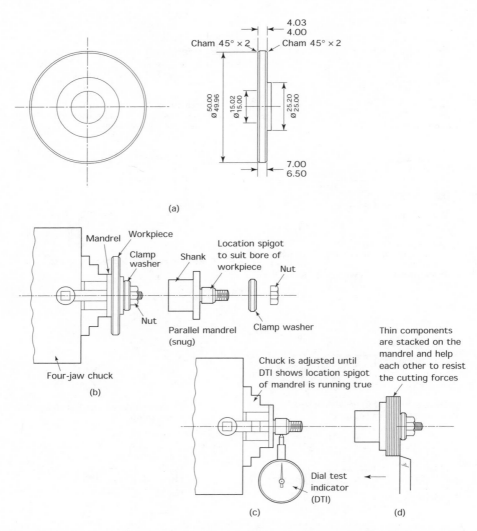

Figure 10.52 *Example of parallel mandrel work: (a) 50 mm diameter to be turned concentric with the bore (dimensions in millimetres); (b) use of parallel mandrel; (c) setting the parallel mandrel; (d) use of the parallel mandrel for thin work*

used for very thin components. These can be mounted side by side in a batch as shown in Fig. 10.52(d). This not only increases the productivity but the components support each other, so preventing distortion resulting from the cutting forces.

10.25.5 Four-jaw chuck

Figure 10.53(a) shows a component that has to be reversed and reset for the second operations. The initial turning can be done in a three-jaw, self-centring chuck so that it appears as shown in Fig. 10.53(b). However, when it is reversed for the second operations it has to be held in a four-jaw chuck so that it can be 'clocked up' to run true with a DTI.

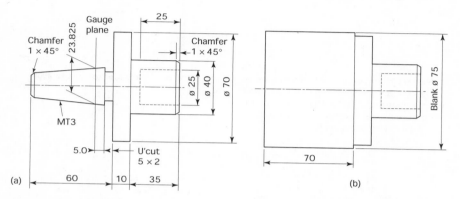

Figure 10.53 *Component requiring second operation machining: (a) finished component; (b) component as turned in three-jaw chuck ready for second operation work (dimensions in millimetres)*

The sequence for the *second operations* to make this component is shown in Fig. 10.54. Had a batch of these components been required, then all the first operations would have been completed in a three-jaw chuck for the entire batch. The three-jaw chuck would then have had its hard jaws replaced by a set of *soft jaws* and these would have been bored out to suit the component as discussed earlier in this chapter. Since the jaws would have been turned to size *in situ*, the work mounted in them would run true without adjustment and without having to 'clock up' each individual component. For a batch of components this saves time over using a four-jaw chuck.

10.25.6 Faceplate

The faceplate is used when the axis of the turned component has to be perpendicular (at right angles) to the datum surface as shown in Fig. 10.55(a). In this example the 50 mm diameter has to be rebored to take a replacement bearing. The new bore has to be concentric with the existing bore and perpendicular to the face AA. The component is lightly clamped to a faceplate and trued up using a DTI as shown in Fig. 10.55(b) by gently tapping the component into position with a soft faced hammer or mallet. It is then clamped tightly to resist the cutting forces and rechecked to ensure it hasn't moved. Finally it is rebored and checked for size.

Exercises   **10.1**   *Safety in the use of machine tools*
    (a)   Describe FIVE important personal safety precautions that should be taken when operating a centre lathe.

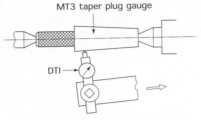

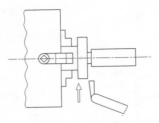

1 Set MT3 taper plug gauge between centres
Set over compound slide so that DTI shows a
  constant reading along the full length of taper
Compound slide is kept at this setting up to
  and including operation 5

4 Undercut using a cranked tool to avoid
fouling the flange

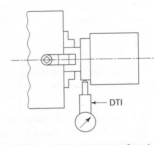

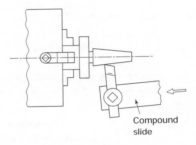

2 Remove centres and mount four-jaw chuck
Hold on ø40 mm in four-jaw chuck
Set to run true using a DTI bearing on the
  previously turned ø70 mm

5 Turn taper using compound slide.
  Remember, this was set to correct angle
  in operation 1 using a 3MT plug gauge.
  Check workpiece taper using a stepped,
  3MT ring gauge

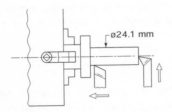

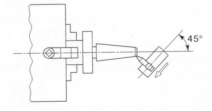

3 Turn maximum diameter for MT3 taper
(ø24.1 mm) and face to length (60 mm)

6 Reset compound slide to 45°. Chamfer
end of taper

Figure 10.54 *Operation sequence for component requiring second operation machining*

    (b)   Name FIVE important safety features that should be provided
on all centre lathes.

    (c)   Describe five safety rules that should be observed when oper-
ating a centre lathe.

10.2 *The centre lathe*

    (a)   Figure 10.56 shows an outline drawing of a centre lathe. Copy
the drawing and name the features shown.

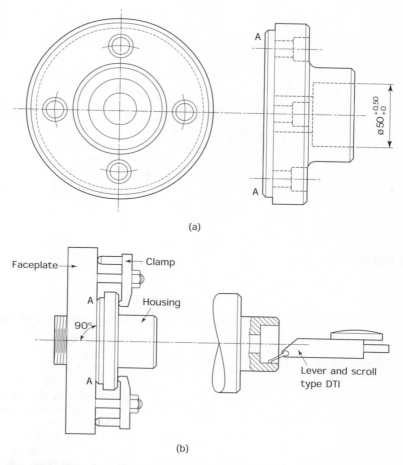

Figure 10.55 *Bearing housing to be rebored (a), method of clamping bearing housing onto a faceplate and setting it to run true (b)*

(b) List the advantages and limitations of a quick change tool post compared with a four-way turret tool post.
(c) With the aid of sketches, describe how the following surfaces can be generated on a centre lathe.
  (i) Cylindrical surfaces.
  (ii) Plane surfaces.
  (iii) Conical (tapered) surfaces (one method only need be shown).

10.3 *Spindle noses*
Select and sketch three types of spindle nose and list their relative advantages and limitations. State which one is most likely to be found on a modern industrial lathe.

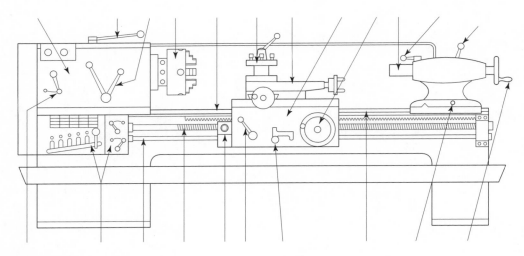

Figure 10.56 *Exercise 10.2(a)*

10.4 *Workholding*

(a) When turning between centres, explain why:

(i) The headstock centre must be checked for true running.

(ii) The tailstock centre must be eased from time to time when using a solid centre.

(iii) Work that should be cylindrical may be tapered. Also state how you would check for this inaccuracy and how you would correct it.

(iv) Slender work is sometimes the correct size at each end but oversize in the middle (barrel shaped). Explain how you would prevent this happening.

(b) Work is sometimes held between centres on a taper mandrel. Explain why this is necessary and what precautions you would take to prevent the work becoming loose.

(c) When holding work in a three-jaw, self-centring chuck:

(i) Describe the precautions that should be taken to keep the chuck in good condition and prolong its initial accuracy.

(ii) Explain why separate internal and external jaws are required.

(iii) Explain why soft jaws may sometimes be used.

(d) With reference to the four-jaw chuck:

(i) List its advantages and limitations compared with a three-jaw, self-centring chuck.

(ii) Sketch a component that needs to be made in a four-jaw chuck.

(e) List the advantages and limitations of using collets compared with using a three-jaw chuck.

(f) Sketch a typical component that needs to be turned on a faceplate rather than in a chuck. Also show how the component would be attached to the faceplate.

10.5 *Concentricity and eccentricity*

(a) Explain briefly with the aid of sketches what is meant by the terms:
   (i) Concentricity.
   (ii) Eccentricity.

(b) Explain briefly with the aid of sketches how concentricity between various internal and external diameters can be maintained:
   (i) When turning from the bar.
   (ii) When setting for second operation work.

10.6 *Miscellaneous operations*

(a) Describe THREE ways of producing holes and bores on a lathe and list the relative advantages and limitations of each of the methods chosen.

(b) (i) Describe how you would use taps and dies to produce screw threads on a lathe.
   (ii) Describe the precautions you would take when using taps and dies on a lathe to ensure an accurate thread is produced.

(c) With the aid of sketches describe ONE method of taper turning and list the advantages and limitations of the method chosen.

10.7 *Turning tools and chip formation*

(a) Figure 10.57 shows four typical turning tools. Describe, with the aid of sketches, typical applications for these tools.

(b) Explain:
   (i) what is meant by the term continuous chip;
   (ii) what is meant by the term non-continuous chip;
   (iii) the conditions under which these different types of chip may be produced;
   (iv) what a chip-breaker is and why it may be used.

(c) Explain, with the aid of sketches, how the following tool angles are applied to single point turning tools.
   (i) Rake angle.
   (ii) Clearance angle.
   (iii) Secondary clearance angle (boring tool).
   (iv) Wedge angle.
   (v) Plan approach angle.

(d) Explain, with the aid of sketches:
   (i) the difference between positive and negative rake cutting as applied to turning tools;

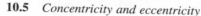
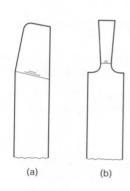
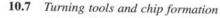
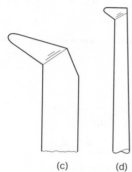

(a)   (b)

(c)   (d)

Figure 10.57 *Exercise 10.7(a)*

(ii) the difference between *oblique* and *orthogonal* cutting.

(e) List the essential requirements of a cutting fluid for general turning operations.

(f) Describe the precautions that should be taken when mixing and using a soluble cutting fluid.

(g) List the advantages and disadvantages of using a cutting fluid when turning.

(h) Calculate the spindle speed, to the nearest rev/min, for turning a 50 mm diameter at a cutting speed of 40 m/min.

(i) Using the spindle speed calculated in (h) above, calculate the time taken to take a cut 75 mm long at a feed rate of 0.15 mm/rev.

10.8 *Turning operations*

(a) Describe with the aid of sketches the production of the component shown in Fig. 10.58. Pay particular attention to the method of workholding. List the tools and equipment used.

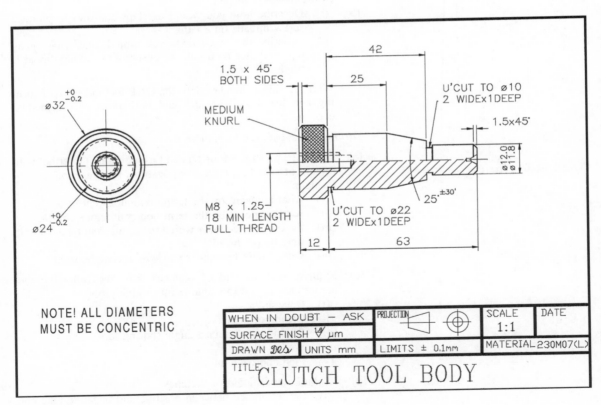

Figure 10.58 *Exercise 10.8(a)*

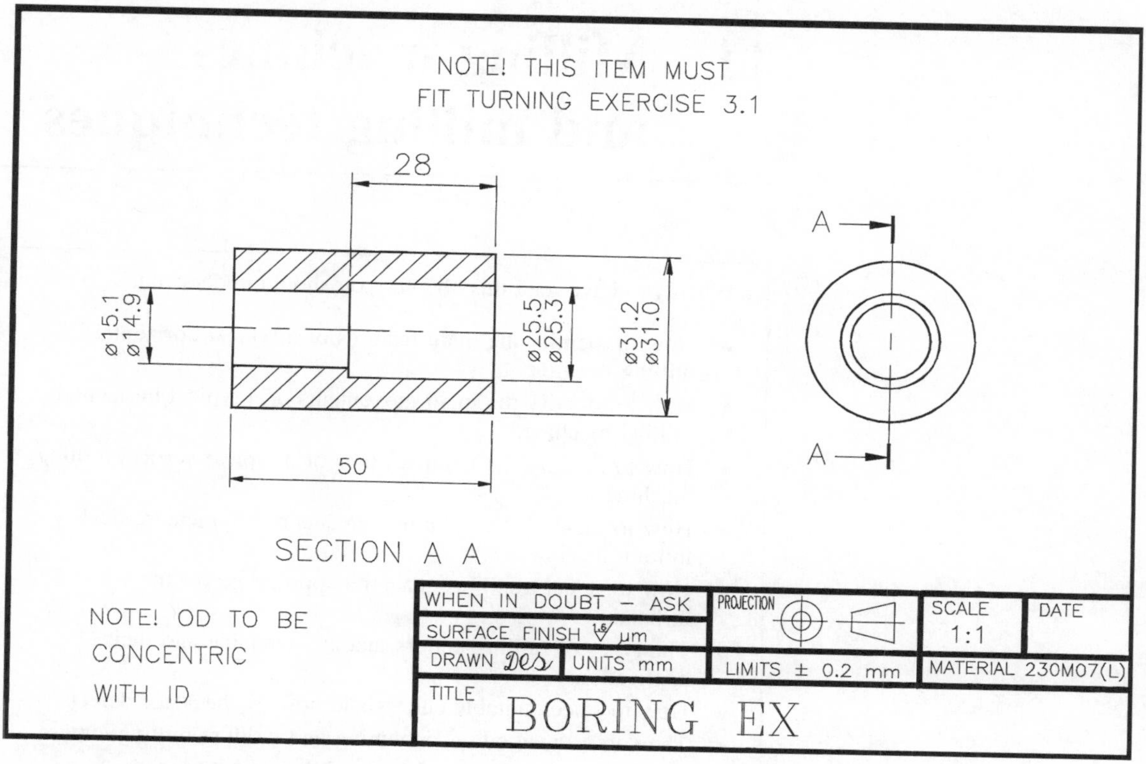
NOTE! THIS ITEM MUST
FIT TURNING EXERCISE 3.1
28
ø15.1
ø14.9
ø25.5
ø25.3
ø31.2
ø31.0
50
A
A
SECTION A A
NOTE! OD TO BE
CONCENTRIC
WITH ID
WHEN IN DOUBT – ASK
SURFACE FINISH 1.6 µm
DRAWN DES
UNITS mm
PROJECTION
LIMITS ± 0.2 mm
SCALE
1:1
DATE
MATERIAL 230M07(L)
TITLE
BORING EX

Figure 10.59 *Exercise 10.8(b)*

(b) Describe with the aid of sketches the production of the component shown in Fig. 10.59. Pay particular attention to the method of workholding. List the tools and equipment used.

11 Milling machines and milling techniques

When you have read this chapter you should understand:

- How to identify the main features of a typical horizontal milling machine.
- How to identify the main movements of a typical horizontal milling machine.
- How to identify the main features of a typical vertical milling machine.
- How to identify the main movements of a typical vertical milling machine.
- How to select a milling machine appropriate for the work in hand.
- The types of milling cutters that are available and their applications.
- How to select suitable cutters and how to check for defects.
- The correct methods of mounting and holding milling cutters.
- The available methods of workholding and setting.
- How to use milling machines to produce vertical, horizontal and angular faces and slots.

11.1 Safety

Milling machines are classified as *especially dangerous machines*. In addition to the normal requirements of the Health and Safety at Work Act, these machines are also subject to the Horizontal Milling Machine Regulations. Copies of these Regulations are available in the form of a wall chart which is supposed to be hung up near to where such machines are being used.

The main danger associated with milling machines is the cutter. Therefore:

- Make sure the cutter guard is in place before starting the machine.
- Do not remove swarf with a brush whilst the cutter is revolving.
- Do not wipe away coolant from the cutting zone with a rag whilst the cutter is revolving.
- Do not take measurements whilst the cutter is revolving.
- Do not load or unload work whilst the cutter is revolving.

- Do not put your hands anywhere near the cutter whilst it is revolving.

Figure 11.1(a) shows a typical cutter guard as used by skilled operators in toolrooms, prototype workshops and jobbing workshops where the machine is being frequently reset.

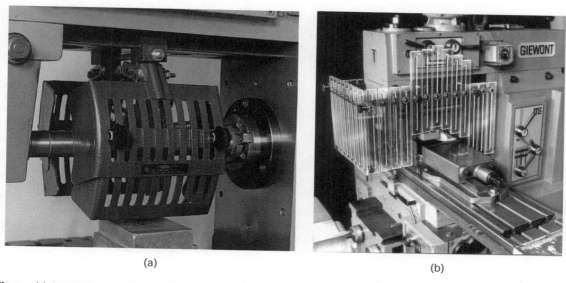

(a)   (b)

Figure 11.1 *Milling machine guards: (a) toolroom type cutter guard; (b) production type cutter guard*

Figure 11.1(b) shows a production type guard suitable where only semi-skilled labour is employed to operate the machine. The whole of the cutting zone is guarded and loading and unloading of the workholding fixture takes place safely outside the guard.

11.2 The milling process

Milling machines are used to produce parallel, perpendicular and inclined plain surfaces using multi-tooth cutters. These cutters are rotated by the machine spindle, and it is from the plane in which the axis of the spindle lies that determines the name of the machine. The geometry of a single point cutting tool as considered in the previous chapters is shown in Fig. 11.2(a), whilst Fig. 11.2(b) shows how these angles are applied to a milling cutter tooth. The additional secondary clearance angle prevents the heel of the tooth catching on the workpiece as the tool rotates. It also provides chip clearance. Figure 11.2(c) shows an actual milling cutter. Because of the large number of teeth used, the surface produced is virtually a plain surface free from ripples. The surface can be improved even further by cutting the teeth with a helix angle as shown in Fig. 11.2(d)

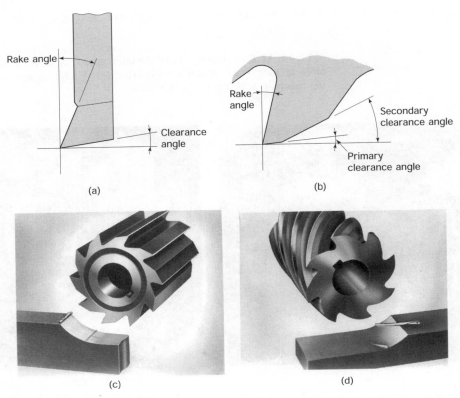

Figure 11.2 *Milling cutter tooth angles: comparison of cutter angles for a single point cutting tool (a) and a milling cutter tooth (b); (c) orthogonal cutting (straight tooth) cutter; (d) oblique cutting (30° helical tooth cutter) (photographs reproduced courtesy of Cincinatti Milacron Ltd)*

instead of straight across the cutter. This also evens out the forces acting on the machine transmission system since one tooth is starting to cut before the previous tool has finished cutting.

As for turning, modern practice favours the use of carbide-tipped milling cutters for production milling where high rates of material removal are required or when high strength materials are being machined. These can have brazed-on tips as shown in Fig. 11.3(a) or inserted, disposable tips as shown in Fig. 11.3(b). Nowadays, cutters with disposable carbide and coated carbide tips are widely used on production and even for the prototype machining of high strength, hard and abrasive materials.

It would appear from the above comments that the more teeth a cutter has got, the better will be the finish and the faster the cutter will be able to remove metal. This is true only up to a point. For any cutter of a given circumference, increasing the number of teeth reduces the space between the teeth. This makes the teeth smaller and weaker and it also reduces the room for the chips so that the teeth tend to clog easily and break.

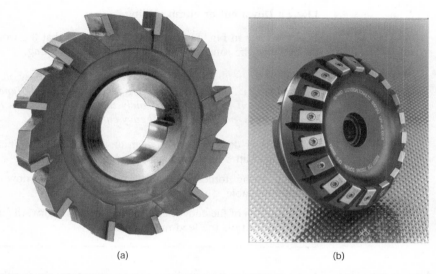

(a)　　　　　　　　　　(b)

Figure 11.3 *Carbide-tipped milling cutters: (a) brazed tip cutter; (b) inserted disposable tip cutter (reproduced courtesy of Richard Lloyd (Galtona) Ltd)*

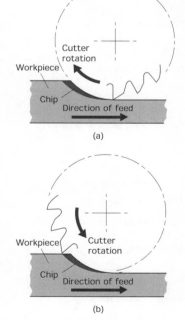

Figure 11.4 *Chip formation when milling: (a) up-cut milling; (b) down-cut milling*

When choosing a milling cutter for a particular job, the spacing (pitch) of the teeth should be kept as wide as possible for a given class of work in order to provide adequate strength and chip clearance. Thus coarse pitch cutters should be used for roughing out robust work as they have more efficient material removal characteristics and are more economical in the cutting power required. Finer pitch cutters should be used with light cuts where fragile work is involved and a fine finish is required.

11.2.1 Up-cut or conventional milling

This is shown in Fig. 11.4(a). You can see that the work is fed towards the cutter against the direction of rotation.

- This prevents the work being dragged into the cutter if there is any backlash in the feed mechanism.

- Unfortunately this technique causes the cutting edges to rub as each tooth starts to cut and this can lead to chatter and blunting of the cutting edge.

- The cutting action tends to lift the work off the machine table.

- For safety this is the technique you should always adopt unless your instructor advises you to the contrary because he or she knows that your machine is equipped to operate safely using the following technique.

11.2.2 Down-cut or climb milling

This is shown in Fig. 11.4(b). Here you can see that the work is fed into the cutter in the same direction as the cutter is rotating.

> *Safety: The climb milling technique can be used only on machines fitted with a 'backlash eliminator' and which are designed for this technique. If it can be used safely this technique has a number of advantages, particularly for heavy cutting operations.*

- The cutter does not rub as each tooth starts to cut. This reduces the risk of chatter and prolongs the cutter life.

- The cutting forces keep the workpiece pressed down against the machine table.

- The action of the cutter helps to feed the work forward and takes most of the load off the feed mechanism.

11.3 The horizontal spindle milling machine

The *horizontal milling machine* gets its name from the fact that the axis of the spindle of the machine, and therefore the axis of the arbor supporting the cutter, lies in a horizontal plane as shown in Fig. 11.5. The more important features and controls are also named in this figure.

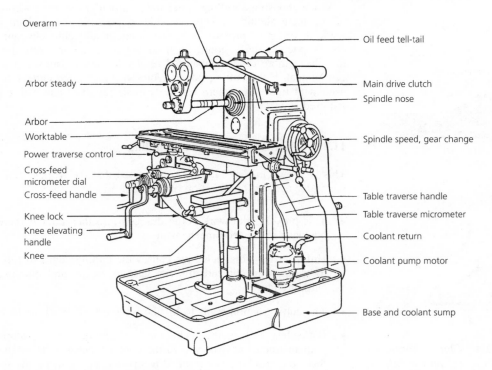

Figure 11.5 *Horizontal spindle milling machine*

11.3.1 Basic movements and alignments of a horizontal spindle milling machine

The basic alignments and movements of a horizontal milling machine are shown in Fig. 11.6. The most important alignment is that the spindle axis, and therefore the arbor axis, is parallel to the surface of the worktable. The depth of cut is controlled by raising the knee and table subassembly. The position of the cut is controlled by the cross-slide and the feed is provided by a lead screw and nut fitted to the table and separately driven to the spindle. Unlike the feed of a lathe which is directly related to the spindle speed and measured in mm/rev, the feed of a milling machine table is independent of the spindle speed and is measured in mm/min.

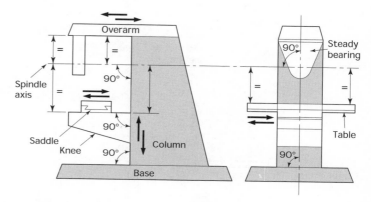

Figure 11.6 *Horizontal spindle milling machine: movements and alignments*

The horizontal milling machine can produce surfaces that are parallel to the worktable as shown in Fig. 11.7(a). It can also produce surfaces that are perpendicular to the worktable as shown in Fig. 11.7(b). The use of a side and face is shown in Fig. 11.7(c). It can be seen that for this latter cutter the depth of cut is limited by the relative diameters of the cutter and the arbor spacing collars.

11.4 The vertical spindle milling machine

The *vertical milling machine* gets its name from the fact that the axis of the spindle of the machine, and therefore the axis of the cutter being used, lies in the vertical plane as shown in Fig. 11.8. The more important features and controls are also named in this figure.

11.4.1 Basic movements and alignments of a vertical spindle milling machine

The basic alignments and movements of a vertical milling machine are shown in Fig. 11.9. The most important alignment is that the spindle axis, and therefore the cutter axis, is perpendicular to the surface of the

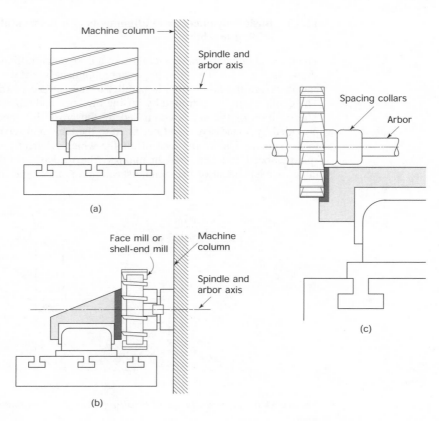

Figure 11.7 *Surfaces parallel and perpendicular to the worktable (horizontal milling machine): (a) use of a slab mill to machine a surface parallel to the milling machine table; (b) use of a face mill or a shell-end mill to machine a surface perpendicular to the milling machine table; (c) use of a side and face milling cutter to machine a surface perpendicular to the milling machine table – the depth of the perpendicular surface is limited by the relative diameters of the cutter and spacing collars*

worktable. The depth of cut is controlled by raising the knee and table subassembly or, for some operations raising or lowering the spindle. For maximum rigidity, the spindle is normally raised as far as possible. The position of the cut is controlled by the cross-slide and the feed is provided by a lead screw and nut fitted to the table and separately driven to the spindle. As for horizontal milling, the feed of a vertical milling machine table is independent of spindle and is measured in mm/min.

Vertical milling machines produce surfaces parallel to the worktable by means of face milling cutters mounted directly on the spindle end as shown in Fig. 11.10(a). Compared with the rate of metal removal that can be removed with a slab or roller mill on a horizontal machine, larger surfaces can be covered in one pass at greater rates of material removal with a face mill on a vertical spindle machine. Surfaces perpendicular to the worktable are produced by the side of an end milling cutter as shown

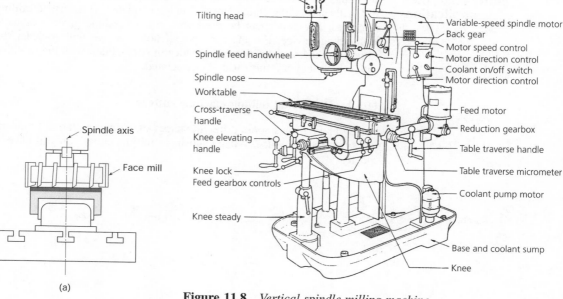

Figure 11.8 *Vertical spindle milling machine*

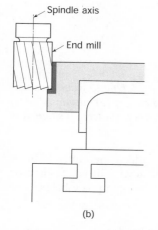

(a)

(b)

Figure 11.10 *Surfaces parallel and perpendicular to the work-table (vertical milling machine): (a) use of a face mill to machine surfaces parallel to the work-table; (b) use of an end mill to machine surfaces perpendicular to the machine table*

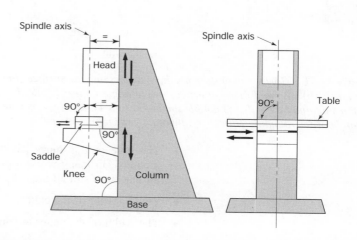

Figure 11.9 *Vertical spindle milling machine: movements and alignments*

in Fig. 11.10(b). Since the cutter is supported as a cantilever by its shank alone, the load that can be put on it is limited and only relatively low rates of material removal can be removed in this way.

<table>
<tr><td>

11.5 Types of milling cutters and their applications

</td><td>

Although side and face milling cutters and slab (roller) milling cutters are usually associated with horizontal milling machines, and end mills, slot drills and facing cutters are normally associated with vertical milling machines, any cutter can be used with either machine given a suitable toolholding device. For the time being, however, we will consider the cutters and the surfaces that the produce in conjunction with the machine with which they are most usually associated.

</td></tr>
</table>

11.5.1 Horizontal milling machine cutters

Figure 11.11 shows some different shapes of milling cutter and the surfaces that they produce. When choosing a milling cutter you will have to specify:

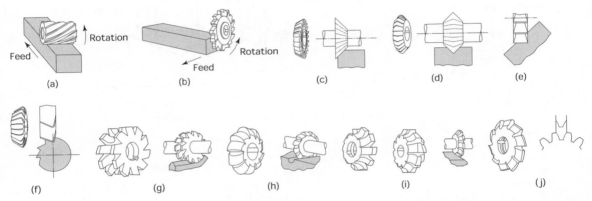

Figure 11.11 *Horizontal milling machine cutters and the surfaces they produce: (a) slab milling cutter (cylinder mill); (b) side and face cutter; (c) single-angle cutter; (d) double equal-angle cutter; (e) cutting a V-slot with a side and face mill; (f) double unequal-angle cutter; (g) concave cutter; (h) convex cutter; (i) single and double corner rounding cutters; (j) involute gear tooth cutter*

- The bore of this must suit the arbor on which the cutter is to be mounted. In many workshops one size of arbor will be standard on all machines and all the cutters will have the appropriate bores.
- The diameter of the cutter.
- The width of the cutter to suit the work in hand.
- The shape of the cutter.
- The tooth formation.

11.5.2 Vertical milling machine cutters

A selection of milling cutters suitable for a vertical milling machine is shown in Fig. 11.12 and some typical applications are shown in Fig. 11.13. Note that only *slot drills* can be used for making pocket cuts

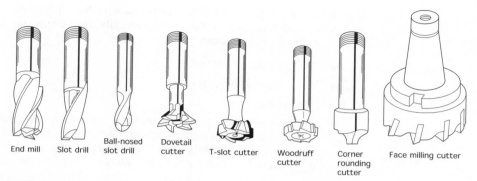

Figure 11.12 *Typical milling cutters for vertical spindle milling machines*

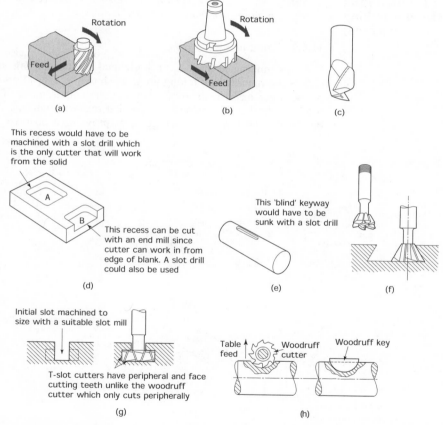

Figure 11.13 *Vertical milling machine cutters and the surfaces they produce: (a) end milling cutter; (b) face milling cutter; (c) slot drill; (d) recess A would need to be cut with a slot drill because it is the only cutter that will work from the centre of a solid; recess B could be cut using a slot drill or an end mill because it occurs at the edge of the solid; (e) this blind keyway would have to be sunk with a slot drill; (f) dovetail (angle) cutter; (g) T-slot cutter; (h) Woodruff cutter*

from the solid. All the other cutters have to be fed into the workpiece from its side as they cannot be fed vertically downwards into the work. When choosing a cutter you will need to specify:

- The diameter of the cutter.

- The length of the cutter.

- The type of cutter.

- The type of shank. Some cutters have solid shanks integral with the cutter for holding in a chuck, whilst other cutters are made for mounting on a separate stub arbor. Some large face milling cutters are designed to bolt directly onto the spindle nose of the machine.

11.6 Cutter mounting (horizontal milling machine)

Safety: Make sure the machine is electrically isolated before attempting to remove or mount arbors and cutters.

11.6.1 Long arbor

For most milling operations on horizontal spindle milling machines the cutters are mounted on a long arbor as shown in Fig. 11.14(a). One end of the arbor has a taper for locating in the spindle nose of the milling machine. It also has a slotted flange that registers with the driving dogs on the spindle nose. This arrangement provides a positive drive to the

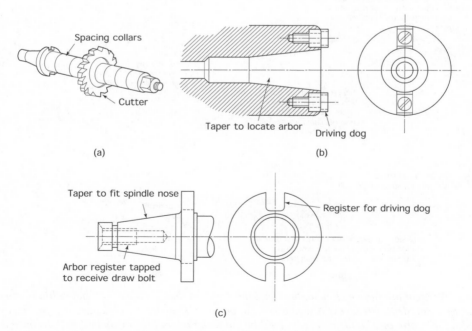

Figure 11.14 *Horizontal milling machine arbor: (a) long arbor for horizontal milling machine; (b) milling machine spindle nose; (c) taper register of arbor to fit spindle nose*

arbor and no slip is possible. Details of the spindle nose are shown in Fig. 11.14(b) and details of the taper on the arbor end are shown in Fig. 11.14(c). The taper of a milling machine spindle nose is not self-holding like the morse taper of a drill shank. Milling machine arbors have to be held in place by a threaded drawbar that passes through the whole length of the spindle. Tightening the drawbar into the end of the arbor pulls it tightly into the spindle nose.

The outer end of the arbor is supported in a *steady*. The steady itself is supported by the milling machine *overarm* as shown in Fig. 11.15. The forces acting on a milling cutter when it is removing metal rapidly are very great. Therefore the cutter arbor must be adequately supported and the cutter correctly positioned to avoid inaccuracies, chatter and, at worst, a bent arbor. In Fig. 11.15(a) the cutter is incorrectly mounted. There is excessive overhang from the points of support.

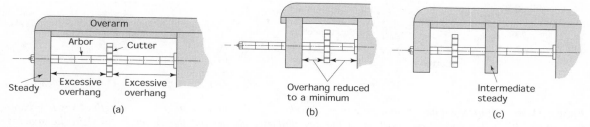

Figure 11.15   *Correct use of overarm steady: (a) bad mounting; (b) and (c) good mounting*

In Fig. 11.15(b) the overarm and steady bearing have been repositioned to provide support as close to the cutter as possible. Also the cutter itself has been mounted as close to the spindle nose as possible. Thus any overhang has been reduced to a minimum and the cutter is supported with the maximum rigidity.

Sometimes the shape and size of the work prevents the cutter being mounted close to the spindle nose. Figure 11.15(c) shows how an additional, intermediate steady can be positioned on the overarm to support the arbor immediately behind the cutter. This again reduces the overhang to a minimum.

11.6.2   Mounting cutters on a long arbor

The following description assumes that the machine has been left in a clean condition without a cutter on the arbor but with the spacing collars in position on the arbor and the locknut only finger tight to prevent it and the collars from getting lost.

* Remove the locknut from the spindle end and slide the bearing bush and the spacers off the arbor.

* Carefully clean the arbor and check for scoring or other damage. Report any such damage to your instructor/supervisor. In severe cases of damage the arbor may have to be replaced.

- Estimate by eye the position of the cutter from the size and shape of the work and the position of the cut and slide as many collars onto the shaft as are needed to ensure the cutter will be in the correct position.

- Inspect the cutter for blunt cutting edges, chipped teeth and damage to the bore. If these or any other defects are found, return the cutter to the stores to be exchanged for one in good condition.

- Clean the sides of the cutter and its bore and slide this onto the arbor as shown in Fig. 11.16(a). Milling cutter teeth are very sharp, particularly at the corners. Protect your hands by wearing leather gloves or holding the cutter in a thick cloth wiper.

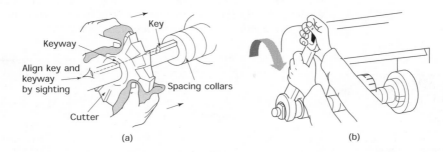

(a)   (b)

Figure 11.16 *Mounting a cutter on a long arbor: (a) keying the cutter to the arbor – length of key is greater than the width of the cutter, any portion of the key that extends beyond the cutter is 'lost' in the spacing collars which also have keyways cut in them; (b) tightening the arbor nut – the steady must be in position when tightening or loosening the arbor nut to prevent bending the arbor*

- Insert a key into the keyway of the arbor to drive the cutter. This prevents the cutter slipping and scoring the arbor. Also, if the cutter stops rotating whilst the table feed is engaged, the arbor will be bent. Although you will see people not bothering with a key, so that they just rely on friction to drive the cutter; this is not good practice for the reasons already mentioned.

- Slide additional spacing collars onto the arbor as required to bring the bearing bush in line with the steady bearing. These spacing collars should be kept to a minimum to avoid excessive overhang and to ensure maximum rigidity as previously mentioned.

- Position the overarm and the steady bearing as shown in Fig. 11.16(b) and tighten their clamping nuts.

- It is now safe to tighten the arbor locknut. This must be tightened or loosened only with the steady in position. This prevents the leverage of the spanner bending the arbor.

- Set the machine to a moderate speed and start it up. Out-of-true running can result from a warped cutter, incorrect grinding and lack of cleanliness in mounting the cutter. If it runs out of true, switch off the machine, remove the cutter, check for cleanliness and remount.

- If the cutter still runs out, seek the assistance of your instructor.

11.6.3 Straddle and gang milling

These techniques are more associated with production milling than with toolroom and prototype work. However, since they are associated with the use of horizontal milling machines they are included here.

Straddle milling

Straddle milling is used to machine two sides of a component at the same time as shown in Fig. 11.17(a). Solid spacing collars are used to take up most of the space between the cutters and an adjustable collar is used for the final adjustment.

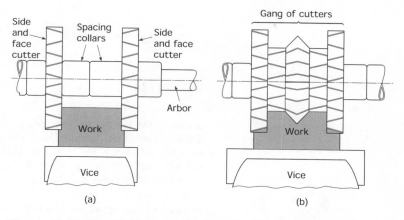

Figure 11.17 *Straddle and gang milling: (a) straddle milling; (b) gang milling*

Gang milling

Gang milling is even more ambitious and involves milling all the sides and faces of the component at the same time as shown in Fig. 11.17(b). To maintain the correct relationships between the cutters, they are kept together as a set on a spare mandrel and are all reground together when they become blunt.

11.7 Cutter mounting (vertical milling machine)

Safety: Make sure the machine is electrically isolated before attempting to remove or mount arbors and cutters.

11.7.1 Stub arbor

Figure 11.18(a) shows an 'exploded' view of a stub arbor and a shell end milling cutter. The cutter is located on a cylindrical spigot and is driven positively by dogs. It is retained in position by a recessed bolt. To

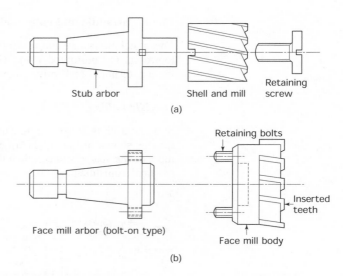

Stub arbor   Shell and mill   Retaining screw

(a)

Retaining bolts

Inserted teeth

Face mill arbor (bolt-on type)   Face mill body

(b)

Figure 11.18 *Use of stub arbors: (a) shell end mill; (b) face mill*

maintain the correct fit, the spigot and register must be kept clean and the cutter must be tightened onto the arbor so that there is no movement between the cutter and the arbor during cutting. Figure 11.18(b) shows a small face mill and its arbor. In both cases the arbor is located in the taper bore of the spindle nose and it is retained in position by the threaded drawbar that passes through the length of the machine spindle. *Note:* Stub arbors and their associated cutters can also be used on horizontal spindle milling machines.

Another type of stub arbor is shown in Fig. 11.19. This allows the cutters normally associated with a horizontal milling machine to be used on a vertical spindle milling machine. Because the stub arbor is supported only at one end, it is not as rigid as the horizontal milling machine arbor and this restricts the size of the cutter that can be used and the rate of metal removal that can be employed.

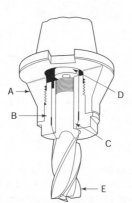

Figure 11.20 *Collet chuck for screwed-shank solid end mills: A – main body of collet chuck; the locking sleeve B positions the collet C and mates with the taper nose of the collet to close the collet on the cutter shank; the collet is internally threaded to prevent the cutter E being drawn out of the chuck whilst cutting; the male centre D anchors the shank end of the cutter and ensures true running*

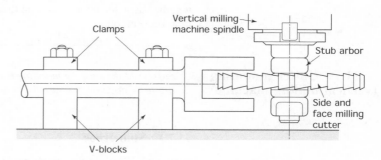

Clamps   Vertical milling machine spindle   Stub arbor   Side and face milling cutter   V-blocks

Figure 11.19 *Stub arbor for use with cutters normally associated with horizontal milling machines*

11.7.2 Collet chuck

Basically a collet is a hardened and tempered steel sleeve with a parallel bore on the inside and a tapered nose on the outside. It is slit at regular intervals around its circumference so that it can close onto the shank of the cutter when the outer sleeve is tightened. Concentric tapers are used to ensure true running and to compensate for wear. Figure 11.20 shows a section through a typical collet chuck.

- The shank of the cutter has a threaded portion at its end that screws into the rear end of the collet. This prevents the forces acting on the flutes of a cutter with positive rake from drawing the cutter out of the collet.

- The hardened and ground conical centre serves to locate the rear of the cutter and also to act as an end stop and prevents the cutter and the collet being pushed up into the chuck body.

11.8 Workholding

The work to be machined on a milling machine may be held:

- In a machine vice.

- Clamped directly onto the machine table.

- Clamped to an angle plate that is itself clamped to the machine table.

- In a milling fixture for production work. To save time pneumatic clamping is often employed.

In this chapter only the first two methods will be considered.

11.8.1 Machine vice (plain)

Figure 11.21(a) shows a plain machine vice. It has two sets of fixing holes so that it can be set with its jaws either parallel to the travel of the machine table as shown in Fig. 11.21(b), or it can be set with its jaws perpendicular to the travel of the machine table as shown in Fig. 11.21(c). To facilitate setting, the underside of the vice body has slots machined in it both parallel and perpendicular to the fixed jaw. *Tenon blocks* can be secured into these slots. The tenon blocks stand proud of the slots so that they also locate in the T-slots of the machine table as shown in Fig. 11.21(d).

To maintain positional accuracy of the vice:

- Check the tenons are a close slide fit in the tenon slots in the vice body and also in the T-slots of the machine table.

- Check that the tenons are clean and free from burrs and bruises.

- Clean the tenon slots and insert the tenon blocks, securing them with socket head cap screws.

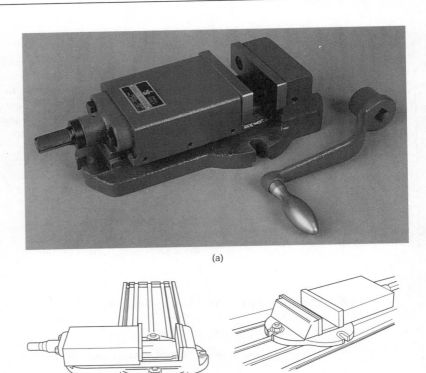

Figure 11.21 *Mounting and setting a plain machine vice: (a) plain machine vice; (b) vice set with jaws parallel to T-slots; (c) vice set with jaws perpendicular to T-slots; (d) use of tenon block to align vice with the T-slots*

- Check that the T-slots in the machine table are clean and free from burrs and bruises.
- Lower the vice carefully onto the machine table and locate the tenons in the appropriate T-slot.
- Secure the vice to the machine table with suitable T-bolts. Ordinary hexagon bolts should not be used as their heads do not fit properly and they can work loose.
- The vice should now be ready to hold the work.

11.8.2 Machine vice (swivel base)

If the machine vice has a swivel base as shown in Fig. 11.22(a), or it is a plain vice without tenons, then it will have to be set either parallel or

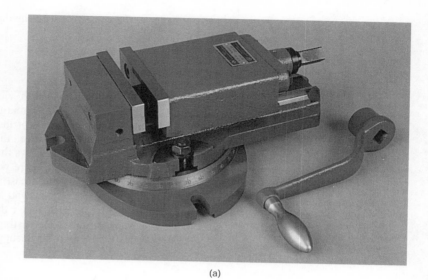

(a)

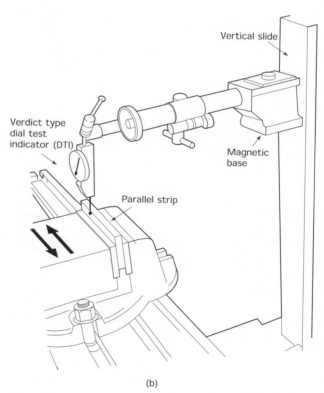

(b)

Figure 11.22 *Setting swivel base machine vices and plain vices without tenons: (a) swivel base machine vice; (b) setting a machine vice*

perpendicular to the worktable with the dial test indicator (DTI) as shown in Fig. 11.22(b).

11.8.3 Direct mounting

Work that is too large to hold in a vice or is of inconvenient shape can be clamped directly to the machine table as shown in Figs 11.23(a) and 11.23(b). Sometimes the shape of the casting or forging is such that a jack or wedge is required to level the work ready for cutting. The example shown in Fig. 11.23(c) shows that the opposite end to the clamp is supported on a packing piece. There will, of course, be clamps at both ends of the workpiece. Sometimes castings are slightly warped but not sufficiently to allow the use of jacks and wedges. Thin packing and pieces of shim steel should be inserted under the casting to remove any 'rock' and to provide support under the casting where clamps are to be used. Tightening clamps down onto an unsupported part of the casting could cause it to crack.

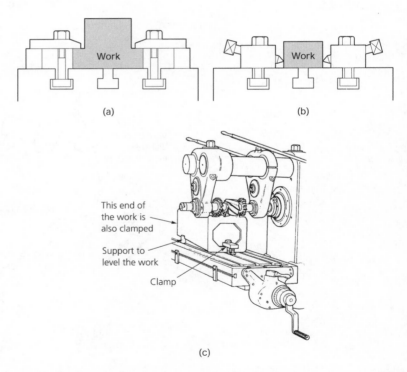

(a)   (b)

(c)

Figure 11.23 *Holding larger work: (a) use of clamps; (b) use of table dogs; (c) levelling work*

Angle plates as described in Section 7.3.2 can also be used for locating and supporting work on the milling machine table.

11.8.4 Dividing head (simple indexing)

Sometimes you will need to make a series of cuts around the periphery of a component; for example, when cutting splines on a shaft or teeth on a gear wheel. Such an operation requires the work to be rotated through a given angle between each cut. This rotation of the work through given angles between the cuts is called indexing. Figure 11.24 shows a *simple (direct) dividing head*. The index plate locates the spindle of the head directly without any intermediate gearing. In the example shown there are only two rows of holes for clarity. In practice there would be many more rows to give a bigger range of possible spacings.

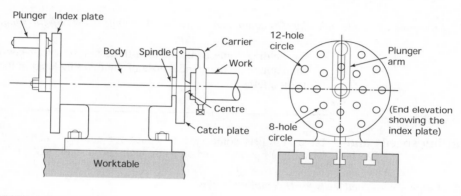

Figure 11.24 *Simple dividing head*

For example, we can index through 120° between the cuts so as to give us three equally spaced slots. We would use the 12 hole circle in the index plate since this is divisible by three, and we would move the plunger arm through a distance of four holes between the cutting of each slot.

If we had wanted four slots we have a choice, we could have rotated the work through three holes in the 12 hole circle between each cut, or we can rotate the work through two holes in the eight hole circle. The result would be the same. Figure 11.25(a) shows a typical component where three equally spaced slots are to be cut.

- The blank would be turned and bored to size ready for milling.

- The blank would then be mounted on a mandrel and supported between the dividing head and its tailstock as shown in Fig. 11.25(b).

- The work is centred under the cutter and cutting takes place.

- For rigidity, cutting should take place towards the diving head and towards the 'plus' end of the mandrel so that the blank cannot work loose.

- You can either complete each slot before indexing to the next one, or you can index from slot to slot for each increase in the depth of cut so that all the slots are finished together.

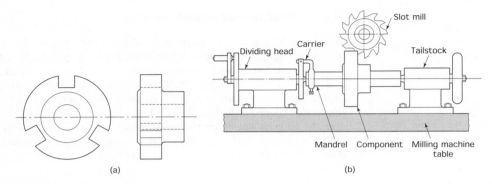

Figure 11.25 *Example of simple indexing: (a) component requiring indexing; (b) set-up for simple indexing*

- For holding some components a three-jaw or a four-jaw chuck may be mounted on the spindle nose of the dividing head in the same way as on a lathe.

11.9 Cutting speeds and feeds

Table 11.1 lists some typical values for cutting speeds and feed rates for milling operations when using high-speed steel (HSS) milling cutters.

TABLE 11.1 *Cutting speeds and feeds for HSS milling cutters*

Material being milled	Cutting speed (m/min)	Feed per tooth (chip thickness) (mm)					
		Face mill	Slab mill	Side & face	Slotting cutter	Slitting saw	End mill
Aluminium	70–100	0.2–0.8	0.2–0.6	0.15–0.4	0.1–0.2	0.05–0.1	0.1–0.4
Brass (alpha) (ductile)	35–50	0.15–0.6	0.15–0.5	0.1–0.3	0.07–0.15	0.035–0.075	0.07–0.3
Brass (free-cutting)	50–70	0.2–0.8	0.2–0.6	0.15–0.4	0.1–0.2	0.05–0.1	0.1–0.4
Bronze (phosphor)	20–35	0.07–0.3	0.07–0.25	0.05–0.15	0.04–0.07	0.02–0.04	0.04–0.15
Cast iron (grey)	25–40	0.1–0.4	0.1–0.3	0.07–0.2	0.05–0.1	0.025–0.05	0.05–0.2
Copper	35–45	0.1–0.4	0.1–0.3	0.07–0.2	0.05–0.1	0.025–0.05	0.05–0.2
Steel (mild)	30–40	0.1–0.4	0.1–0.3	0.07–0.2	0.05–0.1	0.025–0.05	0.05–0.2
Steel (medium carbon)	20–30	0.07–0.3	0.07–0.25	0.05–0.15	0.04–0.07	0.02–0.04	0.04–0.15
Steel (alloy – high tensile)	5–8	0.05–0.2	0.05–0.15	0.035–0.1	0.025–0.05	0.015–0.025	0.025–0.1
Thermosetting plastic*	20–30	0.15–0.5	0.15–0.5	0.1–0.3	0.07–0.15	0.035–0.075	0.07–0.3

*Low speed due to abrasive properties.
Notes:
1. The *lower* speed range is suitable for heavy, roughing cuts.
   The *higher* speed range is suitable for light, finishing cuts.
2. The feed is selected to give the required surface finish and rate of metal removal.

These are only an approximate guide and you should consult the manufacturers' data sheets, manuals or wall charts for more specific information. When using carbide and coated carbide-tipped cutters it is important to use the manufacturers' data sheets for speeds and feeds in order to obtain the maximum benefit from these more expensive cutters.

Cutting speed calculations on milling machines using high-speed steel cutting tools are the same as those we considered for the centre lathe. We still have to calculate the spindle speed in rev/min given the cutting speed for the material of the workpiece but this time we use the diameter of the cutter not the diameter of the workpiece. Again, the machine is set to the nearest spindle speed *below* the calculated value to avoid damage through overheating. This is particularly important for milling cutters as they are expensive and more difficult to regrind than single point lathe tools, to avoid damage to the cutter.

Example 11.1   *Calculate the spindle speed in rev/min for a milling cutter 125 mm in diameter, operating at a cutting speed of 30 m/min for low carbon (mild) steel. For this example take $\pi = 3$ since we work only to the nearest speed on the gearbox anyway.*

$$N = \frac{1000S}{\pi D}$$

where: N = spindle speed
S = 30 m/min

$$= \frac{1000 \times 30}{3 \times 125}$$

$$= \textbf{80 rev/min}$$

Calculations for the table feed rate for milling are somewhat different to the feed calculations associated with centre lathe turning. In centre lathe turning you calculated the feed rate as the distance moved by the tool per revolution of the work in rev/min. When calculating feed rates for milling machines, this is stated as the distance moved by the machine table per minute based on the rate per tooth of the cutter and the number of teeth. The cutting speeds and feeds given in manufacturers' handbooks and wall charts are a useful guide. However, as in all machining operations, the actual speeds and feeds chosen will depend upon:

- The surface finish required.
- The rate of metal removal required.
- The power of the machine.
- The rigidity of the machine.
- The rigidity of the work.
- The security of the workholding device.
- The material from which the work is made.

364 Engineering Fundamentals

- The type of cutter, the material from which it is made, and its tooth form.
- Whether or not a coolant is used and the flow rate if a coolant is used.

Example 11.2 *Calculate the table feed rate in mm/min for a 12 tooth cutter revolving at 80 rev/min (see Example 5.3) when the feed per tooth is 0.1 mm.*

$$\text{Feed/rev} = \text{feed/tooth} \times \text{number of teeth}$$

$$= 0.1 \text{ mm} \times 12$$

$$= \textbf{1.2 mm/rev}$$

$$\text{Table feed} = \text{feed/rev} \times \text{rev/min for cutter}$$

$$= 1.2 \text{ mm/rev} \times 80 \text{ rev/min}$$

$$= \textbf{96 mm/min}$$

So the cutter will rotate at 80 rev/min and the table and workpiece will move past it at a feed rate of 96 mm/min.

We can also use this information to determine the cutting time taken to machine a particular surface, as in the following example.

Example 11.3 *Using the following data, calculate the time taken to complete a 270 millimetre long cut using a slab mill (roller mill). Take π as 3.*

$$\text{Diameter of cutter} = 125 \text{ mm}$$

$$\text{Number of teeth} = 6$$

$$\text{Feed/tooth} = 0.05 \text{ mm}$$

$$\text{Cutting speed} = 45 \text{ m/min}$$

$$N = \frac{1000S}{\pi D} \qquad \text{where: } N = \text{spindle speed (rev/min)}$$
$$S = 45 \text{ m/min}$$
$$= \frac{1000 \times 45}{3 \times 125} \qquad \qquad \pi = 3$$
$$D = 125 \text{ mm}$$

$$= \textbf{120 rev/min} \ldots (1)$$

$$\text{Feed/rev} = \text{feed/tooth} \times \text{number of teeth}$$

$$= 0.05 \text{ mm/tooth} \times 6$$

$$= \textbf{0.3 mm/rev}$$

$$\text{Table feed} = \text{feed/rev} \times \text{number of teeth}$$

$$= 0.05 \text{ mm/rev} \times 120 \text{ rev/min (from 1)}$$

$$= \textbf{36 mm/min} \ldots (2)$$

$$\text{Time to complete 270 mm cut} = \frac{\text{length of cut}}{\text{table feed}}$$

$$= \frac{270 \text{ mm}}{36 \text{ mm/min}} \quad \text{(from 2)}$$

$$= \textbf{7.5 min}$$

11.10 Squaring up a blank on a horizontal milling machine

Before finding out how to square up a blank on a milling machine we must consider a problem that can occur when holding work in a machine vice. Like all machine vices we use the fixed jaw as a datum surface perpendicular to the machine worktable and the slideways of the vice as a datum surface parallel to the machine worktable. The moving jaw slides along the slideways machined into the body of the vice. For the jaw to slide there has to be clearance and, in time, wear will also take place. Since the clamping forces are offset they form a *couple* that tends to rotate the moving jaw as shown in Fig. 11.26(a). This tends to lift the work off its seating and tilt it causing loss of parallelism in the workpiece as shown in Fig. 11.26(b). To prevent this happening the vice must be kept in good condition. If there is difficulty in getting the work to seat properly on the parallel strips due to vice wear, a piece of steel rod of circular cross-section can be placed between the moving jaw and the workpiece as shown in Fig. 11.26(c). Any lift in the moving jaw, as

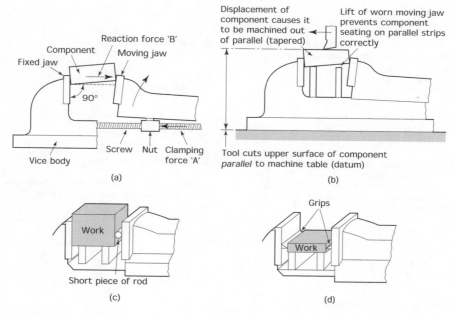

Figure 11.26 *Effect of wear in a machine vice: (a) forces A and B form a 'couple' that tries to rotate the moving jaw; if the slides are worn the moving jaw will lift and displace the component being held, as shown; (b) lack of parallelism due to worn vice; (c) use of cylindrical packing; (d) use of grips*

the vice is tightened, results in the rod rolling up the side face of the workpiece which remains tightly clamped against the datum surfaces of the vice. Grips as shown in Fig. 11.26(d) may be used where it is more important to pull the work down onto the parallels than to keep it against the fixed jaw. The side and bottom faces of the triangular grips are just over 90° so that as the vice is tightened up the grips pull down on the workpiece and hold it tightly against the parallel strips.

To square up the blank, the vice jaws are set parallel to the worktable with a DTI as shown in Fig. 11.27. The work is held down on the parallel strips using grips as just described and the first face is machined. This

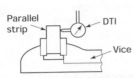

1 Set vice jaws parallel to table using a DTI
   When vice is correctly set the DTI reading should
   be constant as it travels along the parallel strip

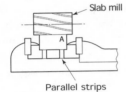

2 Set sawn blank in vice using grips
   Mill surface 'A' using a slab (roller) mill

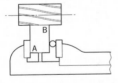

3 Turn job through 90° so that previously
   machined surface (A) is against fixed jaw
   of vice; this ensures surface (A) and (B)
   are perpendicular to each other
   Machine surface 'B'

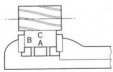

4 Turn job through 90° and machine surface
   'C' until 40 mm thick; check thickness at
   each end of job to ensure parallelism

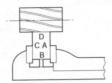

5 Turn job through 90° again and machine
   surface 'D' until job is 65 mm wide; check
   width at each end to ensure parallelism

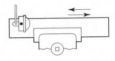

6 Turn vice through 90° and check with DTI
   parallel to spindle axis

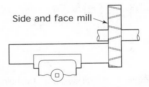

7 Use side and face milling cutter to machine
   end square
   Wind table across and machine to length;
   check length with vernier calliper

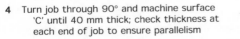

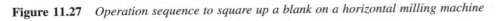

Figure 11.27 *Operation sequence to square up a blank on a horizontal milling machine*

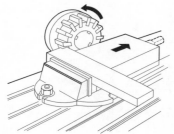

Figure 11.28 *Machining the ends of larger blanks*

face is then used as a datum surface and is held against the fixed jaw using a piece of round rod to prevent the work lifting as the vice is tightened. The next cut is taken and we now have two surfaces machined at right angles to each other. The remaining faces can be machined to size and the work is square. Finally, the vice is reset with its fixed jaw perpendicular to the machine worktable using a DTI as shown. The ends of the blank are then machined using a side and face milling cutter. For large work a face mill can be mounted directly into the machine spindle as shown in Fig. 11.28.

11.11 Milling a step (horizontal milling machine)

The sequence for milling a step is shown in Fig. 11.29. Let's assume that the blank has already been squared up by one or other of the techniques already described. We will also assume that the position of the step has been marked out and that the marking-out lines have been preserved with dot punch marks. Figure 11.29 shows the work being roughed out using the scribed lines as a guide.

- Do not work right up to the lines but leave some metal for finishing to size.

- Check the depth of the roughed-out slot using a depth micrometer or a vernier depth gauge.

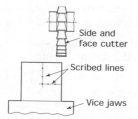

1 Set up blank in a machine vice under a side and face cutter as shown so that outer side of the cutter is just clear of the work

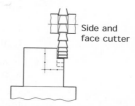

2 Take a series of cuts until the step produced is just clear of the scribed line showing the bottom of the step

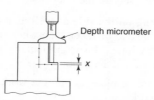

3 Use a depth micrometer or the depthing leg of a vernier caliper to measure actual depth of the step
[*x* = required depth – reading]

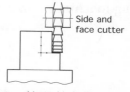

4 Raise milling machine table by the distance *x* as shown by the micrometer dial on the knee elevating screw
Take final cut which should 'split' the witness marks on the scribed line; the cutter is now at the correct depth

Figure 11.29 *Machining a step using a horizontal milling machine*

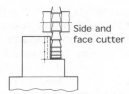

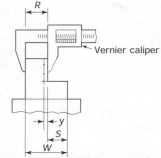

5   Keeping the depth setting constant take a series
    of cuts until the step approaches the vertical
    scribed line

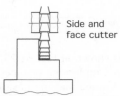

6   Use a vernier caliper or a micrometer
    caliper to measure the width of the
    component.
    Let R = vernier reading
    Then $S = W - R$
    and y = required width of step -S

7   Move the milling machine table over by a
    distance y as shown and take the final cut;
    this is achieved using the micrometer dial
    on the cross-traverse screw
    The final cut should 'split' the witness marks
    on the scribed line; the step is now complete

Figure 11.29 *(continued)*

- Use the micrometer dials of the machine to increase the depth of cut to within a few 'thou' (inch measurements) or a few hundredths of a millimetre (metric measurement) and check again.

- Use the micrometer dial of the knee elevating screw of the machine to increase the cut to the finished depth.

- Now repeat this procedure to set the width of the step. This time you will use either a micrometer caliper or a vernier caliper to take the measurements. The machine will be set using the micrometer dial of the saddle cross traverse screw.

11.12   Milling a step (vertical milling machine)

The process is the same as just described except that an end mill or a shell end mill will be used. Remember that:

- You will be cutting on the side as well as the end of the end mill so lighter cuts will have to be taken than when using a side and face mill on a horizontal machine. This is particularly true if a 'long reach' end mill is being used for a deep step.

- An end mill cannot be plunged into the work; it has to be fed in from the side of the work.

11.13   Milling a slot (horizontal milling machine)

Sometimes you cannot work steadily up to a scribed line and finish the cut to size using measuring instruments and the micrometer dials of the machine. For example, when cutting a slot with a slitting saw or a slot mill whose thickness is equal to the width of the slot, you can have only 'one bite at the cherry'. The work has to be positioned under the cutter in the correct position first time. The technique for positioning the cutter is shown in Fig. 11.30. Only light cuts should be taken to avoid overloading the cutter. Also, do not allow the cutter to become clogged with metal swarf. A good flow of coolant will help to wash the swarf away.

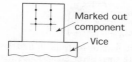

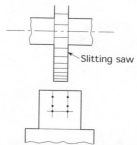

1   The machine vice is set on the milling machine work table with its fixed jaw parallel to the spindle axis (perpendicular to the table traverse)
The workpiece is mounted in the vice

3   Lower the machine table until the cutter is clear of the work and move the table across using the cross traverse handwheel on the knee of the machine
The amount the machine table is moved over is: *x* + thickness of the feeler gauge

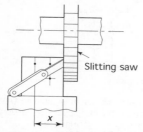

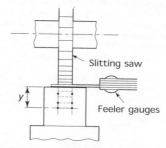

2   The table is raised and the cutter is brought gently up to the side of the workpiece so that a convenient size feeler gauge blade can just be slid between the cutter and workpiece

4   The machine table is raised until a feeler gauge can just be inserted between the work and the cutter; successively deeper cuts are taken until the depth of the slot is reached
This is: *y* + thickness of the feeler gauge

Figure 11.30   *Machining a slot on a horizontal milling machine*

11.14   Milling an angular surface

First of all the blank is squared up. Then it is marked out and mounted in the machine vice at a suitable angle so that the V-shape is clear of the vice jaws. A series of cuts can then be taken either using a side and face cutter on a horizontal spindle milling machine or a shell end mill on a vertical spindle milling machine.

Figure 11.31 shows how a bevel protractor is used to set the work to the required angle. In this example a side and face milling cutter is being used on a horizontal milling machine. A series of cuts is taken until the

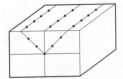

1 Mark out position of 'V' on the end and top
face of the blank

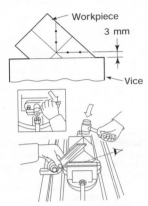

2 Mount the marked out blank in the machine vice
as shown with the lines of the 'V' vertical and
horizontal; the horizontal line should be 3 mm
above the jaws for cutter clearance
The blank setting at 45° can be checked by
means of a bevel protractor as shown

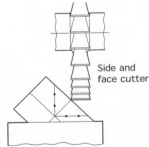

3 Select a side and face cutter of sufficient
diameter that it can cut to the bottom of
the 'V' without the arbor collars fouling the
workpiece
Position the work using the knee cross-traverse
and elevating controls; the corner of the
cutter should just touch on the centre marked
out line. Zero the micrometer dials

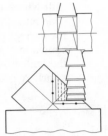

4 Remove the surplus material in a series of even
cuts until the cutter approaches the scribed lines
Note:
  • Since the workpiece is only held by friction
    only light cuts can be taken or the workpiece
    may be dislodged
  • Check the angle of the workpiece again with
    the protractor before taking the finishing cuts
    and adjust if necessary

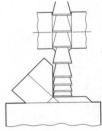

5 Gently raise the machine table so that the face
of the cutter just splits the horizontal marked
out line on the workpiece
Remove the metal in even cuts as previously until
the side of the cutter splits the vertical marked
out line on the workpiece
Note:
  • The V-block is now complete and can be
    removed from the vice
  • Remove all sharp corners and burrs with a
    fine file

Figure 11.31 *Machining angular surfaces on a horizontal milling machine*

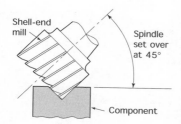

Shell-end mill

Spindle set over at 45°

Component

Figure 11.32 *Milling a V-slot using a shell end mill on a vertical milling machine*

marked-out lines are 'split'. Proof of the lines being split is provided by the dot punch 'witness' marks. Half the dots should remain if the line has been split accurately. The sequence of operations to produce the V-shaped slot is shown in Fig. 11.31.

Figure 11.32 shows an alternative way of producing the 'V' by using a shell end milling cutter in a vertical milling machine with the head and spindle inclined at 45°. This enables the work to be set in the vice in the normal way. Further, because the blank is resting on the bottom of the vice or on parallel packing strips, it is more rigidly supported and is less likely to be disturbed by the action of the cutter.

Exercises

11.1 *Safety*
  (a) Describe FOUR safety precautions that should be taken when using a milling machine.
  (b) Sketch any horizontal milling machine cutter guard with which you are familiar.

11.2 *Milling cutters*
  (a) With the aid of a sketch show how the following cutting angles are applied to the tooth of a milling cutter.
    (i) Rake angle.
    (ii) Clearance angle.
  (b) With the aid of a sketch explain why milling cutter teeth have to have secondary clearance.
  (c) With the aid of sketches show how the teeth of some milling cutters cut orthogonally whilst others can cut obliquely.
  (d) With the aid of sketches explain the essential differences between *up-cut* and *down-cut* (climb) milling techniques. List the advantages and limitations of both techniques.

11.3 *Milling machines*
  (a) With the aid of sketches, explain the essential differences between horizontal and vertical milling machines.
  (b) With the aid of sketches show how a horizontal milling machine can produce surfaces that are:
    (i) parallel to the surface of the worktable;
    (ii) perpendicular to the surface of the worktable;
    (iii) perpendicular to the surface of the worktable but using a face milling cutter.
  (c) With the aid of sketches show how a vertical milling machine can produce surfaces that are:
    (i) parallel to the surface of the worktable;
    (ii) perpendicular to the surface of the worktable;
  (d) Explain how the spindle speeds and feed rates for milling machines are related and how this relationship differs from that for centre lathes.

11.4 *Selection of milling machines and milling cutters*
  (a) Figure 11.33 shows some simple components that require milling operations during their manufacture. For each

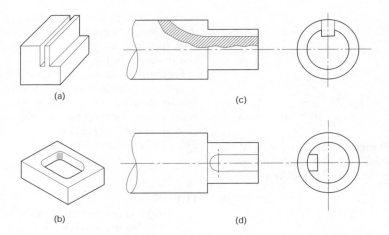

(a) (c) (b) (d)

Figure 11.33   *Exercise 11.4(a)*

example, state the most suitable type of machine that should be used, giving the reasons for your choice.

(b) Figure 11.34 shows some typical milling cutters. With the aid of sketches indicate a suitable application for each of the cutters.

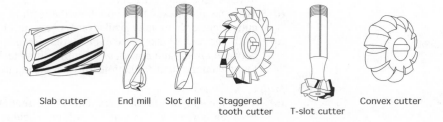

Slab cutter   End mill   Slot drill   Staggered tooth cutter   T-slot cutter   Convex cutter

Figure 11.34   *Exercise 11.4(b)*

(c) When ordering a cutter from the stores:
 (i) state FOUR essential factors that must be specified to ensure you get the correct cutter;
 (ii) state FOUR cutter defects for which you should check for before using the cutter.

11.5 *Mounting milling cutters*
 (a) Briefly describe:
  (i) the purpose of the overarm steady;
  (ii) how the overarm steady should be positioned.
 (b) With the aid of sketches briefly describe TWO typical applications of a stub arbor.
 (c) With the aid of sketches briefly explain the difference between *straddle milling* and *gang milling*.

11.6 *Workholding on a milling machine*

    (a)   Small components are usually held in machine vices mounted on the worktable of the machine.

        (i)   State which jaw and which horizontal surface of a machine vice form the datum surfaces from which the workpiece is set.

        (ii)   Explain why machine vices are sometimes fitted with tenon blocks to engage the T-slots of the worktable.

        (iii)   Explain how you would set a machine vice NOT fitted with tenon blocks so as to ensure correct alignment.

    (b)   When holding rough castings, clamped directly to the worktable of the machine, describe the precautions that should be taken to allow for inaccuracies in the cast surfaces and also to prevent damage to the machine table.

    (c)   Sketch the set-up for machining the hexagon on the component shown in Fig. 11.35, using a direct indexing simple dividing head as previously described in this chapter. The component will be supplied turned ready for milling.

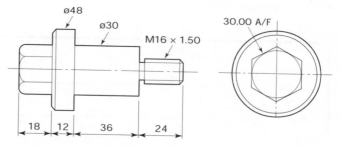

Figure 11.35   *Exercise 11.6(c)*

11.7 *Speeds and feeds*

    (a)   Calculate the spindle speed in rev/min for a milling cutter 150 mm in diameter operating at a cutting speed of 25 m/min.

    (b)   Calculate the table feed rate in mm/min for a 14 tooth cutter revolving at the speed calculated in (a) above when the feed per tooth is 0.1 mm.

    (c)   Combining the results from (a) and (b) above, calculate the time taken to take a cut 250 mm long.

11.8 *Milling operations*

    (a)   With the aid of sketches describe the manufacture of the component shown in Fig. 11.36, paying particular attention to the selection of the machine and cutter(s) and the method of workholding. List the equipment (other than spanners and keys) that you would require.

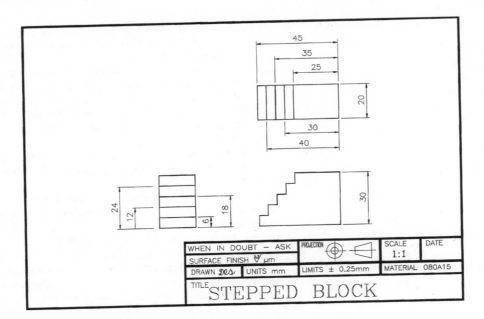

Figure 11.36 *Exercise 11.8(a)*

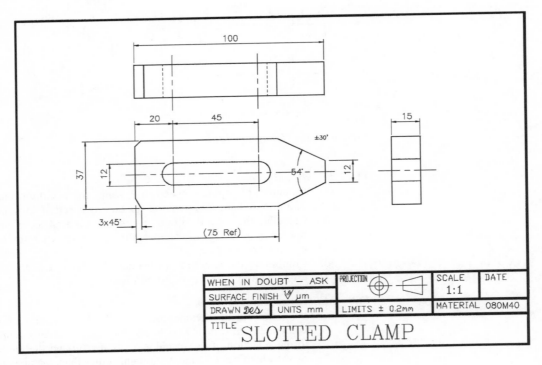

Figure 11.37 *Exercise 11.8(b)*

(b) With the aid of sketches describe the manufacture of the component shown in Fig. 11.37, paying particular attention to the selection of the machine and cutter(s) and the method of workholding. List the equipment (other than spanners and keys) that you would require.

12 Grinding machines and processes

When you have read this chapter you should understand:

- The main features of typical surface grinding machines.
- The main movements of typical surface grinding machines.
- How to care for surface grinding machines in order to maintain their accuracy and alignments.
- The selection of a surface grinding machine appropriate to the work in hand.
- The setting and securing of a workpiece on a magnetic chuck.
- The correct setting and operation of a surface grinding machine.

12.1 Safety when grinding

The abrasive wheels used in grinding processes are relatively fragile and can be easily broken. If an abrasive wheel breaks whilst rotating at high speeds it can do considerable damage and cause serious accidents. For this reason great care must be taken in:

- Storing and handling abrasive wheels.
- Mounting and balancing abrasive wheels.
- Guarding abrasive wheels (burst containment).
- Truing and dressing abrasive wheels.
- Using abrasive wheels.

Because of their potential danger there are additional regulations that apply specifically to the use of abrasive wheels and grinding processes. We will now examine some of the more important provisions of the *Abrasive Wheel Regulations*.

12.1.1 Training and appointment of persons to mount wheels

Abrasive Wheel Regulation 9 states that no person shall mount an abrasive wheel unless that person:

- Has been trained in accordance with the training schedule of these regulations.

- Is competent to carry out that duty.

- Has been properly appointed and that the appointment has been confirmed by a signed and dated entry in the appropriate register. This entry must carry particulars of the class or description of the abrasive wheels that person is appointed to mount. Any such appointment can be revoked by the company by a signed and dated entry in the register.

- A copy of that entry or a certificate has been given to the appointed person and this must also indicate the particulars of the class or description of the abrasive wheels that person is appointed to mount.

The above comments do not apply to a person undergoing training in the work of mounting abrasive wheels, providing they are working directly under the supervision of a competent person (instructor) who has himself or herself been trained and appointed under these regulations. A trainee must be certified as soon as the training module has been satisfactorily completed.

12.1.2 Guards

Regulation 10 requires that a guard shall be provided and kept in position at every abrasive wheel unless the nature of the work absolutely precludes its use. An abrasive wheel guard has two main functions.

- To contain the broken pieces of the wheel in the event of it bursting.

- To prevent the operator, as far as possible, from coming into contact with the rapidly rotating wheel.

To achieve these aims, the wheel should be enclosed to the greatest possible extent, the opening being as small as possible consistent with the nature of the work being performed. Apart from certain guards for portable grinding machines, all abrasive wheel guards should be capable of adjustment. This is so that the whole wheel, except for that part necessarily exposed, can be enclosed. As the wheel wears down, the guard should be adjusted from time to time so as to maintain maximum protection.

The guard should be securely bolted or otherwise attached to the frame or body of the machine. On portable machines the guard should be attached by a clamp of unit construction, the clamp to be closed on the machine frame by a single high tensile bolt.

Except for very small machines, cast iron or similar brittle materials should not be used for abrasive wheel guards. Because of the magnitude of the forces involved when a wheel bursts, the sheet metal used for most cutter guards is unsuitable, and abrasive wheel guards should be fabricated by welding from substantial steel plate.

12.1.3 Wheel speeds

The overspeeding of abrasive wheels is a common cause of failure by bursting. For this reason the manufacturer's specified *maximum permissible speed* must never be exceeded. Regulation 6 requires that every abrasive wheel having a diameter of more than 55 mm shall be marked with the maximum permissible speed at which it can safely be used, the speed, as specified by the manufacturer, to be stated in revs/min. The speed of smaller wheels shall be stated in a notice. In the case of mounted wheels and points, the overhang at the specified speed must also be stated in the notice.

12.1.4 Spindle speeds

Regulation 7 requires that the maximum working speed or speeds of every grinding machine shall be specified in a notice attached to the machine. This enables the person who is mounting an abrasive wheel on the machine to check that the speed of the spindle does not exceed the maximum permissible speed of the wheel.

12.1.5 Selection of wheels

Regulation 13 requires that in selecting a wheel, due account shall be taken of the factors that affect safety. Selecting the correct wheel for the workpiece is equally important for both safety and efficient production. As a general rule, soft wheels are selected for grinding hard workpiece materials. Similarly hard wheels are usually selected for the grinding of soft workpiece materials. The selection of abrasive wheels will be considered more fully in Section 12.4.

12.1.6 Misuse of the abrasive wheel

Wheel breakage can occur if the operator presses the workpiece against the abrasive wheel with excessive pressure. This may occur if the:

- Wheel is running slower than its recommended speed and is not cutting satisfactorily.
- Wrong wheel has been selected for the job in hand.
- Wheel has become loaded or glazed (see below and also Section 12.5).

Particular care must be taken when grinding on the sides of straight sided wheels. Such a technique is dangerous when the wheel is appreciably worn or if a sudden or excessive pressure is applied.

12.1.7 Truing and dressing

The wheel should be dressed when it becomes loaded or glazed. Loading and glazing prevent the wheel from cutting satisfactorily and can cause overheating of the work and also overheating of the abrasive wheel. Overheating of the wheel results in weakening of the bond and failure of the wheel. It also tempts the operator into pressing the work harder onto the wheel which can result in wheel failure (bursting).

Correct dressing of the abrasive wheel keeps the wheel running concentric with the spindle axis. This is essential:

- For maintaining wheel balance and preventing vibration patterns on the surface of the workpiece.

- For preventing vibration damage to the machine bearings.
- For accurate dimensional control.
- When off-hand grinding since it allows the workrest to be kept close to the periphery of the wheel. This prevents the work from being dragged down between the wheel and the workrest.

12.1.8 Eye protection

Persons carrying out dry grinding operations (no cutting fluid being used) and truing or dressing abrasive wheels are required to be provided with and to wear approved eye protectors (goggles) and dust masks.

12.2 Fundamental principles of grinding

Grinding is the name given to those processes which use abrasive particles for material removal. The abrasive particles are made by crushing hard, crystalline solids such as aluminium oxide (emery) and silicon carbide. Grinding wheels consist of large numbers of abrasive particles, called *grains*, held together by a *bond* to form a multi-tooth cutter similar in its action to a milling cutter. Since the grinding wheel has many more 'teeth' than a milling cutter and, because this reduces the 'chip clearance' between the teeth, it produces a vastly improved surface finish at the expense of a slower rate of material removal. The fact that the cutting points are irregularly shaped and randomly distributed over the active face of the tool enhances the surface finish produced by a grinding process. Figure 12.1 shows the dross from a grinding wheel highly magnified. It will be seen that the dross consists of particles of abrasive material stripped from the grinding wheel together with metallic chips that are remarkably similar in appearance to the chips produced by the milling process.

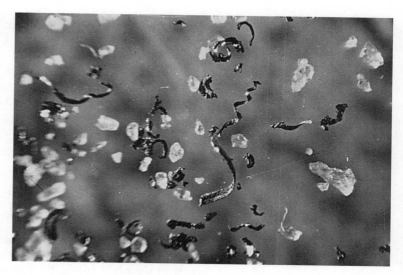

Figure 12.1 *Grinding wheel dross*

The grains at the surface of the wheel are called *active grains* because they are the ones that actually perform the cutting operation. In peripheral grinding, each active grain removes a short chip of gradually increasing thickness in a similar way to the tooth of a milling cutter as shown in Fig. 12.2. As grinding proceeds, the cutting edges of the grains become dulled and the forces acting on the grains increase until either the dulled grains fracture and expose new cutting surfaces, or the whole of the dulled grains are ripped from the wheel exposing new active grains. Therefore, grinding wheels have self-sharpening characteristics.

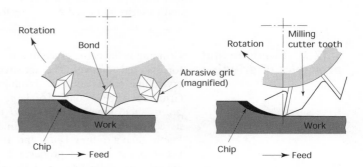

Figure 12.2   *Cutting action of abrasive wheel grains*

12.3 Grinding wheel specification

A grinding wheel consists of two constituents:

* The *abrasive* grains that do the cutting.

* The *bond* that holds the grains together.

The specification of a grinding wheel indicates its construction and its suitability for a particular operation. For example, let's consider a wheel carrying the marking:

38A60-J5V

This is interpreted as follows:

* 38A is the *abrasive type* (see Table 12.1).

* 60 is the *grit size* (see Table 12.2).

* J is the *grade* (see Table 12.3).

* 5 is the *structure* (see Table 12.4).

* V is the *bond material* (see Table 12.5).

Therefore a wheel carrying the marking 38A60-J5V has an aluminium oxide type abrasive, the abrasive grit has a medium to fine grain size, the grade of the wheel is soft, the structure has a medium spacing, and the grains are held together by a vitrified bond.

12.3.1 Abrasive

This must be chosen to suit the material being cut. As a general classification:

- 'Brown' aluminium oxide is used for grinding tough materials.
- 'White' aluminium oxide is used for grinding hard die steels and high-speed steel cutting tools.
- Silicon carbide (green grit) is used for very hard materials such as tungsten carbide tool tips.

Table 12.1 indicates how the abrasive type may be coded using the British Standard (BSI) marking system. The British Standard marking system calls only for 'A' for aluminium oxide abrasives or 'C' for silicon carbide abrasives. However, it does permit the use of a prefix to the A or the C so that specific abrasives can be identified within each broad classification. Table 12.2 compares the British Standard marking system with that of the Norton Abrasive Company.

TABLE 12.1 *British Standard abrasive marking system*

Abrasive			
Aluminium oxide		*Silicon carbide*	
Aloxite	A	Silicon carbide	C
Alundum	A	Black crystolon	37C
Bauxilite	A	Unirundum	C
Blue aloxite	BA	Green silicon carbide	GC
Mixed bauxilite	MA	Green crystolon No. 39	39C
Pink aloxite	PA		
White aloxite	AA		
White alundum	38A		
White bauxilite	WA		

TABLE 12.2 *Abrasive types (Norton abrasives)*

Manufacturer's type code	BS code	Abrasive	Application
A	A	Aluminium oxide	A high strength abrasive for hard, tough materials
32A	A	Aluminium oxide	Cool; fast cutting, for rapid stock removal
38A	A	Aluminium oxide	Light grinding of very hard steels
19A	A	Aluminium oxide	A milder abrasive than 38A used for cylindrical grinding
37C	C	Silicon carbide	For hard, brittle materials of high density such as cast iron
39C	C (green)	Silicon carbide	For very hard, brittle materials such as tungsten carbide

12.3.2 Grain size (grit size)

The number indicating the grain or grit size represents the number of openings per linear 25 mm in the sieve used to size the grains. The larger the grain size number, the finer the grain. Table 12.3 gives a general classification. The sizes listed as *very fine* are referred to as 'flours' and are used for polishing and super-finishing processes.

TABLE 12.3 *Grit size*

Classification	Grit sizes
Coarse	10, 12, 14, 16, 20, 24
Medium	30, 36, 40, 46, 54, 60
Fine	70, 80, 90, 100, 120, 150, 180
Very fine	220, 240, 280, 320, 400, 500, 600

12.3.3 Grade

This indicates the strength of the bond and therefore the 'hardness' of the wheel. In a *hard* wheel the bond is strong and securely anchors the grit in place, thus reducing the rate of wear. In a *soft* wheel the bond is weak and the grit is easily detached, resulting in a high rate of wear.

The bond must be carefully related to the use for which the wheel is intended. Too hard a wheel will result in dull, blunt grains being retained in the periphery of the wheel causing the generation of excessive heat at the tool/wheel interface with the resultant softening (blueing) of the tool being ground. Too soft a wheel would be uneconomical due to rapid wear and would also result in lack of control of dimensional accuracy in the workpiece when precision grinding. Table 12.4 gives a general classification of hardness using a letter code.

TABLE 12.4 *Grade*

Classification	Letter codes
Very soft	E, F, G
Soft	H, I, J, K
Medium	L, M, N, O
Hard	P, Q, R, S
Very hard	T, U, W, Z

12.3.4 Structure

This indicates the amount of bond between the grains and the closeness of adjacent grains. In milling cutter parlance it indicates the '*chip clearance*'. An open structured wheel cuts freely and tends to generate less heat in the cutting zone. Therefore an open structured wheel has '*free-cutting*' and rapid material removal characteristics. However, it will not produce such a good finish as a closer structured wheel. Table 12.5 gives a general classification of structure.

TABLE 12.5 *Structure*

Classification	Structure numbers
Close spacing	0, 1, 2, 3
Medium spacing	4, 5, 6
Wide spacing	7, 8, 9, 10, 11, 12

12.3.5 Bond

There is a wide range of bonds available and care must be taken to ensure that the bond is suitable for a given application, as the safe use of the wheel is very largely dependent upon this selection.

- *Vitrified bond*. This is the most widely used bond and is similar to glass in composition. It has a high porosity and strength, producing a wheel suitable for high rates of material removal. It is not adversely affected by water, acid, oils or ordinary temperature conditions.

- *Rubber bond*. This is used where a small amount of flexibility is required in the wheel, such as in thin cutting-off wheels and centreless grinding control wheels.

- *Resinoid (bakelite) bond*. This is used for high-speed wheels where the bursting forces are great. Such wheels are used in foundries for dressing castings. Resinoid bond wheels are also used for the larger sizes of cutting-off wheels. They are strong enough to withstand considerable abuse.

- *Shellac bond*. This is used for heavy duty, large diameter wheels, where a fine finish and cool cutting is required. Such wheels are used for grinding mill rolls.

- *Silicate bond*. This is little used for precision grinding. It is mainly used for finishing cutlery (knives) and edge tools such as carpenters' chisels.

Table 12.6 lists the literal code used to specify the bonding materials discussed above.

TABLE 12.6 *Bond*

Classification	BS code
Vitrified bond	V
Resinoid bond	B
Rubber bond	R
Shellac bond	E
Silicate bond	S

12.4 Grinding wheel selection

The correct selection of a grinding wheel depends upon many factors and in this section of the chapter it is possible to give only general 'guide-lines'. Manufacturers' literature should be consulted for more precise information.

12.4.1 Material to be ground

- *Aluminium oxide* abrasives should be used on materials with relatively high tensile strengths.
- *Silicon carbide* abrasives should be used on materials with relatively low tensile strengths.
- A fine grain wheel can be used on hard, brittle materials.
- A coarser grain wheel should be used on soft, ductile materials.
- When considering the *grade*, a general guide is to use a soft grade of wheel for a hard workpiece, and a hard grade of wheel for a soft workpiece.
- When considering the *structure*, it is permissible to use a close structured wheel on hard, brittle materials, but a more open structured wheel should be used for soft, ductile materials.
- The *bond* is seldom influenced by the material being ground. It is usually selected to suit the process.

12.4.2 Rate of stock removal

- A coarse grain wheel should be used for rapid stock removal, but it will give a comparatively rough finish. A fine grain wheel should be used for finishing operations requiring low rates of stock removal.
- The structure of the wheel has a major effect on the rate of stock removal; an open structured wheel with a wide grain spacing being used for maximum stock removal whilst providing cool cutting conditions.
- It should be noted that the performance of a grinding wheel can be appreciably modified by the method of dressing (see Section 12.5) and the operating speed.

12.4.3 Bond

As explained in Section 12.3, the bond is selected for its mechanical properties. It must achieve a balance between:

- sufficient *strength* to resist the rotational, bursting forces and the applied cutting forces; and
- the requirements of cool cutting together with the controlled release of dulled grains and the exposure of fresh cutting edges.

12.4.4 Type of grinding machine

A heavy, rigidly constructed machine can produce accurate work using softer grade wheels. This reduces the possibility of overheating the workpiece and 'drawing' its temper (i.e. reducing its hardness) or, in extreme cases, causing surface cracking of the workpiece. Furthermore, broader wheels can be used and this increases the rate of metal removal without loss of accuracy.

12.4.5 Wheel speed

Variation in the surface speed of a grinding wheel has a profound effect upon its performance. Increasing the speed of the wheel causes it to behave as though it were of a harder grade than that marked upon it. Conversely, reducing the surface speed of a grinding wheel causes it to behave as though it were of a softer grade than that marked upon it.

Care must be taken when selecting a wheel to ensure that the bond has sufficient strength to resist the bursting effect of the rotational forces. Table 12.7 lists the recommended speeds for off-hand, toolroom, and light production grinding. *Never exceed the safe working speed marked on the wheel.*

TABLE 12.7 *Recommended wheel speeds*

	Wheel speed range (m/s)	Surface coverage range (feet/min)
Cylindrical grinding (vitrified or silicate bond)	33–25	6500–5000
Internal grinding	25–20	5000–4000
Surface grinding	33–20	6500–4000
Tool and cutter grinding	30–23	6000–4500

12.5 Grinding wheel defects

A clear understanding of grinding wheel defects is essential for safe working. A wheel that is loaded or glazed will not cut freely and if excess force is used the wheel may shatter. This is extremely dangerous.

12.5.1 Loading

When a soft material, such as a non-ferrous metal, is ground with an unsuitable wheel, the spaces between the grains become clogged with metal particles. Under such circumstances the particles of metal can often be seen embedded in the wheel. This condition is referred to as loading and is detrimental to the cutting action of the grinding wheel. Loading destroys the clearance between the grains, causing them to rub rather than to cut.

This results in excessive force having to be used to press the work against the wheel in an attempt to make the wheel cut. This in itself may be sufficient to fracture the wheel. In addition, considerable heat is generated by the wheel rubbing instead of cutting and this may not only adversely affect the hardness of the component, but it may cause the wheel to overheat, the bond to weaken, and the wheel to burst.

12.5.2 Glazing

A wheel consisting of relatively tough grains, strongly bonded together, will exhibit the self-sharpening action (see Section 12.2) only to a small degree and will quickly develop a shiny, or *glazed*, appearance. This is due to the active grains becoming blunt and shiny over a large area. Like any other blunt cutting tool, a glazed wheel will not cut properly and this will lead to overheating of the workpiece and the wheel. Grinding under these conditions is inefficient and the force required to make the wheel cut may be sufficiently excessive to cause the wheel to burst. The only permanent remedy for glazing is the use of a softer grade of wheel.

12.5.3 Damage

If you find the abrasive wheel of a grinding machine you are about to use is damaged or defective in any way *do not attempt to start up the machine*. Report the damage immediately to your instructor or your supervisor. Damage may consist of the wheel being chipped, cracked, worn unevenly or dressed on the side until it is dangerously thin. Vibration caused by lack of balance or worn spindle bearings should also be reported. In addition to wheel faults, report any missing or faulty guards or incorrectly adjusted work rests. These must be corrected or replaced by a qualified person before you use the machine.

12.6 Grinding wheel dressing and truing

To make a 'glazed' or 'loaded' abrasive wheel serviceable or to 'true' the wheel so that its circumference is concentric with the spindle axis, the wheel must be *dressed*. There are various devices used to dress grinding wheels but they all have the same aims. These are:

- To remove blunt grains from the matrix of the bond.
- To fracture the blunt grains so that they exhibit fresh, sharp cutting edges.
- To remove any foreign matter that may be embedded in the wheel.
- To ensure the periphery of the wheel is concentric (running true) with the spindle axis.

12.6.1 Huntington type wheel dresser

This is shown in Fig. 12.3. The star wheels dig into the wheel and break out the blunt grains and any foreign matter that may be clogging the wheel. Since the star wheels rotate with the grinding wheel little abrasive

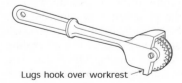

Lugs hook over workrest

Figure 12.3 *Huntington wheel dresser*

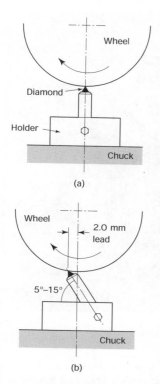

Figure 12.4 *Diamond wheel dresser: (a) incorrect – tip of diamond will wear flat, this will blunt the new abrasive grains as they are exposed; (b) correct – diamond leading wheel centre and trailing direction of rotation, the diamond will keep sharp and dress cleanly*

action takes place and wear of the star wheels is minimal. This type of wheel dressing device is widely used for pedestal type, off-hand grinding machines, but it is not suitable for dressing and truing the wheels of precision grinding machines.

12.6.2 The diamond wheel dresser

This is shown in Fig. 12.4. Generally, Brown Burt stones from Africa are used since these are useless as gem stones and are, therefore, relatively cheap. The diamond cuts the wheel to shape and is used for dressing and truing the wheels on precision grinding machines, such as surface and cylindrical grinding machines. The diamond holder should be rotated from time to time to maintain the shape of the stone and prevent it from becoming blunt.

- Figure 12.4(a) shows the diamond being used incorrectly. Used in this way, the diamond will develop a 'flat', and this will blunt the new grains as they are exposed.

- Figure 12.4(b) shows the correct way to use the diamond. It should trail the direction of rotation of the wheel by an angle of 5° to 15°, but lead the centre of rotation slightly. This will maintain the shape of the diamond so that it will keep sharp and dress cleanly.

The effective structure of the wheel can also be controlled to some extent by the way in which the wheel is dressed. Traversing the diamond rapidly across the face of the wheel has the effect of opening the structure, whilst a slow traverse has the effect of making the wheel cut as though it had a close structure.

12.6.3 The dressing stick

This consists of a stick of coarse abrasive crystals bonded together. It is used for removing the sharp corners from grinding wheels and for dressing small, mounted wheels. It is also used for relieving the sides of grinding wheels when working up to a shoulder.

12.7 Grinding wheel balancing

Precision grinding machines make provision for balancing the grinding wheel and its hub. An out-of-balance wheel produces vibration, causing a 'chessboard' pattern on the finished surface and, if allowed to continue, causing wear and damage to the spindle bearings. Large and heavy grinding wheels also need to be balanced, since the out-of-balance forces can be very considerable and may cause the wheel to burst.

Unlike pedestal and bench type off-hand grinding machines where the wheel has a lead bush and is mounted directly onto the spindle of the machine, the abrasive wheels of precision grinding machines do not have a lead bush but are mounted directly onto a separate hub. This, in turn, is mounted on the machine spindle. To effectively carry out the balancing of the grinding wheel a balancing stand of the type shown in Fig. 12.5

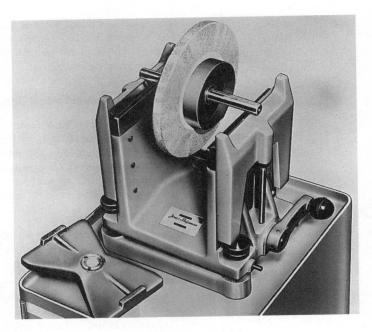

Figure 12.5   *Grinding wheel balancing stand*

should be used. The hardened steel knife edges can be levelled by means of two adjusting screws. A levelling plate with a sensitive bubble level is positioned temporarily across the knife edges and indicates when they are level in all directions.

The hub usually contains adjustable balance weights and the procedure for the static balancing of a grinding wheel and hub assembly is as follows.

- After mounting, the grinding wheel should be trued on the machine before balancing and it may require rebalancing from time to time as it wears down.

- Position the three balance segments (weights) equidistant around the face of the flange as shown in Fig. 12.6(a). Grub screws are provided

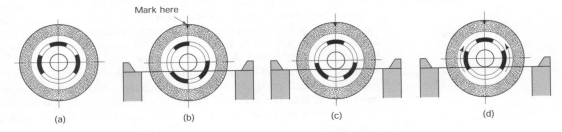

Figure 12.6   *Balancing procedure (reproduced courtesy of Jones and Shipman plc)*

for clamping the balance weight in position when the balance point is reached.

- To balance the wheel and hub they are first mounted on a mandrel which, in turn, is supported on the knife edges of the balancing stand. Allow the wheel and hub to turn freely. The wheel will roll back and forth until it stops with the heaviest part of the assembly at the bottom. When stationary, mark the top centre of the wheel with chalk as shown in Fig. 12.6(b).

- Move the segments equally round the flange until one segment is aligned with the mark as shown in Fig. 12.6(c).

- If movement still occurs, move the other two segments gradually towards the mark, as shown in Fig. 12.6(d) until the wheel and hub remain stationary in any position.

The grinding wheel and hub are removed from the mandrel and are carefully mounted on the grinding machine spindle, where the wheel is retrued ready for use.

12.8 The double-ended off-hand grinding machine

Figure 12.7(a) shows a typical double-ended, off-hand grinding machine widely used in workshops for sharpening single point cutting tools. It uses plain cylindrical grinding wheels of the type shown in Fig. 12.7(b).

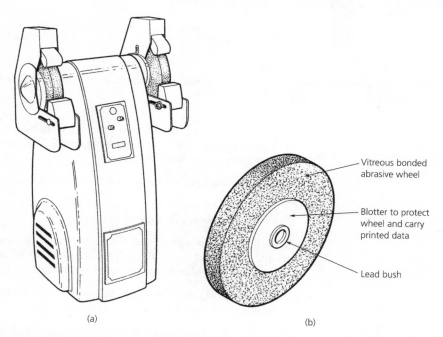

Vitreous bonded abrasive wheel

Blotter to protect wheel and carry printed data

Lead bush

(a)

(b)

Figure 12.7 *Double-ended, off-hand grinding machine*

Because of its apparent simplicity, this type of grinding machine comes in for more than its fair share of abuse. For *safe* and *efficient* cutting the grinding wheel must be correctly mounted and correctly used. Let's now consider the correct way to mount a grinding wheel on this type of machine. Remember that under the Abrasive Wheel Regulations already discussed in this chapter, only certificated personnel and trainees under the direct supervision of a certificated person may change a grinding wheel.

For the following notes on mounting a new grinding wheel, refer mainly to Figs 12.8, 12.9 and 12.10.

- For the names of the parts of the wheel mounting assembly see Fig. 12.8(a).

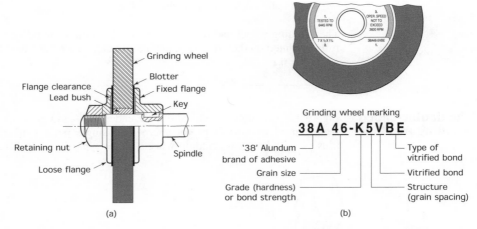

(a)

(b)

Figure 12.8 *Mounting a grinding wheel (stage 1): (a) the wheel mounting; (b) checking the new wheel (reproduced courtesy of Norton Grinding Wheel Co.)*

- Remove the securing nut. Viewed from the front of the machine, the left-hand wheel nut will have a left-hand thread. The right-hand wheel nut will have a right-hand thread.

- Remove the outer (loose) flange and the wheel that is to be discarded.

- Clean the spindle and wheel flanges to remove any trace of the old wheel and any burrs that may be present.

- Check that the new wheel is of suitable size and type for the machine and the work it is to perform. This information is printed on the 'blotters' on each side of the wheel as shown in Fig. 12.8(b).

- Check particularly that the operating speed is correct. Remember that the spindle speed must be marked on the machine.

- Check that the wheel is not cracked or faulty by 'ringing' it as shown in Fig. 12.9(a). To do this the wheel is freely suspended on stout twine

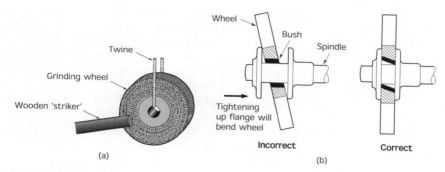

Figure 12.9 *Mounting a grinding wheel (stage 2): (a) 'ringing' a grinding wheel; (b) fitting the bush: incorrect – if the lead bush in the centre of the wheel is too tight a fit on the spindle, there is a danger that the wheel will crack as the flanges are tightened up; correct – the bush is eased out with a three-square scraper until the wheel can float on the spindle, it will then pull up square with the fixed flange without cracking. (Note: The misalignment of the bush has been exaggerated for clarity)*

and *lightly* tapped with a wooden rod. If the wheel is free from cracks or manufacturing faults, such as voids, it will 'ring' with a clear note.

- Slip the wheel onto the spindle. The lead bush in the centre of the wheel should be an easy fit on the spindle. If it is tight the abrasive wheel may twist and crack as the flanges are tightened up. Tight bushes should be opened up with a three-square scraper so that the wheel can float into position as shown in Fig. 12.9(b). The error in the bush has been exaggerated for clarity.

- Replace the 'loose' flange and check that the 'blotters' on the sides of the abrasive wheel are slightly larger than the flanges. The blotters

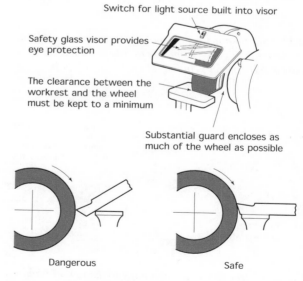

Figure 12.10 *Setting the wheel guard and workrest adjustment*

prevent the sharp edges of the flanges from biting into the wheel and starting a crack. The diameter of the flanges should be at least half the diameter of the wheel to give it adequate support.

- Replace the securing nut on the spindle and tighten it up. Use only the minimum of force to secure the wheel. Excessive tightening will crush and crack the wheel.
- Replace the wheel guard and adjust the visor and workrest as shown in Fig. 12.10.
- Test the wheel by running it up to speed. *DO NOT stand in front of the wheel whilst testing it in case it shatters.*
- Finally, true the wheel ready for use.

12.9 Resharpening hand tools and single point cutting tools

The off-hand grinding machine just described is used mainly for resharpening workshop hand tools and single point tools such as lathe tools and shaping machine tools. We will now look at some examples of how this should be done.

12.9.1 Chisels

These are ground as shown in Fig. 12.11(a). The cutting edge should be slightly radiused by rocking the chisel from side to side as shown.

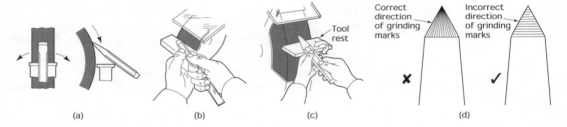

(a)   (b)   (c)   (d)

Figure 12.11 *Sharpening bench tools: (a) sharpening a cold chisel – the cutting edge should be slightly radiused by rocking the chisel from side to side as indicated; (b) removing a 'mushroomed' head; (c) sharpening a centre punch; (d) correct grinding of centre punch point*

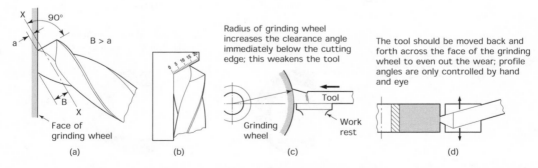

(a)   (b)   (c)   (d)

Figure 12.12 *Sharpening drills and lathe tools: (a) off-hand grinding a drill point; (b) twist drill point angle and lip length gauge; (c) grinding the clearance angle; (d) grinding the plan profile*

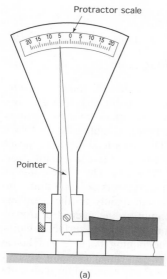

(a)

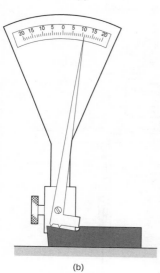

(b)

Figure 12.13 *Lathe tool protractor: (a) checking the clearance angle; (b) checking the rake angle*

Take care not to overheat the chisel so that the cutting edge becomes discoloured. This will indicate that the chisel edge has become soft and useless. Any 'mushrooming' of the chisel head must be removed as shown in Fig. 12.11(b).

12.9.2 Centre punches and dot punches

Centre punches and dot punches are sharpened as shown in Fig. 12.11(c). The punch is held against the grinding wheel at the required angle and rotated between the thumb and forefinger to generate the conical point. Again, care must be taken not to soften the point of the punch by overheating it. The grinding marks must run from the point and not around it. This is shown in Fig. 12.11(d). Incorrect grinding will weaken the point causing it to crumble away.

12.9.3 Twist drills

These are most easily ground against the flat side of the grinding wheel as shown in Fig. 12.12(a). The straight cutting lip of the drill should lie vertically against the side of the wheel, and the drill should be gently rocked against the wheel about the axis XX to produce the point clearance. When the drill has been ground it should be checked on a drill point gauge as shown in Fig. 12.12(b). This ensures that the angles are equal and correct. It also ensures that the lips of the drill are of equal length. This is essential for efficient cutting and the production of accurately sized holes. Again care must be taken not to overheat the tool and soften it.

12.9.4 Single point tools

Lathe and shaping machine tools can also be ground on the off-hand grinding machine. Figure 12.12(c) shows the front clearance angle being ground, and Fig. 12.12(d) shows the plan trailing angle being ground. The tool shown is a straight nosed roughing tool for a lathe. Again care must be taken not to overheat the tool and soften it.

Experienced centre-lathe operators usually judge the cutting angles by 'eye' based on years of experience. However, more consistent results can be obtained by using a lathe tool protractor as shown in Fig. 12.13.

12.10 Surface grinding machine

Surface grinding machines can be divided into four categories:

- Horizontal spindle – reciprocating table.
- Horizontal spindle – rotary table.

- Vertical spindle – reciprocating table.

- Vertical spindle – rotary table.

12.10.1 Horizontal spindle – reciprocating table

In this book we are concerned only with the horizontal spindle, reciprocating table type of machine as used in toolrooms for precision grinding. A typical example is shown in Fig. 12.14, and names its main features. As well as manual table traverse, it has a powered table traverse that is infinitely variable from zero to 25 m/min. The cross-feed may be adjusted manually or automatically. The automatic cross-feed rate is variable from about 0.2 mm to about 5 mm per pass of the wheel. The vertical in-feed of the wheel is very precisely controlled in increments of 0.005 mm. This type of machine uses grinding wheels that cut mainly on the periphery and, if wheel wear is to be kept to a minimum in the interest of dimensional accuracy, stock removal is rather limited. Precision surface grinding wheels are normally mounted on hubs containing balance weights as described in Section 12.7. Usually the surface grinder operator keeps a number of wheels of different specifications ready mounted on spare hubs so that they can be quickly interchanged as required.

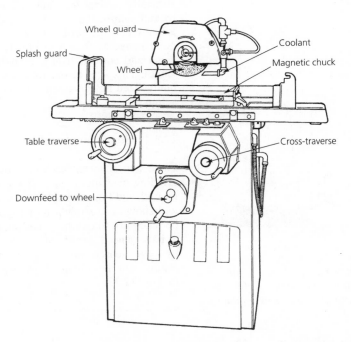

Figure 12.14 *Typical toolroom type surface grinding machine*

Figure 12.15 shows the relative geometrical movements and alignments for a horizontal spindle, reciprocating table grinding machine. You can see

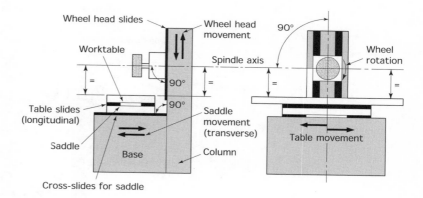

Figure 12.15 *Surface grinding machine: movements and alignments*

that they have a close similarity to those of a horizontal milling machine. This is not surprising since both machines are designed to produce plain surfaces using a cylindrical, rotating cutter whose axis is horizontal. The important difference is that whereas the milling machine is concerned with high rates of material removal, the surface grinding machine is designed to produce a surface of high dimensional accuracy and to a high standard of surface finish but with a low rate of material removal. Surface grinding is essentially a finishing process.

Most cutting takes place on the periphery of the wheel but shallow steps can be ground using the side of the wheel as well. Since the grinding wheel is relatively weak with respect to side forces, great care must be taken when working on the side of the wheel. Special attachments are available for dressing the grinding wheel to different shapes so that it can grind radii or other profiles.

12.11 Workholding

Workholding on surface grinding machines is usually effected by means of a magnetic chuck. However, this is possible only if a workpiece made from a ferromagnetic material such as steel is to be ground. Alternatively any of the techniques associated with the milling machine may be used. For example, direct clamping to the machine table, the use of vices of various types and also grinding fixtures.

12.11.1 Magnetic chucks

Most chucks employ permanent magnets. Figure 12.16(a) shows the construction of a standard chuck, and Fig. 12.16(b) shows the construction of a fine pole chuck for holding thinner components.

Figure 12.17(a) shows a section through a standard chuck in the 'ON' position. It will be seen that the lines of magnetic flux pass through the workpiece which must be made of a magnetic material. The magnets are mounted in a grid which can be offset by the operating handle. When this

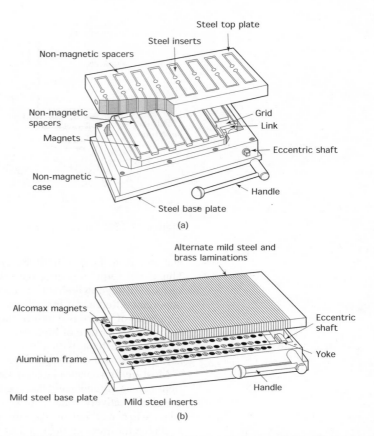

Figure 12.16 *The magnetic chuck: (a) standard type chuck; (b) fine pole type chuck (reproduced courtesy of Eclipse Magnetics Ltd)*

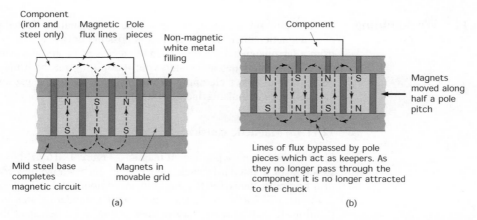

Figure 12.17 *The magnetic chuck: principle of operation: (a) chuck 'on' – lines of flux pass through component; (b) chuck 'off' – lines of flux bypassed by pole pieces (reproduced courtesy of Eclipse Magnetics Ltd)*

is moved to the 'OFF' position as shown in Fig. 12.17(b), the magnetic flux field is bypassed through the pole pieces. In this position the pole pieces act as 'keepers' which prevent the magnets from losing their magnetism. In the OFF position no magnetic flux passes through the workpiece and, therefore, the workpiece is no longer attracted to the chuck. The flux field does not hold the component against the cutting forces directly, but provides a friction force between the component and the chuck. It is the friction that prevents the component from moving.

Hard steels tend to become magnetized and to hold their magnetism after they have been removed from the chuck. Demagnetizing is a simple operation. Figure 12.18 shows a typical *demagnetizer*. The top surface of this device consists of the two pole pieces of an electromagnet. The gap between them is filled by a soft, non-magnetic material. With the demagnetizer switched on, the magnetized workpiece is simply 'wiped' across the pole pieces. The alternating flux of the demagnetizer removes any residual magnetism in the workpiece material.

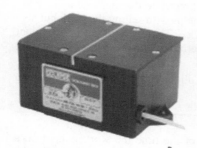

Figure 12.18 *Typical demagnetizer (reproduced courtesy of Eclipse Magnetics Ltd)*

12.11.2 Mechanical clamping

For the general purpose workholding of non-magnetic materials on surface grinding machines and the holding of awkwardly shaped components of any metal, various mechanical workholding techniques can be used similar to the techniques used for milling. These can be:

- Workholding in a plain machine vice which, in turn, is mounted on the magnetic chuck as shown in Fig. 12.19(a).

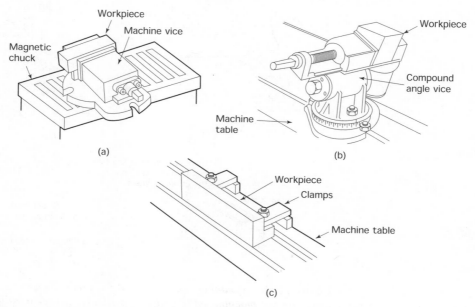

Figure 12.19 *Mechanical clamping: (a) use of machine vice on a magnetic chuck; (b) use of a compound angle vice bolted directly to the machine table; (c) work clamped directly to machine table*

- Workholding in a swivelling and tilting vice when a surface has to be ground at an angle to the machine table as shown in Fig. 12.19(b). Usually this type of vice is bolted directly to the machine table using the T-slots provided. This not only helps with setting the work but also compensates for the height of the vice. There would not be sufficient 'daylight' for it to pass under the grinding wheel if it was raised by the thickness of a magnetic chuck.

- The workpiece can also be clamped directly to the table of the machine as shown in Fig. 12.19(c).

12.12 Mounting a magnetic chuck on the worktable

Except for production grinding, most of the time the work is held on a permanent magnet chuck of the type described in the previous section, so let's now see how such a chuck is mounted on the machine table and trued up.

- Clean the table of the machine and the base of the chuck. Check for and carefully remove any burrs with a flat smooth oil stone.

- Seat the chuck centrally on the machine table, check that there is no rock. Absolute cleanliness is essential, there must be no oil or solid dirt particles between the table and the chuck.

- Lightly clamp into position as shown in Fig. 12.20(a).

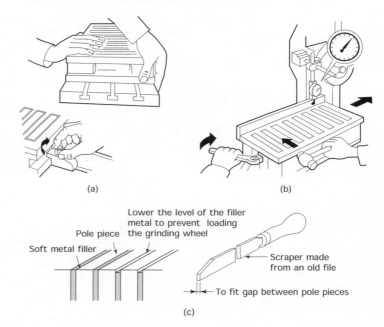

Figure 12.20 *Mounting and setting a magnetic chuck: (a) place the chuck on the machine table and clamp lightly; (b) set parallel to table traverse and tighten clamps; (c) relief of soft filler metal between pole pieces*

- Raise the backplate and, using a DTI as shown in Fig. 12.20(b), set the chuck so that the backplate is parallel to the direction of traverse.

- Note that the backplate is used as a datum when grinding stepped components.

- When correctly set the DTI should show a constant reading along the whole length of the backplate.

- Now tighten the clamps and check again to make sure the chuck hasn't moved.

- When finally installed the top plate of the chuck should be ground *in situ*. The soft metal filling between the pole pieces will clog the grinding wheel, so remove with a scraper as shown in Fig. 12.20(c). Remove only the minimum amount of filler metal but sufficient so that the level of the filler metal is still *just below* the level of the pole pieces when grinding is complete.

- Lower or remove the backplate so that the wheel can clear the sides of the chuck whilst initial grinding is taking place.

- Set the cross-slide and table traverse stops so that the wheel clears each side and end of the chuck. Start up the machine and dress the wheel for rough grinding. That is, traverse the diamond across the face of the wheel rapidly.

- *Check that the chuck is turned OFF whilst this initial grinding is in progress otherwise grinding dross will accumulate between the pole pieces.*

- Start the traverse and lower the wheel carefully until it is just touching the high spots on the chuck.

- Turn on the coolant.

- Apply a cut of 0.015 mm, engage the cross traverse and grind the top surface of the chuck.

- Disengage the traverse, stop the machine, turn off the coolant, and examine the chuck. If it is not ground all over, lower the wheel by another 0.015 mm and take another cut. Repeat until the surface of the chuck has been ground all over.

- Check that the soft filler metal is still below the level of the pole pieces and remove more metal if necessary.

- Redress the wheel for fine grinding (slow traverse of the diamond across the wheel face). Take a finishing cut of 0.005 mm and check that the whole surface of the chuck is finished ground. Listen to the wheel whilst it is grinding. Any change in, or interruption of, the sound indicates that a further cut may be necessary.

- Disengage the traverse, stop the machine, and wind the wheel clear of the chuck, remove sharp edges and clean down.

- The chuck is now ready for use.

12.13 Grinding a flat surface

Safety: Keep your hands and any wipers away from the rapidly revolving wheel at all times.

12.13.1 Setting up

- Check that the wheel is of a suitable type for the material being cut and the finish required.

- Dress the wheel according to the material being cut and the finish required. Rapid traversing of the diamond produces an 'open' structure for roughing cuts and soft materials. Slow traversing of the diamond produces a 'closed' structure for finishing cuts and hardened materials. It may be necessary to take one or more roughing cuts followed by a finishing cut for final sizing.

- Check the drawing to see which faces are to be ground and the finished size. In this example we are assuming that both faces need to be ground.

- Check the thickness of the work so that you can assess the grinding allowance. Try to arrange the grinding process so that half the allowance is taken from both faces.

- Place the work centrally on the chuck and check for 'rock'.

- If there is any rock due to distortion during hardening or poor initial machining, place non-magnetic shims (paper or thin card) under the work until it seats solidly. Otherwise the chuck may spring the work flat when it is switched on and the work will return to its original shape when the chuck is switched off.

- Make sure that the workpiece covers as many pole pieces as possible and that the chuck is turned ON.

- Set the table and cross-slide traverse stops so that the wheel just clears the work in all directions.

12.13.2 Grinding the first face

- Switch on the machine and start the traverse.

- Hand feed the wheel down carefully until you have visual and audible indications that the wheel is just touching the high spots of the work.

- Turn on the coolant.

- Engage the automatic cross-feed and grind the whole area of the workpiece.

- Stop the traverse, turn off the coolant, and wind the work clear of the grinding wheel using the cross traverse handle.

- Examine the surface of the work. It is unlikely it will have cleaned up all over at this first pass.

- Increase the downfeed by another 0.05 mm and take a second cut as shown in Fig. 12.21(a).

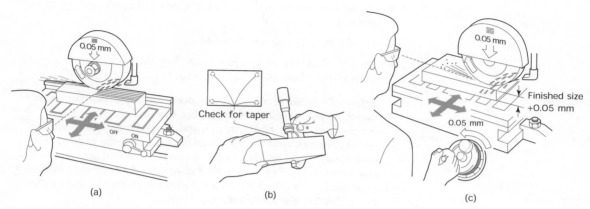

(a)   (b)   (c)

Figure 12.21 *Grinding a flat component*

- Again wind the work clear of the wheel and examine the surface. When the wheel is cutting all over the surface, stop the machine and prepare to grind the opposite face.

- You should have removed no more than half of the grinding allowance at this stage.

12.13.3 Grinding the second face

- With the machine switched off, turn the chuck off and remove the workpiece and any shims you may have used.

- Clean the workpiece and the surface of the magnetic chuck. Remove any sharp corners.

- Check the thickness of the workpiece so that you can assess the amount of metal that is to be removed as shown in Fig. 12.21(b).

- Replace the work on the chuck. Check for 'rock'. If your first surface is correctly ground there should be no rock unless there is a particle of abrasive between the work and the chuck. Reclean and try again.

- When the work is correctly seated, switch on the chuck and start up the machine.

- Repeat the procedure for the first surface. The second surface should clean up without using up all the grinding allowance. You need some for the finishing cuts (see Fig. 12.21(c)).

- Stop the machine, remove the work and clean the work and the chuck.

- Redress the wheel for finishing using a light cut and traversing the diamond slowly across the wheel.

- Check how much metal is left on the job.

- Replace it on the chuck and take a skim across the first surface.

- Again reverse the work, check the remaining amount of metal to remove.

- Restart the machine and finish to size.

- Switch off the machine, remove and clean the work, remove any sharp corners and clean down the machine.

Safety: To avoid accidents it has been suggested that you should switch off the machine whilst loading and unloading the work. For trainees this is the safest way to work. However, for some machines this is not possible since they need the wheel spindle to be running continuously to maintain its operating temperature if accurate work is to be produced. In this case the traverse hand wheels must be used to position the work as far from the wheel as possible when loading and unloading the work. Take great care.

Exercises   **12.1**   *Safety when using abrasive wheel grinding machines*

(a)   State the requirements of Regulation 9 of the Abrasive Wheel Regulations concerning persons allowed to mount abrasive wheels on grinding machines and the circumstances under which a trainee may change an abrasive wheel.

(b)   Describe the essential differences between an abrasive wheel guard and a milling cutter guard and explain the need for these differences.

(c)   List the defects for which you should check before using an off-hand, double-ended grinding machine to sharpen a chisel or other cutting tool.

12.2   *Abrasive wheels*

(a)   Explain what is meant by the following terms related to abrasive (grinding) wheels:
  (i)   active grains;
  (ii)   grit;
  (iii)   bond;
  (iv)   grade;
  (v)   structure.

(b)   An abrasive wheel carries a British Standard marking of 39C120-K4V. What does this signify? A speed in rev/min should also be marked on the wheel. What does this signify?

(c)   Explain what is meant by the terms *glazing* and *loading* as applied to abrasive wheels. How can these conditions be rectified?

(d)   Explain the essential difference between *dressing* and *truing*. With the aid of sketches describe how these operations may be performed.

(e)   Explain in general terms:

(i) How the material being ground influences the selection of a suitable grinding wheel.
(ii) How the rate of stock removal influences the selection of a suitable grinding wheel.

(f) Precision grinding machines have their abrasive wheels mounted on hubs that contain balance weights.
(i) Why do the wheels of precision grinding machines have to be balanced?
(ii) Why would a toolroom grinding machine operator keep a variety of wheels available ready mounted and balanced on their hubs.

12.3 *Grinding machines*
(a) Sketch a typical pedestal type double-ended, off-hand grinding machine and label its essential features.
(b) Describe briefly, with the aid of sketches, how a magnetic chuck should be set up on the table of a horizontal spindle, reciprocating table, surface grinding machine and how the chuck should be prepared ready for use.

12.4 *Grinding operations*
(a) Describe, with the aid of sketches, how the following jobs should be carried out on a double-ended, off-hand grinding machine.
(i) Sharpening a cold chisel and removing any mushrooming from its head.
(ii) Regrinding a lathe parting-off tool.
(iii) Sharpening a centre punch.
(b) Describe, with the aid of sketches, how the component shown in Fig. 12.22 can be finished ground all over on a horizontal spindle, reciprocating table, toolroom surface grinding machine.

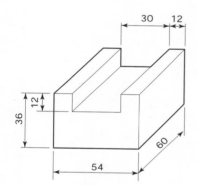

Figure 12.22 *Exercise 12.4(b)*

Index